Annette Schaub (ed.)

New Family Interventions and
Associated Research in Psychiatric Disorders

Gedenkschrift in Honor of
Michael J. Goldstein

SpringerWienNewYork

Dipl. Psych. Dr. Annette Schaub
Department of Psychiatry, Ludwig–Maximilian
University of Munich, Germany

© 2002 Springer-Verlag/Wien

Typesetting: Scientific Publishing Services, Madras, India
Printing: Manz Crossmedia GmbH, A-1051 Wien
Binding: Papyrus, A-1100 Wien
Cover Illustration: Peter Pongratz "Lob der Schizophrenie 1964–65"
Reproduction with kind permission

SPIN: 10842640

With 16 Figures

CIP-data applied for

ISBN 3-211-83700-0 Springer-Verlag Wien New York

Contents

Gedenkschrift in Honor of Michael J. Goldstein

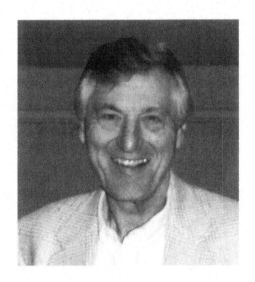

Part I
1 Introduction

Annette Schaub

This book is to honor **Michael J. Goldstein Ph.D.**, Professor of Psychology and Psychiatry at the University of California, who passed away in 1997. Mike was known for his caring, humanistic, and hope-inspiring approach to helping patients and their relatives cope with severe psychiatric illnesses, and for the support, warmth, and open-mindedness he showed in his relationships with colleagues and visitors from all over the world. Mike's humor, his optimism that social science could be used to better the human condition, and his conviction that patients, relatives, and clinicians could work collaboratively to manage psychiatric illness and improve the lives of all involved, were an inspiration to everyone he touched. Furthermore, because of the nature of Mike's work, his research has had a tremendous influence on many who never knew him, and the clinical innovations he helped develop have improved the lives of countless patients and families, and will no doubt continue to help many in the future. While Mike's work lives on, we and many others will miss his friendship and uplifting spirit he engendered in all of us.

On April 28, 1997, the faculty center at the University of California, Los Angeles organized a program in memory of Mike. After this meeting it was suggested that a symposium be dedicated to Mike at the next World conference. He had initiated, organized and supported many studies in clinical psychology and psychiatry, so it seemed fitting that one should be organized in his memory.

The papers included in this book were mainly presented at this symposium of the VI World Congress, World Association for Psychosocial Rehabilitation (WAPR), May 2–5, 1998, Hamburg, Germany. The symposium in remembrance of Mike focused on new family interventions and associated research in psychosis.

This book begins with an overview by **Kurt Hahlweg** of Mike's significant contributions to research on psychosis. Mike's research interests included family factors related to schizophrenia and other mental disorders, as well as clinical psychopharmacological studies. However, his main focus was on developing and evaluating psychoeducational family interventions for schizophrenia and bipolar disorder. He pioneered the use of short-term psychoeducational family therapy in schizophrenia and combined it with different antipsychotic treatment options in order to minimize relapses. More recently, he and his colleagues developed one of the first family interventions for bipolar disorder. In 1997 Mike posthumously received the Gerald Klerman Award for Biopsychosocial Research for his 40 years of extraordinary contributions to the assessment, prevention and treatment of patients with schizophrenia and bipolar disorder.

The structure of this book follows Mike's footsteps in this domain and is subdivided into family factors in severe mental illness, as well as intervention strategies for severe psychiatric disorders.

Don H. Linszen and **Peter M. Dingemans** give a detailed overview of the historical background of the concept of schizophrenia, the role of the family, and different family intervention strategies. The authors describe an application and extension of Goldstein's crisis intervention model (Goldstein, Rodnick, Evans, May, and Steinberg, 1978) with families who are trained to recognize and support patients with a first episode of schizophrenia. This work is based on the hypothesis that recognition and intervention at the earliest possible stage of florid psychosis in schizophrenia and related disorders could contribute to earlier resolution of psychotic and negative symptoms as well as prevention of subsequent relapses and of further psychosocial deterioration. The primary goal of this intervention is to create a working alliance between the patient, the family and the professionals leading to a treatment plan that includes strategies for managing the illness and for helping patients achieve personal goals (Linszen, Dingemans, Scholte, Van der Does, Nugter, Lenior, and Goldstein, 1996).

There is growing evidence that social factors contribute to the course and outcome in schizophrenia. During his long career, Mike never failed to acknowledge the importance of family transactions with respect to psychopathology. Mike proposed a complex transactional model to understand how family attitudes evolve during the course of a relatives' schizophrenic disorder. It therefore seems fitting that, in a book of papers written in his honor, the focus is on family aspects of different psychiatric illnesses, including borderline personality disorder.

Even with continuous long-term neuroleptic treatment that has been shown to be effective in preventing further episodes, about 40% of patients relapse during the first year of discharge from the hospital. The high rate of relapse has stimulated research on contributing factors. Apart from medication non-compliance, social stressors, in particular life events and/or a family environment are important.

In their heuristic model, Nuechterlein and Dawson (1984) predict overt psychotic behavior as the results from an interaction between vulnerability factors, stressors and protective factors. The model comprises four major categories: a) enduring vulnerability characteristics (e.g., disturbance of information processing), b) external environmental stressors, and c) development of psychotic symptoms, and d) protective factors such as medication and psychosocial interventions. This model not only stimulated research, but has also influenced the development of effective psychosocial approaches in schizophrenia.

In the context of the vulnerability-stress-coping model of schizophrenia (e.g., Zubin and Spring, 1977; Nuechterlein and Dawson, 1984), specific communication patterns such as high Expressed Emotion (EE, Leff and Vaughn, 1985) and negative Affective Style (AS, Doane, West, Goldstein, Rodnick, and Jones, 1981) are conceived as specific stressors which impinge on biological vulnerability, precipitating relapses. Numerous studies (e.g., from the "Family Research Group" at UCLA) have demonstrated the important relationship between negative family communication and increased risk of relapse (e.g., Goldstein, 1987).

Because Expressed Emotion is a valid construct that can be measured (e.g., by the Camberwell Family Inventory, Vaughn and Leff, 1976a; Five Minute Speech Sample, Magana, Goldstein, Karno, Miklowitz, Jenkins, and Falloon, 1986), it provides one way to explore hypotheses about the effects of family factors on psychiatric illness. The literature on EE provides ample evidence that family characteristics such as criticism, hostility, and emotional overinvolvement predict poor clinical outcomes in disorders such as schizophrenia, unipolar depression and bipolar disorder (e.g., Miklowitz, Goldstein, Nuechterlein, Snyder, and Mintz, 1988).

In several studies, Mike and his colleagues showed that critical attitudes on the part of relatives were correlated with similarly negative behaviors during family interaction problem solving tasks (Miklowitz, Goldstein, Falloon, and Doane, 1984; Strachan, Leff, Goldstein, Doane, and Burtt, 1986). Physiological data suggest that patients react with higher levels of arousal to the presence of high versus low EE relatives. Detailed analysis demonstrated that the patient contributes to the development and maintenance of negative communication just as much as the relatives (Hahlweg, Goldstein, Nuechterlein, Magana, Mintz, Doane, Miklowitz, and Snyder, 1989).

Several studies have examined the congruence between patients' and relatives views of family climate (e.g., Tompson, Goldstein, Lebell, Mintz, Marder, and Mintz, 1995). **Martha C. Tompson** and **Amy G. Weisman** examined whether patients' perceptions of their family members correlated with their psychiatric symptoms. Other studies from Mike's group showed that certain nonverbal signs of subclinical psychopathology and other nonsymptomatic behaviors elicit high EE attitudes, as well as result from them (e.g., Rosenfarb, Goldstein, Mintz, and Nuechterlein, 1995; Woo, Goldstein, Nuechterlein, 1997; Rosenfarb, I. S., Nuechterlein, K. H., Goldstein, M. J., and Subotnik, K. L., 2000). Patients from high-EE families showed more hostile and unusual behavior with relatives than those from low EE-homes, who, in contrast showed more anxious behavior. The results support a transactional model in which odd and/or hostile patient behaviors may lead to negative familial attitudes (or EE), which are perceived by patients and lead to negative/hostile patient behaviors towards the relatives, which in turn increases negative familial attitudes and behaviors (Goldstein, Rosenfarb, Woo, and Nuechterlein, 1994).

Peter M. Dingemans, **Don H. Linszen** and **Maria E. Lenior** focus on the state of art in research on patients' psychopathology and parental EE. In their study with young recent onset patients with schizophrenia they examine the relationship between EE and attributions (e.g., negative symptoms as volitional signs of unwillingness compared to positive symptoms as illness symptoms). They also discuss whether EE is rather dependent on psychotic processes than trait characteristics. They recommend psychoeducational programs to be more tailored to meeting family's needs rather than narrowly focusing on reducing parental EE (Linszen et al., 1996).

In this context **Andreas Altorfer** and **Marie-Luise Käsermann** focus on the psychophysiological evaluation of interactions during conversations between psychotic patients and their relatives. There is a lack of information regarding the immediate physiological effects of stressors. Therefore Altorfer and Käsermann developed specific approaches that allow for measuring nonverbal behavior and psychophysiological variables online during conversations. The method is a powerful instrument for gaining insight into the processes by which stress influences communication.

Nuechterlein, Ventura, Snyder, Gitlin, Subotnik, Dawson, and Mintz (1998) investigated the predictors of the early course of schizophrenic and schizoaffective patients. Patients were treated with fluphenazine, individual case management, skills-focused group therapy and family education. The contribution of **Subotnik**, **Nuechterlein** and **Ventura** addresses predictors of relapse in recent-onset schizophrenia. This prospective study showed both high EE and occurrence of independent life events were predictive of psychotic relapse. During a period of ongoing antipsychotic medication and psychosocial intervention, discrete stressful life events, high EE and more severe symptoms predicted relapses. The predictive role of these psychosocial stressors was not accounted for by genetic factors (family history, neurocognitive vulnerability factors), suggesting that environmental stress operates through separate processes.

Similar to Mike's study in 1978 (Goldstein et al., 1978) antipsychotics were efficient to prevent relapses. Maintenance antipsychotic medication raised the threshold for return of psychotic symptoms, such that a psychotic relapse was less likely unless major environmental stressors occurred. Several consequences for prevention of relapse with schizophrenic patients ensue from this model and from the results of EE research: neuroleptic medication helps to control positive symptoms of the disorder, probably by lowering autonomic hyperarousal, while psychosocial interventions modify unfavorable familial factors.

Jill M. Hooley and **George M. Dominiak** focus on family interactions of patients with borderline personality, following Mike's approach in this area. Contrary to what is typically found for samples of patients with schizophrenia and mood disorders, high levels of family criticism and hostility were not associated with poor clinical outcome for the borderline patients. However and even more striking, the patients in families with emotional overinvolvement had a better clinical course of their illness. The authors conclude that regardless of whether family members of borderline patients are directly or indirectly involved in the development of the disorder, they need to be helped in order to collaborate with the treatment team.

Basic research on psychosocial factors in schizophrenia and bipolar disorder led to the development of family intervention strategies. Mike did not intend to blame families for high EE behavior, but instead wanted to focus on the role of the family in the course and treatment of psychiatric illnesses, and to provide crisis-oriented and psychoeducational treatment when needed. Two main consequences emerge from the research mentioned above: the findings clearly indicate that there are interactive communication patterns in familes that may worsen or improve the course of patients' psychiatric illness. In order to be able to modify the behavior of all family members simultaneously, the patient should be included in family counseling.

The next section involves family interventions in schizophrenia, depression and bipolar disorder.

Kurt Hahlweg and **Georg Wiedemann** outline the principles and results of psychoeducational family programs in schizophrenia. In spite of some differences, these programs are all based on long-term interventions on areas such as problemsolving, and treatment with antipsychotics. They are all directed at problems of the patient as well as at reducing the whole family's burden. In the Munich treatment study the combined effects of behavioral family management (BMF) and standard dose (SD) or targeted neuroleptic medication (TM) on relapse and social functioning of the patient as well as coping and burden of the family were investigated. Psychoeducational family therapy in combination with standard dose medication proved to be highly effective in preventing relapse in schizophrenia. These results are in line with findings of Anglo-American studies and call for a more widespread application of these psychosocial approaches in order to provide the best services available for the chronically ill schizophrenic patient and their families.

Goldstein's study (1978) on the effectiveness of family interventions appeared two years after Vaughn and Leff's (1976a) replication of the association between relatives EE and the outcome of schizophrenia (Brown, Birley, and Wing, 1972). Their study on the specificity of the EE effect with patients suffering from depressive neurosis, excluding patients with psychotic symptoms of any sort, showed that critical comments also predicted relapse of depression, although at a lower threshold from schizophrenia (Vaughn and Leff, 1976b). In **Julian Leff's** chapter he describes a controlled trial of couple therapy versus antidepressant medication for depressed patients with a critical partner, investigating the possible causal link between critical comments, self-esteem and depressive symptoms and the mechanisms by which this might operate. The drop-out rate for couple therapy was much lower than for drug treatment and the treatment effects were more favourable and lasting, even throughout the second year.

In the final stages of his carreer Mike turned his attention to understanding the impact of family psychoeducation on the course of bipolar disorder. Together with David Miklowitz he developed a family-focused intervention program for bipolar disorder based on the behavioral family management model of Falloon, Boyd, and McGill (1984). Compared to patients with schizophrenia, patients with bipolar disorders have good premorbid social adjustment and they are less severely ill between episodes. These patients are more overtly emotional and demanding in family interactions, more psychologically minded and more likely to resist and challenge a didactic approach to treatment. The family focused program was designed to be more flexible and less didactic to meet the different needs of families with a member who has bipolar disorder.

Mike and his research group compared the effectiveness of either family intervention or individual therapy for bipolar disorder in conjunction with standard medication management in Los Angeles. Preliminary findings of the study by Rea, Goldstein, Tompson, and Miklowitz (1998) indicate that participants who received family treatment had fewer symptoms of mania and depression during the study. Further, individuals receiving family treatment were hospitalized less during the year of participation in the study as well as during the following year.

In Boulder the comparison group was a standard care crisis management condition with all patients receiving mood-stabilizing medication. Results of the one-year outcome are presented in **Richards** and **Miklowitz's** chapter. Bipolar patients recovering from a recent episode fared better in family treatment than did those who received standard crisis management care. They had less severe overall affective symptoms, especially depression, during the course of the first year following the episode.

Kim T. Mueser, **Lindy Fox** and **Carolyn Mercer** outline the importance of involving family members in the treatment of patients with severe mental illness and substance use disorders and describe a family intervention model for dual disorders. Alcohol and drug use disorders are a major problem that plagues the lives of many persons with severe mental illness, and may have a deterious effect on the course of psychiatric illness. Working with the families of dually diagnosed patients may be beneficial as relatives are often the most important social relationships in their lives. Their competencies are strengthened by psychoeducation about the interactions between substance use and mental illness, as well as by applying motivational strategies. Reducing family tension due to substance abuse may decrease clients' vulnerability to relapse.

Annette Schaub gives an overview of illness self-management programs in schizophrenia, bipolar disorder and depression. During the last 15 years, psychoeducational and coping-oriented treatment programs combined with pharmacotherapy have gained prominence in the treatment of schizophrenia and depression. Whereas there used to be a reluctance to inform patients with schizophrenia about their illness, education about schizophrenia is now offered to the patients themselves in individual or group settings. Providing information about a specific mental illness, such as schizophrenia, and its treatment based on the vulnerability-stress-coping model demystifies the illness and develops a more constructive understanding of its course and treatment. Several controlled treatment studies document the effectiveness of psychoeducational and coping-oriented treatment.

Hans-Jürgen Möller reviews current developments in the pharmacological treatment of schizophrenia, with particular focus on atypical neuroleptics. The multifactorial etiology of schizophrenia calls for a multidimensional therapy approach integrating psychopharmacological and psychosocial interventions. The efficacy of antipsychotics for both treatment of the acute phase and relapse prevention has been well demonstrated. Psychoeducational approaches are important to increase patients' and families' understanding of the illness and its treatment, including the role of medication. Due to their more benign side effects and somewhat greater impact on negative symptoms, compliance with atypical neuroleptics may be higher than with conventional neuroleptics, thereby improving the long-term prognosis of schizophrenia.

The hope of the editor in bringing together basic research and therapeutic applications is that this volume will stimulate research aimed at understanding the complex interactional components that influence the course of psychiatric illness. The further hope is to encourage further research on treatment designed to ameliorate the symptoms, stigma, and disability experienced by patients with severe mental illness, and the stress and suffering experienced by caregivers. These hopes and goals are consonant with Mike's contributions to these areas and reflect his enduring influence on our collective efforts to better understand and treat severe mental illness.

Acknowledgement

The author would like to thank Mrs. Sandra Rose Malik for her valuable help in completing Michael J. Goldstein's vita and Vida Goldstein for her presence at this symposium at Hamburg and her support. She also wants to thank the pharmaceutical company Lilly. Homburg, for supporting the publication of this book.

References

Brown, G.W., Birley, J.L.T., and Wing, J.K. (1972): Influence of family life on the course of schizophrenic disorders: a replication. British Journal of Psychiatry 121: 241–258

Doane, J.A., West, K.L., Goldstein, M.J., Rodnick, E.H., and Jones, J.E. (1981): Parental communication deviance and affective style: Predictors of subsequent schizophrenia spectrum disorders in vulnerable adolescents. Archives of General Psychiatry 38: 679–685

Falloon, I.R.H., Boyd, J., and McGill, C. (1984): Family Care of Schizophrenia. New York: Guilford Press

Goldstein, M.J. (1987): The UCLA high-risk project. Schizophrenia Bulletin 13: 505–514

Goldstein, M.J., Rodnick, E.H. Evans, J.R., May, P.R.A., and Steinberg, M. (1978): Drug and family therapy in the aftercare and treatment of acute schizophrenia. Archives of General Psychiatry 35: 1169–1177

Goldstein, M.J., Rosenfarb, I., Woo, S., and Nuechterlein, K.H. (1994): Intrafamilial relationships and the course of schizophrenia. Acta Psychiatrica Scandinavica 90 (Suppl. 384): 60–66

Hahlweg, K., Goldstein, M.J., Nuechterlein, K.H., Magana, A.B., Mintz, J., Doane, J.A., Miklowitz, D.J., and Snyder, K.S. (1989): Expressed emotion and patient-relative interaction in families of recent onset schizophrenics. Journal of Consulting and Clinical Psychology 57: 11–18

Leff, J. and Vaughn, C. (1985): Expressed emotion in families. New York: Guilford Press

Linszen, D.H., Dingemans, P.M., Scholte, W.F., Van der Does, J.W., Nugter, M.A. Lenior, M.E., and Goldstein, M.J. (1996): Treatment, expressed emotion and relapse in recent onset schizophrenic disorders. Psychological Medicine 26: 333–342

Magana, A.B., Goldstein, M.J., Karno, M., Miklowitz, D.J., Jenkins, J., and Falloon, I.R.H. (1986): A brief method for assessing expressed emotion in relatives of psychiatric patients. Psychiatry Research 17: 203–212

Miklowitz, D.J., Goldstein, M.J., Falloon, I.R.H., and Doane, J.A. (1984): Interactional correlates of expressed emotion in the families of schizophrenics. British Journal of Psychiatry 144: 482–487

Miklowitz, D.J., Goldstein, M.J., Nuechterlein, K.H., Snyder, K.S., and Mintz, J. (1988): Family factors and the course of bipolar affective disorder. Archives of General Psychiatry 45: 225–231

Nuechterlein, K.H., and Dawson, M.E., (1984): A heuristic vulnerability/stress model of schizophrenic episodes. Schizophrenia Bulletin 10: 300–312

Nuechterlein, K., Ventura, J., Snyder, K., Gitlin, M., Subotnik, K., Dawson, M., and Mintz, J. (1998) The Role of Stressors in Schizophrenic Relapse: Longitudinal Evidence and Implications for Psychosocial Interventions. Proceedings of the VI World Congress, World Association for Psychosocial Rehabilitation (WAPR) (p. 114), Hamburg, Germany

Rea, M.M., Goldstein, M.J. Tompson, M.C., and Miklowitz, D.J. (1998): Family and Individual Therapy in Bipolar Disorder: Outline and First Results of the UCLA Study. Proceedings of the VI World Congress, World Association for Psychosocial Rehabilitation (WAPR) (p. 115), Hamburg, Germany

Rosenfarb, I.S., Goldstein, M.J., Mintz, J., and Nuechterlein, K.H. (1995): Expressed emotion and subclinical psychopathology observable within the transactions between schizophrenic patients and their family members. Journal of Abnormal Psychology 104(2): 259–267

Rosenfarb, I.S., Nuechterlein, K.H., Goldstein, M.J., and Subotnik, K.L. (2000): Neurocognitive vulnerability, interpersonal criticism, and the emergence of unusual thinking during family transactions in patients with schizophrenia. Archives of General Psychiatry 57: 1174–1179

Strachan, A.M., Leff, J.P., Goldstein, M.J., Doane, J.A., and Burtt, C. (1986): Emotional attitudes and direct communication in the families of schizophrenics: A cross-national replication. British Journal of Psychiatry 149: 279–287

Tompson, M.C., Goldstein, M.J., Lebell, M.B., Mintz, L.I., Marder, S.R., and Mintz, J. (1995): Schizophrenic patients' perceptions of their relatives' attitudes. Psychiatry Research 57: 155–167

Vaughn, C., and Leff, J.P. (1976a): The measurement of expressed emotion in families of psychiatric patients. British Journal of Social and Clinical Psychology 15: 157–165

Vaughn, C., and Leff, J.P. (1976b): The influence of family and social factors on the course of psychiatric illness: a comparison of schizophrenic and depressed neurotic patients. British Journal of Psychiatry 129: 125–137

Woo, S.M., Goldstein, M.J., and Nuechterlein, K.H. (1997): Relatives' expressed emotion and nonverbal signs of subclinical psychopathology in schizophrenic patients. British Journal of Psychiatry 170: 58–61

Zubin, J., and Spring, B. (1977): Vulnerability-a new view of schizophrenia. Journal of Abnormal Psychology 86: 103–126

Munich, 2002   *A. Schaub*

2
Michael J. Goldstein's Impact on the Field

Kurt Hahlweg

When Michael J. Goldstein died on March 13, 1997, the scientific community and in particular Clinical Psychology lost an outstanding teacher, creative therapist, internationally renowned scholar and a wise, humorous and caring friend. Michael Goldstein is survived by his wife Vida, his two daughters, Janet and Ellen, his son Peter, and four grandchildren Fiona, Natalia, Robert and Jacob. He also leaves an important legacy in the lives of his doctoral students in the US and Europe and of his research fellows.

Mike Goldstein was born in New York City on June 28, 1930. He attended the State University of Iowa, where he obtained a bachelor of art degree in Speech Pathology. In 1953 he obtained a master of science degree in Clinical Psychology from Washington State University and in 1957 he received a doctor of philosophy degree in Clinical Psychology from the University of Washington. He began his academic career at the University of California, Los Angeles in 1957. In 1968 he attained the rank of Full Professor and remained at UCLA until his death. While at Franz Hall, he developed the Family Laboratory and devoted his professional life to the study of family factors in schizophrenia and bipolar disorder as well as to the development of effective psychoeducational family treatment interventions for these disorders.

During the course of his career, Mike was the recipient of many honors and awards. He was a Fulbright Research Professor at the University of Copenhagen (1960–1961), where he and his family became familiar with the European life style, resulting in many visits to Europe. In 1989, he was a visiting Professor at Nagasaki University, Japan, and in 1992 he was awarded with the Spinoza

Chair of the Department of Psychiatry, University of Amsterdam. Mike Goldstein was honored by election as Fellow of the American College of Neuropsychopharmacology and the American Psychological Association, and the Distinguished Scientist Award from SSCP and APA. He was appointed as member, chairman, and consultant of many NIMH grant review committees as well as a consultant for WHO. In 1997 he received posthumously the Gerald Klerman Award for Biopsychosocial Research for his 40 years of extraordinary contributions to the assessment, prevention and treatment of patients with schizophrenia and bipolar disorder.

From 1956 onwards, he published *128 empirical articles, 55 book chapters, 7 authored books, and served as editor or coeditor of 6 books*. His reference list is attached as an appendix to this chapter.

The coherence and continuity of his research enterprise is underscored by the fact that his research received NIMH support without interruption from 1964 until his death; in 1989 he received the NIMH MERIT award. His main research interest were:

A. Family factors related to schizophrenia and other mental disorders
B. Research and practise in Family Therapy

In the following Mike Goldstein's major research contributions will be summarized.

Family Factors Related to Schizophrenia and Other Mental Disorders

The UCLA High-risk Project (Goldstein, 1985, 1987)

The association between observed disturbances in family relationships in which a member has been diagnosed as having schizophrenia had let to the conclusion that these disturbances may have preceded the onset of illness and contributed to it. These hypothesis owed much to the impact of Psychoanalysis and Family Therapy, particularly after 1950. Despite frequent reports in the literature of disordered relationship systems in families with a schizophrenic relative, it was difficult to separate those relationships reactive to the psychotic relative from those antedating the onset of the disorder. Unless it can be demonstrated that such relationships precede the onset of the disorder, either in its prodromal or full-blown state, it is difficult to accept the hypothesis that disturbed family relationships play a contributory role in the development of the disorder. This issue can be answered only within a high-risk design in which the hypothesized intrafamilial risk factors are measured prospectively and the offspring followed throughout the risk period for the disorder.

The UCLA high-risk longitudinal-prospective study was designed to establish whether certain characteristic patterns of family relationships were risk markers for the subsequent development of schizophrenia and related disorders such as schizotypal, paranoid, and borderline personality disorders. It is the landmark study in this field, and the only up to date, in which the contribution of familial factors was investigated in a prospective study. The study is to praise for its methodological rigor, the development and refinement of the family measures, the stamina of Mike Goldstein to successfully conduct this 20 year study, and for the impact, the results had on our understanding of the family factors in psychopathology.

The study was designed by Goldstein and Rodnick and began in 1965 (see Goldstein et al., 1968) with a cohort of 64 families, each of whom with a mild to moderately disturbed teenager. Each family had applied for help for their teenager at the UCLA based psychology clinic. The cohort was believed to include a number of individuals at risk for subsequent schizophrenia and schizophrenia-linked disorders because of the hypothesis, that disturbances in adolescence increased the likelihood of more severe psychopathology in adulthood.

Design

All families studied were intact at the time of the initial assessment. The families were predominantly Caucasian, of middle- to upper middle-class status, and above average in intelligence. None of the adolescents were considered psychotic or borderline psychotic, at the time of admission. The families agreed to participate in a six-session series of family assessment procedures designed to reveal characteristic patterns of family interaction. The family assessment consisted of two main elements – individual assessment of the parents and index person, and family assessment in which the family was observed discussing a series of conflictual family problems. The working hypothesis was that early signs of maladjustment in an adolescent, coupled with the presence of disturbances in communicational and affective climate within the family, would increase the risk for schizophrenia or schizophrenia-spectrum disorders in the offspring.

Dimensions of family behavior. There are obviously many aspects of family behavior that have been hypothesized to be relevant to the development of schizophrenia. Goldstein and his colleagues relied on measures that had been well operationalized and had been found empirically valid in systematic studies of families with a schizophrenic offspring. These measures are: *communication deviance (CD), expressed emotion (EE), and affective style (AS).*

Communication Deviance. CD is derived from the work of Wynne and colleagues (1977) and refers to parent's inability to establish and maintain a shared focus of attention during transactions with another person. Typically, this measure is derived from transactions between a parent and an examiner during the administration of a projective technique, usually the Rorschach or Thematic Apperception Test (TAT).

In this study, the individual TATs administered to each parent were used to rate CD. Parental units were classified into three levels of CD: *High, Intermediate* or *Low* CD.

Expressed Emotion (EE). This is a construct reflecting *attitudes* of criticism and/or emotional overinvolvement expressed during a tape-recorded interview with an examiner, the Camberwell Family Interview (CFI, Vaughn and Leff, 1976). A modified version of the CFI was used in this study with the parents. Parents were categorized as high or low EE, based largely on the criticism criterion (>6 criticisms expressed = high EE), and then classified into parental groups as follows: *dual high* EE, both parents high; *mixed,* one parent high, the other low; and *dual low* EE, both parents are low EE.

Affective Style. The second measure of affective attitudes was termed negative affective style and derived from *directly* observed interactions during which family members discussed conflictual problems. These interactions were coded with the Affective Style (AS) measure that resemble the EE dimension as they might be expressed transactionally (Doane et al., 1981). Families were classified as negative, intermediate, or benign in affective style.

Follow-up procedures. Five years after the initial contact, the young adult index persons were interviewed with a structured psychiatric interview and diagnosed by Research Diagnostic Criteria (RDC) by a clinician without knowledge of any other data on the case. Ten years after this diagnostic assessment, the process was repeated again, although the data from the 15-year assessment were categorized according to DSM-III. The earlier RDC diagnoses were converted to the closest DSM-III equivalent. Data from $N = 54$ index cases could be used for the data analysis.

Results

To establish the predictive validity of the three family measures, it was necessary to group the diagnosis into clusters. As with the family predictors, a trichotomy was used, based on the notion of the extended schizophrenia spectrum suggested originally in the Danish Adoption Studies (Kety et al., 1968): *Schizophrenia Spectrum Disorder*, that included schizophrenia, schizotypal, paranoid personality disorder, borderline and schizoid personality disorder; "Other" psychiatric disorder, and No Mental Illness (NMI) over the 15-year period.

The three family predictors then were entered into a log linear analysis to evaluate:

(1) how they related to the three outcome categories as independent factors, and (2) how well they related when the variance in the other two predictors was partialled out.

The distributions of outcomes are presented first for each predictor taken by itself, as shown in Table 1.

When the log linear procedure was used to test the contribution of each variable with overlapping variance with the others removed, probabilities for the partial association were 0.002 for CD, 0.001 for AS, but a clearly nonsignificant 0.789 for EE. Thus, when both affective measures are in the log linear analysis, EE no longer reaches a significant contribution to the prediction of outcome.

Discussion

The main conclusion from this study is, that the adolescent at risk for schizophrenia-spectrum disorders comes from a home environment characterized by high CD and a strongly negative affective climate. The behavioral indicator of affective attitude, AS type, proved to be a better addition to CD than the attitudinal measure of EE. It is

Table 1. The UCLA High Risk Project: Distribution of Outcome (Goldstein, 1987, p. 509)

	Communication deviance (CD)			Affective style (AS)			Expressed emotion (EE)		
	NMI	Other	Spectrum	NMI	Other	Spectrum	NMI	Other	Spectrum
Low[1]	8	3	1	11	11	1	5	12	1
Intermiate	3	11	5	1	6	2	6	5	6
High	3	7	10	4	4	12	1	4	7
		(p<.002)			(p<.0008)			(p<.04)	

Note: NMI = no mental illness; Other = other psychiatric disorder than schizophrenia spectrum; Spectrum = extended schizophrenia spectrum, broad grouping.
[1] For AS, comparable categories are benign, intermediate, and negative; or EE, dual low, mixed, and dual high EE.

interesting to note that the only difference between the intermediate and negative AS profiles was the presence of a minimum of one supportive statement by a parent in the context of critical AS behaviors. While it is hard to imagine that one such positive remark could make such a notable difference in a 10-minute, emotionally loaden interaction, it may reflect tendencies towards compromise or a latent positive attitude towards the adolescent largely masked by the conflict of the moment, a quality that may be totally lacking in the negative AS profile family.

The results of this study indicate that measures such as CD, AS, and EE are effective in identifying family units whose offspring are at greater than normal risk for subsequent schizophrenia and related disorder. However, they appear to have predictive validity in the context of a family unit with at least one child who is having behavioral difficulties. Future studies need to establish that these variables are true risk markers in the absence of notable offspring psychopathology. In order to characterize Mike Goldstein's careful, self-critical, and future-oriented methodological thinking, I cite the last paragraph of his 1987 paper:

"The family measures used appear to identify a family unit at risk, but are not helpful in telling who among the offspring is at risk. Obviously, the development of a genetic marker for schizophrenia, either from behavioral or biochemical studies, would greatly facilitate our understanding of who is at risk and in what environmental context the at-risk person manifest a schizophrenic disorder. Lacking such markers, future studies should avoid the error of this study of selecting and assessing only one offspring in the high- and low-risk family units. All offspring must be studied if one is to understand why only some offspring in high-risk family units develop schizophrenia or schizophrenia-spectrum disorders.

Along these lines, it would be helpful if future high-risk studies could incorporate the individual vulnerability markers, uncovered in other high-risk studies, such as deficits in neuropsychological performance, information processing, and social relationships, in projects in which family risk markers are measured as well. The nature of the linkage between intrafamilial transactions and the development of cognitive and social competence is still not well worked out, and future high-risk studies could provide important information about the subtle interplay among them across the life span. Are attentional deficits expressions of the diathesis that interact with intrafamilial processes, or do they arise from deviant patterns of communication and affect expression? These are important issues that only prospective longitudinal studies of high- and low-risk populations can resolve." (p. 513).

Do Relatives Express Expressed Emotion?
(Strachan, Goldstein and Miklowith, 1986)

Since the seventies, levels of family expressed emotion (EE) had been repeatedly found to predict relapse rates in schizophrenic patients 9 or 12 months after hospital discharge (Leff and Vaughn, 1985). These studies showed that the chance of relapse increases by a factor of approximately 2.5 when a patient returns to a family environment marked by high levels of criticism or emotional overinvolvement. In contrast to the 50% relapse rate among high EE families at 9 months, the relapse rate among low EE families averages 20%.

Expressed emotion is coded from the individual Camberwell Family Interview (CFI; Vaughn and Leff, 1976) with a relative of the psychiatric patient, and ratings are based on statements made by the relative about the patient. The number of critical comments (statements of irritation, dislike, or resentment about the patient's behavior or personality, usually expressed with corresponding voice tone) in the interview are counted. The degree of emotional overinvolvement (markedly overconcerned, overprotective, or self-sacrificing attitudes and behavior) is rated on a 6-point scale for the whole interview. Relatives are classified as high EE if they show evidence of excessive criticism or emotional overinvolvement. Generally, this interview is administered while the patient is hospitalized for an index episode of the disorder, and it is assumed that the EE rating reflects the type of family environment that the patient will encounter after discharge.

Studies have shown that the EE measure is relevant not only to schizophrenia but also as a valuable predictor of relapse in depression (Hooley, Orley, and Teasdale, 1986) and in recent-onset mania (Miklowitz, Goldstein, Nuechterlein, Snyder, and Mintz, 1988).

Despite the strong association between EE and relapse, we still know relatively little about the mechanism underlying the correlation between family attitudes and the flaring up of symptoms in psychiatric patients. Because the CFI measures relatives' attitudes towards the patient that are expressed within the context of an interview with a mental health professional we need to know whether and in what ways these attitudes are also expressed in face-to-face contact with the patient. One approach to investigate the construct validity of EE is to systematically analyze the behavior of high EE and low EE relatives as they interact with the patient after the patient has left the hospital and returned home.

In three studies, the relationship between EE attitudes and directly observed interactional behavior has been assessed using a standardized situation to elicit interactional behavior and a coding system to reflect the behavioral analogues of EE attitudes (Strachan, Goldstein, and Miklowitz, 1986). Using a modification of an interaction task developed originally by Goldstein and his colleagues (1968) for their forementioned longitudinal prospective study, investigators asked family members to discuss in the laboratory two emotionally loaded family problems derived from a prior interview. The Affective Style (AS; Doane et al., 1981) coding system was used to measure specific verbal behaviors of relatives during this interaction task. The AS system classifies verbal behavior into categories such as support, benign and personal criticism, guilt induction, and intrusiveness (statements indicating that the relative believes that he or she has knowledge of the patient's inner states beyond what the patient has actually said).

In the first study investigating the association between EE attitudes and interactional behavior (Valone, Norton, Goldstein, and Doane, 1983), 52 families from the UCLA longitudinal prospective study were investigated. High EE parents expressed significantly more criticism towards their disturbed but nonpsychotic offspring in direct interactions than did low EE parents. In the second study with a sample including primarily chronic schizophrenic patients and their families (Miklowitz, Goldstein, Falloon, and Doane, 1984), parents rated as high EE because of criticism (on the CFI) were distinguished by their frequent use of critical comments during the interaction task whereas those rated as high EE on the overinvolvement criteria used more intrusive statements. In the third study, conducted in Great Britain (Strachan, Leff, Goldstein, Doane, and Burtt, 1986), these findings were replicated even though the patients in this study had recent onset schizophrenia and the interactional behavior was assessed from dyadic rather than triadic interactions between patients and relatives.

These studies indicated that, when data were aggregated over a total interaction, high EE families with a mentally ill member were characterized by criticism, intrusion, and high verbal output, whereas low EE families interact in a more neutral fashion. Interestingly, none of these studies reported that low EE relatives used more positive or supportive statements than high EE relatives during the family discussion. This finding may be due to the task itself because it was developed to examine conflictual issues, or it may reflect limitations in the AS coding system, which was specifically designed to capture negative communication behaviors. However, it seemed unlikely that the protective value of low EE behavior derives simply from an absence of negative behavior. Although the associations reported to date between relatives' EE ratings during an interview and during family interaction have been congruent with the EE construct and consistent across studies, there were some limitations.

The mentioned studies compared the CFI rating system for EE, which is based on both the verbal and nonverbal behavior of a respondent during an interview with behavior in a directly observed family discussion coded by a system that relies solely on verbal content (the AS system is used with verbatim transcripts exclusively). Therefore, in a fourth study (Hahlweg et al., 1989), another coding system was applied to the interactional data, the Kategoriensystem für Partnerschaftliche Interaktion KPI (Category System for Partner and Family Interaction). The KPI codes both verbal and nonverbal behavior and the behavior of relatives and patient. Because previous studies had aggregated the relative's data over the whole interaction and had not considered the patient's behavior, it was not possible to study the processes of family interaction as they emerged over time. Whereas the AS method is a critical-incident coding system, the KPI codes all units of interactional behavior in sequential order. It was, therefore, possible to apply techniques of sequential analysis to these data to measure the relative contributions of patients and relatives to the observable family processes and to document whether patterns of interaction discriminate high EE from low EE families.

Forty-three families with a schizophrenic patient were included in the study. All patients (and families) were participants in the UCLA Developmental Processes in Schizophrenic Disorders Project (Nuechterlein, Edell, Norris, and Dawson, 1986), which was an ongoing longitudinal study of the early course of schizophrenia. Patients were recruited in a psychotic state during an index hospitalization.

High-EE critical relatives were characterized by a negative interactional style in that they showed more negative nonverbal affect, more criticism, and more negative solution proposals than either low EE or high EE-overinvolved relatives when discussing an emotionally loaded family problem. Both of the latter groups not only showed a lower rate of negative behaviors but also showed a higher rate of positive and supportive statements than did the high EE-critical relatives. Patients who had high EE-critical relatives showed more negative nonverbal affect and more self-justifying statements than patients with either low EE or high EE-overinvolved relatives. Patients living with high EE members, irrespective of subgroup, expressed more disagreements than patients living with low EE relatives.

The results for negative behavior were even more apparent when the findings of the sequential analysis were taken into account. High EE-critical families showed long-lasting negative reciprocal patterns in the nonverbal domain, whereas low EE and high EE-overinvolved families had much shorter negative patterns. It made no difference, whether the patient or the parents started a negative sequence. In both instances, the same interaction pattern resulted. This result points to the need to include the patient into psychoeducational family care because he or she contributes in the same way to the style of interaction.

Research and Practise in Family Therapy

The Brief Focal Family Approach (Goldstein, Rodnick, Evans, May, and Steinberg, 1978)

Long before the results of the forementioned studies with regard to family factors in schizophrenia were known, Goldstein and his colleagues (1978) devised a six-session family treatment model for patients who had been discharged home to their families after brief inpatient treatment of acute episodes of schizophrenia. These patients had been included in a controlled study. Patients were often discharged after only the most disturbing symptoms had remitted, and were often still in the restitution phase. It was clear that these patients were at high risk for subsequent relapse. For this reason an intervention that helped the family in understanding the nature of the patient's illness and the need for stress reduction in the period immediately after discharge appeared indicated.

The crisis-oriented method involved six weekly (1-hour) sessions during which a psychologist met with the patient and family members in a problem-focused group. These sessions focused mainly on current and anticipated future stressors. The families discussed ways to reduce their current difficulties and to possibly prevent past difficulties from recurring. Patients and families were encouraged to adopt realistic expectations concerning their full recovery from the illness and to reduce the pressure on the patient to return rapidly to his or her premorbid social status. A gradual return to social functioning was advocated.

Although the sessions were relatively unstructured, the therapists were to focus on the following four target goals in the six sessions: (1) The patient and his or her family were able to accept the fact that he or she had suffered a psychotic illness. (2) They were willing to identify some of the probable precipitating stressors in the patient's life at the time the illness occurred. (3) They tried to generalize from these and to identify future stressors to which the patient and his or her family were likely to be vulnerable. (4) They tried to do some planning on how to minimize or avoid these future stresses.

The first of these aims involved discussion about the nature of schizophrenia, with the therapist educating the patient and family about the association between stressful events and precipitation of the illness, as well as the serious nature of schizophrenia, its prognosis, and the need for drug treatment and stress management to prevent further episodes. Once the family had a clear grasp of the stress-diathesis hypothesis, a problem-solving format was employed to identify stressors, to explore strategies for avoiding or coping with stressful situations, and to plan and evaluate attempts to use stress-management strategies. Dealing with current symptoms of schizophrenia and practical problems of daily living were stressors commonly identified. Some intrafamilial stressors were dealt with, but attempts to restructure family communication patterns were generally avoided.

In a controlled outcome study the effectiveness of this approach was investigated in a population of predominantly first admission patients who were diagnosed on broad-based criteria for schizophrenia. Patients were all maintained on injections of flu-phenazine, either 25 or 6.25 mg every two weeks. Measures of psychopathology and community tenure were collected before treatment, after six weeks, and after six months. This pioneering study was the first investigating the combined effects of family therapy with two different levels of antipsychotics.

Figure 1 presents the percentage of patients who relapsed by the end of the six week controlled trial and at the six-month follow-up point. At six weeks the low-dose-no family therapy (LO-NFT) had a relapse rate of 24% percent while the high-dose family therapy (HI-FT) had no relapse. At six month, the rate of relapse increased to 48% in LO-NFT but remained at 0 percent in HI-FT. Patients treated with family therapy had significantly lower ratings of psychopathology on withdrawal, affective disturbance, and thought disorder factors of the Brief Psychiatric Rating Scale (BPRS). These advantages for family therapy were less pronounced six months after discharge. The importance of optimal neuroleptic treatment in achieving and sustaining the benefits of psychosocial treatments is underscored by this study, at least in the first few months after an acute episode of schizophrenia.

Stimulated by these results four controlled outcome studies were conducted in the eighties (Leff et al., 1982; Falloon et al., 1984; Anderson et al., 1986; Tarrier et al., 1988). Although the individual concepts differed, there were several common components (Gold-

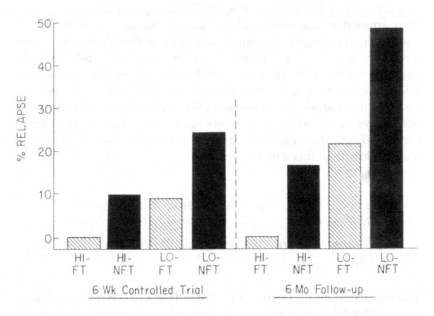

Fig. 1. Relapse of Brief Focussed Family Therapy (Goldstein et al., 1978). Drug condition: High (HI): 1 ml; Low (LO): 1/4 ml; Family therapy (FT); No family therapy (NFT)

stein and Strachan, 1986): i) All approaches were based on the vulnerability-stress model; ii) The patients were on neuroleptic medication; iii) Intervention was relatively brief with about 15 to 25 sessions in the first year; iv) The main focus was on lowering familial stress.

In these studies, the average relapse rate in the first year for patients with standard psychiatric care was about 50% while patients with family psychoeducational treatment had a relapse rate of about 10%. Relapse rates after two years were 70% and 20% respectively. It seems warranted to conclude that the Brief Fokal Family Therapy by Goldstein and his colleagues led the foundation for these very exciting new approaches to the prevention of relapse in schizophrenic patients.

The introduction of lithium in the early 1970 brought great relief to the suffering of bipolar patients and their families. Decades later, however, the illness continues to take a painful pervasive toll: Even patients receiving optimal medication are likely to endure multiple recurrences and to have problems keeping jobs and maintaining relationships. In 1987, Mike Goldstein and David Miklowitz began to study the similarities and differences of the contexts in which schizophrenia and bipolar patients relapse. They then applied to the treatment of bipolar disorder what they had learned from the earlier treatment programs with schizophrenia and developed a 9-month outpatient program designed to help patients and families understand, accept, and manage their illness. In their treatment manual (Miklowitz and Goldstein, 1997) they describe the first treatment approach for bipolar disorder that truly integrates the use of medication and family intervention. The first results of their controlled outcome study are presented in the chapter by Richards and Miklowitz in this volume.

Impact of Family Intervention Programs on Family Communication and the Short-term Course of Schizophrenia (Goldstein and Strachan, 1986)

The replicated finding that some form of family intervention reduces the risk for relapse in patients already on maintenance pharmaco-therapy does not indicate which processes have been modified by the family program. Most family programs, tested in these controlled trials, have been comprehensive in nature, providing education for relatives, support for the family system, as well as specific training in altering intra-familial behavior. A theoretical model that emphasizes the affective climate of the family as a risk factor for relapse would receive greater support if it could be shown that the family programs that reduce relapse do, in fact, modify this component of family life.

However, as Strachan and colleagues (1986) indicated, this merely documents a change in attitudes expressed to an interviewer during a repeated Camberwell Family Interview, but does not indicate that family behaviors have changed. At UCLA, Goldstein and his colleagues attempted this type of evaluation with data from the Falloon et al. (1984) study, which involved a comparison of individual and family therapy for schizophrenic patients maintained on phenothiazine medication. Before each family entered their respective psychosocial treatment program, they participated in a pretreatment family assessment task. This was a direct interaction task described by Strachan and colleagues (1986), in which two problems were discussed with an experimenter present. After the first three months of treatment, this procedure was repeated. The problems discussed were developed in a similar fashion as for the pretreatment assessment. The problems used were those identified as idiosyncratically relevant to each family at the time each assessment took place.

The interactions were audio-recorded, and verbatim transcripts of these discussions were coded blindly by raters using the Affective Style (AS) coding system (Doane et al., 1981). Thirty-three families were included in this analysis. The results showed that there was a greater reduction in the negative affective style codes of criticism and intrusion for parents in family therapy than parents of individually treated patients (see Fig. 2). The analysis of the data on criticisms and intrusions revealed highly significant reductions for both types of negative affective communications for relatives in the family as contrasted with the individual treatment groups.

Since the British work on EE treats criticism and overinvolvement as independent dimensions in defining EE status, the rate of change in criticism separate from the rate of change in intrusiveness was considered. Families were thus classified into three categories: (1) dual increase, in which both criticism and intrusiveness increased from pre- to posttest, (2) dual decrease, in which both declined during the same period, and (3) a mixed group in which one attribute increased while the other decreased. Results showed, that

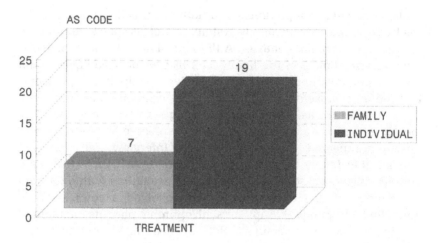

Fig. 2. Total numbers of critical and intrusive statements at 3-month posttest by therapy groups

the dual increase pattern was found in half of the individual therapy families but only rarely in the family therapy group. Conversely, the dual decrease pattern was prominent in the family-treated cases, but less frequent in the individual therapy condition. The frequency of the mixed pattern did not vary by treatment groups. Thus, there was a clear trend for reduction in one or both forms of the negative AS behaviors in the family treatment condition.

The affective climate of the family with a schizophrenic young adult offspring relates to the short-term course of the disorder. Further, when family-based interventions are associated with a longer period of community tenure for the patient, parallel reductions in this negative affective climate are noted in direct observations of family behavior. The optimum results were found when both components of the AS system, criticism and intrusiveness, were reduced in frequency from pre- to a three-month posttest assessment.

Whenever one type of family behavior is reduced in frequency, it naturally raises the question of what characterizes the new pattern of family transactions. A key objective of the study by Falloon et al. was to train family members in a defined set of strategies for dealing with problems inside and outside of the family. A coding system was developed by Doane et al. (1985) for recording instances in the direct family interaction tasks where family members utilized these recommended problem-solving strategies (PSS). When pre- and 3-month direct interaction tasks data were contrasted in the number of PSS behaviors expressed, there was a highly significant difference between treatment conditions at 3 months favoring the family-treated group. Also, when the pattern of change in AS was examined for PSS change levels, sharp differences were found between the dual decrease groups in family therapy and dual increase group in individual therapy in the 3-month data. This means that in the former group there were 20 more instances of PSS behavior than was evident at pretest, while in the latter there was virtually no change from base line. The remaining AS change groups showed slight positive changes in scores that were similar in the two treatment conditions.

These results suggest that a task-centered form of problem solving takes the place of the negative interaction patterns of criticism, blaming, and intrusiveness into the inner state of the patient. When a large reduction in the negative AS behaviors had occurred, a major shift in this more affectively neutral, task-centered behavior is observed; the reverse is noted when heightened levels of both forms of AS are evident. These data suggest a marked reciprocity between uncontrolled negative affective expression focused upon the patient and more controlled, cognitive form of behavior focused upon common family problems.

"Since we have only two points in the Falloon study where direct interaction data were obtained, we cannot speak to the sequential linkage between these two dimensions of family behavior. Does family based intervention first inhibit negative affective expression, thereby permitting the acquisition of problem-solving skills? Or, does the early acquisition of problem-solving skills simply replace negative affective expression without any specific instructions to limit or inhibit these behaviors? Further studies with repeated observations of the family therapy process are needed to tease apart these issues – issues that are critical to understand if we are to plan more effective programs for optimizing family change." (Goldstein and Strachan, 1986, p. 190).

Final Comments

What consequences arise from Mike Goldstein's pioneering and impressive research findings? To me, one of the most important aspects of his work was that he deeply cared about the patients and the family members. Research on family factors and the development of new treatment approaches was not just for scientific purpose but to provide empirically based interventions to reduce their suffering. It seems best to end this chapter with his words:

"... we have not emphasized issues concerning the long-term pharmacotherapy of the patient. We should never forget that all of the successful family programs are built upon a foundation of regular and continuous pharmacotherapy. However, the successful addition of family based intervention programs to regular pharmacotherapy raises the question of whether a potent social therapy permits alteration in the strategy of drug treatment in terms of dose level and pattern of treatment. Given the evidence that a comprehensive family intervention program produces some degree of stabilization of the stress level in the social environment, we can now consider whether this stabilization permits the use of lower dose levels of phenothiazine medication or even more radical strategies, such as intermittent or targeted use of medication. An ironic side effect of an effective family program may be that it permits greater latitude for experimentation in the complementary area of psychopharmacology" (Goldstein and Strachan, 1986, p. 191).

References

Anderson, C.M., Reiss, D.J. and Hogarty, G.E. (1986): Schizophrenia and the family. New York: Guilford Press

Doane, J.A., Falloon, I.R.H., Goldstein, M.J., and Mintz, J. (1985): Parental affective style and the treatment of schizophrenia: Predicting course of illness and social functioning. Archives of General Psychiatry 42: 34–42

Doane, J.A., West, K.L., Goldstein, M.J., Rodnick, E.H., and Jones, J.E. (1981): Parental communication deviance and affective style: Predictors of subsequent schizophrenia spectrum disorder in vulnerable adolescents. Archives of General Psychiatry 38: 679–685

Falloon, I.R.H., McGill, C.W., and Boyd, J.L. (1984): Family care of schizophrenia. New York: Guilford Press

Goldstein, M.J. (1985): Family factors that antedate the onset of schizophrenia and related disorders: The results of a fifteen year prospective longitudinal study. Acta Psychiatrica Scandinavica 71 (Suppl. 319), 7–18

Goldstein, M.J. (1987): The UCLA high-risk project. Schizophrenia Bulletin 13: 505–514

Goldstein, M.J., Judd, L.L., Rodnick, H.E., Alkire, A., and Gould, E. (1968): A method for studying social influence and coping patterns within families of disturbed adolescents. Journal of Nervous and Mental Disease 147: 233–251

Goldstein, M.J., Rodnick, E.H., Evans, J.R., May, P.R.A., and Steinberg, M. (1978): Drug and family therapy in the aftercare and treatment of acute schizophrenia. Archives of General Psychiatry 35: 1169–1177

Goldstein, M.J., and Strachan, A.M. (1986): Impact of family intervention program on family communication and the short-term course of schizophrenia. In: Treatment of schizophrenia: Family assessment and intervention, Goldstein, M.J., Hand, I. and Hahlweg, K. (eds.) pp.185–192. Berlin Heidelberg: Springer

Hahlweg, K.H., Goldstein, M.J., Nuechterlein, K.H., Magana, A.B., Mintz, J., Doane, J.A., Miklowitz, D.J., and Snyder, K.S. (1989): Expressed emotion and patient-relative interaction in families of recent-onset schizophrenics. Journal of Consulting and Clinical Psychology 57: 11–18

Hooley, J.M., Orley, J. and Teasdale, J.D. (1986): Levels of expressed emotion and relapse in depressed patients. British Journal of Psychiatry 148: 642–647

Kety, S.S., Rosenthal, D., Wender, P.H., and Schulsinger, F. (1968): The types and prevalence of mental illness in the biological and adoptive families of adopted schizophrenics. In: The transmission of schizophrenia, Rosenthal, D. and Kety, S.S. (eds.), pp. 345–362. Oxford: Pergamon

Leff, J., Kuipers, L., Berkowitz, R., Eberlein-Vries, R., and Sturgeon, D.A. (1982): A controlled trial of social intervention in the families of schizophrenic patients. British Journal of Psychiatry 141: 121–134

Leff, J. and Vaughn, C. (1985): Expressed emotion in families. New York: Guilford Press

Miklowitz, D., and Goldstein, M.J. (1997): Bipolar disorder. A family focussed treatment approach. New York: Guilford

Miklowitz, D.J., Goldstein, M.J., Falloon, I.R.H., and Doane, J.A. (1984): Interactional correlates of expressed emotion in the families of schizophrenics. British Journal of Psychiatry 144: 482–487

Miklowitz, D.J., Goldstein, M.J., Snyder, K.S., and Mintz, J. (1988): Family factors and the course of bipolar affective disorder. Archives of General Psychiatry 45: 225–231

Nuechterlein, K.H., Edell, W.S., Norris, M., and Dawson, M.E. (1986): Attentional vulnerability indicators, thought disorder, and negative symptoms. Schizophrenia Bulletin 12: 408–426

Strachan, A.M., Goldstein, M.J., and Miklowitz, D.J. (1986): Do relatives express expressed emotion? In: Treatment of schizophrenia: Family assessment and intervention, Goldstein, M.J., Hand, I. and Hahlweg, K. (eds.), pp. 51–58. Berlin Heidelberg: Springer

Strachan, A.M., Leff, J.P., Goldstein, M.J., Doane, J.A., and Burtt, C. (1986): Emotional attitudes and direct communication in the families of schizophrenics: A cross-national replication. British Journal of Psychiatry 149: 279–287

Tarrier, N., Barrowclough, C., Vaughn, C., Bamrah, J.S., Porceddu, K., Watts, S., and Freeman, H. (1998): The community management of schizophrenia: A controlled trial of a behavioral intervention with families to reduce relapse. British Journal of Psychiatry 153: 532–542

Valone, K., Norton, J.P., Goldstein, M.J., and Doane, J.A. (1983): Parental expressed emotion and affective style in an adolescent sample at risk for schizophrenia spectrum disorders. Journal of Abnormal Psychology 92: 399–407

Vaughn, C. and Leff, J.P. (1976): The measurement of expressed emotion in the families of psychiatric patients. British Journal of Social and Clinical Psychology 15: 157–165

Wynne, L.C., Singer, M.T., Bartko, J.J., and Toohey, M.L. (1977): Schizophrenics and their families: Research on parental communication. In: Developments in psychiatric research (Tanner, J.M, ed.), pp. 254–284. London: Hodder and Stoughton

Curriculum vitae

Michael J. Goldstein, Ph.D.
29 June 1930 – 13 March 1997
Place of birth: New York, New York USA
Place of residence: Los Angeles, California USA

Education

1952	State University of Iowa, B.A., with a major in Speech Pathology.
1953	Washington State University, M.S., with a major in Clinical Psychology
1957	University of Washington, Ph.D., with a major in Clinical Psychology
1960	Clinical Psychologist License, PT-2384, August 2, 1960

Professional History

University of California, Los Angeles

1957	Instructor
1958	Assistant Professor
1963	Associate Professor
1968	Professor
1995–1997	Professor Emeritus

Awards and Honors

| 1958 | Fellow, University of Connecticut, Summer Institute in Gerontology, Storrs, Connecticut, USA |
| 1960–1961 | Fulbright Research Professor, University of Copenhagen |

1961	Fellow, American College of Neuropsychopharmacology
1983	UCLA Awardee, Network on Risk and Protective Factors in the Major Mental Disorders, MacArthur Foundation
1984	Fellow, American Psychological Association
1985	Distinguished Contribution to Family Therapy Award, American Family Therapy Association
1987	Cumulative Contribution to Research in Family Therapy Award, American Association for Marriage and Family Therapy
1988	UCLA Distinguished Teaching Award
1989	Visiting Professor, Nagasaki University, Japan
1990	National Institute of Mental Health Merit Award
1991	Spinoza Chair, Department of Psychiatry, University of Amsterdam
1997	Gralnick Foundation Award
1997	Distinguished Contribution Award, Society for the Science of Clinical Psychology
1997	Gerald Klerman Award for Distinguished Biopsychosocial Research, Association for Clinical Psychosocial Research

Research Interests

- Family factors related to schizophrenia and other mental disorders
- Clinical psychopharmacological studies
- Family therapy: Research practice.

Research Support

1976–1997	Principal Investigator: National Institution of Mental Health (NIMH) USPHS Grant MH14584, *Psychological Research on Schizophrenic Conditions*
1989–1997	Principal Investigator: NIMH USPHS Grant MH42556, *Lithium and Family Management of Bipolar Disorder*
1964–1990	Principal Investigator: NIMH USPHS Grant MH08744, *Coping Behavior in Schizophrenia*

1983–1989 Principal Investigator: NIMH UCLA Node Mac-Arthur Foundation Grant, K830902, *MacArthur Network on Risk and Protective Factors in the Major Mental Disorders*

1982–1997 Co-Principal Investigator: NIMH USPHS Grant MH 30911, *Family Assessment and Intervention Laboratory of the UCLA Mental Health Clinical Research Center for the Study of Adult Schizophrenia*

1982–1987 Principal Investigator: NIMH USPHS Grant MH31759, *Consultation in the Risk Research Consortium*

1974–1976 Co-Principal Investigator: The Grant Foundation, *Intrafamilial Transactions and Adolescent Psychology*

1966–1976 Co-Principal Investigator: NIMH USPHS Grant MH 13512, Psychopharmacology Grant, *Phenothiazine Effects in Acute Schizophrenic Behavior*

1966–1972 Co-Principal Investigator: Scottish Rite Committee on Research in Schizophrenia, *Behavioral and Physiological Effects of Phenothiazine Medication*

1967–1969 Co-Principal Investigator: Pornography Research Contract, President's Commission on Obscenity and Pornography

Professional Activities

1969–1974 Member, NIMH Clinical Projects Review Committee

1975–1997 Chair, NIMH Clinical Projects Review Committee

1979–1980 Chair, NIMH Treatment Development and Assessment Review Committee, Panel on Psychosocial Treatments

1979–1997 Consultant, National Institute of Medicine Review of Stress and Illness

1979–1997 Consultant, NIMH, Review of NIMH Study Center

1982–1997 Consultant, NIMH Advisory Committee to Review the Behavioral Sciences Research Program

1977–1981 Member, Dean's Committee, Veteran's Association Hospital, Brentwood, California

1979–1980 Chair, Ad Hoc Panel to Review the NIMH Psychotherapy of Depression Review Committee

1975, 1979 Consultant, WHO, Mental Health Division

1986–1990 Member, NIMH Board of Scientific Counselors

1980–1997 Consultant, NIMH Research Planning Workshops: Children of Psychiatrically Disordered Parents, Office of Prevention, St. Louis, MO, 1980

- Preventative Intervention in Schizophrenia, Conference Organizer and Consultant, Office of Prevention, 1980
- Stress and Related Psychiatric Disorders, Office of Prevention, San Francisco, CA, 1981
- Measurement of Outcome in Chronic Schizophrenia, Center for the Study of Schizophrenia, Portsmouth, NH, 1981
- Stress and Adolescence, Behavioral Sciences Division, Bethesda, MD, 1981
- Preventative Intervention for Relatives with a Mentally-Ill Member, Consultant and Organizer, Prevention Branch and Center for the Study of Schizophrenia, La Jolla, CA, 1982
- Review of a potential collaborative study on combined family and drug therapy for schizophrenia, Center for the Study of Schizophrenia and Biological and Pharmacological Treatments Branch, Washington, DC, 1983
- Healthy Family Functioning, Office of Prevention, La Jolla, CA, 1983
- Member, American Schizophrenia Foundation, Scientific Panel
- Member, Scientific Council, National Alliance for Research on Schizophrenia and Depression (NARSAD), 1987–1997.

Participation in Scientific Journals

1976–1997 Member, Board of Directors, *Family Process*
1983–1994 Corresponding Editor, *Journal of Child Psychology and Psychiatry*
1986–1997 Associate Editor, *Schizophrenia Bulletin*
1976–1980 Member, Editorial Board, *Journal of Abnormal Psychology*
1976–1980 Member, Editorial Board, *Law and Human Behavior*
1987–1997 Associate Editor, *Journal of Family Psychology*
1987–1997 Member, Editorial Board, *Journal of Family Violence*

Publications

Goldstein, M.J. (1956): Perception and acculturation. Davidson Journal of Anthropology 2: 155–164

Goldstein, M.J. (1957): The relationship between coping and avoiding behavior and attitude modification. Dissertation Abstracts 17: 20–64

Barthol, R.P., and Goldstein, M.J. (1959): Psychology and the invisible self. California Management Review 1: 29–35

Goldstein, M.J. (1959): Coping and avoiding behavior and response to fear-arousing propaganda. Journal of Abnormal and Social Psychology 58: 247–252

Goldstein, M.J. (1959): Defensive forgetting and the Taylor scale of anxiety. Journal of Personality 24: 487–496

Goldstein, M.J. (1959): The relationship between coping and avoiding behavior and response to fear-arousing propaganda. Journal of Abnormal and Social Psychology 58: 247–252

Goldstein, M.J. (1960): The social desirability variable in attitude research. Journal of Social Psychology 52: 103–108

Goldstein, J.M., and Barthol, R.P. (1960): Fantasy responses to subliminal stimuli. Journal of Abnormal and Social Psychology 60: 22–26

McNeil, J., and Goldstein, M.J. (1960): Attitude change of students related to anxiety. Research Roundup on Children and Youth. Berkeley, CA: University of California Press

Goldstein, M.J. (1961): The relationship between anxiety and oral word association performance. Journal of Abnormal and Social Psychology 62: 468–471

Goldstein, M.J., and Davis, D. (1961): The impact of stimuli registering outside of awareness upon personal preferences. Journal of Personality 29(3): 247–257

Goldstein, M.J. and Ratleff, J. (1961): The relationship between frequency of usage and ease of recognition with response bias controlled. Perceptual and Motor Skill 13: 171–177

Goldstein, M.J. (1962): A test of the response probability theory of perceptual defense. Journal of Experimental Psychology 63(1): 23–28

Goldstein, M.J. (1962): Intellectual and personality changes accompanying aging. Longevita 67–76. Translation into Italian

Goldstein, M.J. and Himmelfarb, S.Z. (1962): The effects of providing knowledge of results upon the perceptual defense effect. Journal of Abnormal and Social Psychology 64: 143–147

Goldstein, M.J. Himmelfarb, S.Z., and Feder, W. (1962): A further study of the relationship between response bias and perceptual defense. Journal of Abnormal and Social Psychology 64: 56–62

Goldstein, J. and Palmer, J.O. (1963): The Experience of Anxiety. New York: Oxford University Press

Goldstein, J. Jones, R.B., and Kinder, M.I. (1963): A method for the experimental analysis of psychological defenses through perception. Journal of Psychiatric Research 2: 135–146

Goldstein, M.J. (1964): Perceptual reactions to threat under varying conditions of measurement. Journal of Abnormal and Social Psychology 69(5): 563–567

Goldstein, M.J. and Jones, R.B. (1964): The relationships among word association tests, objective personality test scores and ratings of clinical behavior in psychiatric patients. Journal of Projective Techniques and Personality Assessment 28(3): 271–279

Goldstein, M.J. Jones, R.B., Clemens, T.L., Flagg, G.W. and Alexander, F.G. (1965): Coping style as a factor of psychophysiological response to a tension-arousing film. Journal of Personality and Social Psychology 1(4): 290–302

Goldstein, M.J. (1966): Relationship between perceptual defense and exposure duration. Journal of Personality and Social Psychology 3(5): 608–610.

Goldstein, M.J., Acker, C.W., Crockett, J. and Riddle, C. (1966): Psychophysiological reactions to films by chronic schizophrenics: I. Effects of drug status. Journal of Abnormal Psychology 71(5): 335–344

Palmer, J.O. and Goldstein, M.J. (eds.) (1966): Perspectives in Psychopathology. New York: Oxford University Press

Goldstein, M.J. and Acker, C.W. (1967): Psychophysiological reactions to films by chronic schizophrenics: II. Individual differences in resting levels and reactivity. Journal of Abnormal Psychology 72: 23–39

Goldstein, M.J. and Adams, J.N. (1967): Coping style and behavioral response to stress. Journal of Experimental Research in Personality 2(4): 239–251

Goldstein, M.J., Judd, L.L. and Rodnick, E.H. (1967): Effects of social influence patterns of intrafamilial communication and treatment choice. American Journal of Orthopsychiatry 27: 392–394

Goldstein, M.J., Judd, L.L., Rodnick, E.H., Alkire, A.A. and Gould, E. (1968): A method for the study of social influence and coping patterns in the families of disturbed adolescents. Journal of Nervous and Mental Disease 147(3): 233–251

Goldstein, M.J., Held, J.M. and Cromwell, R. (1968): Premorbid adjustment and paranoid-nonparanoid status in schizophrenia. Psychological Bulletin 70(5): 382–386

Goldstein, M.J., Judd, L.L., Rodnick, E.H. and La Polla, A. (1969): Psychophysiological and behavioral effects of phenothiazine administration in acute schizophrenics as a function of premorbid status. Journal of Psychiatric Research 6(4): 271–287

Adams, J.N. and Goldstein, M.J. (1970): A further study of coping style and behavioral response to stress. Personality: An International Journal 1(3): 231–241

Goldstein, M.J. (1970): Premorbid adjustment, paranoid status and patterns of response to phenothiazine in acute schizophrenia. Schizophrenia Bulletin 3: 24–37 reprinted in: Cancro, R (ed.) (1972): Annual review of the schizophrenic syndrome, pp. 457–480. New York: Brunner-Mazel

Goldstein, M.J., Gould, E., Alkire, A., Rodnick, E.H. and Judd, L.L. (1970): Interpersonal themes in the Thematic Apperception Test stories of families of disturbed adolescents. Journal of Nervous and Mental Disease 150(5): 354–365

Goldstein, J.J., Kant, H.S., Judd, L.L., Rice, C.J. and Green, R. (1970): Exposure to pornography and sexual behavior in deviant and normal groups. Technical Reports of the Commission of Obscenity and Pornography, Vol. 7. Washington, DC: United States Government Printing Office

Goldstein, M.J., Rodnick, E.H., Judd, L.L. and Gould, E. (1970): Galvanic skin reactivity among family groups containing disturbed adolescents. Journal of Abnormal Psychology 75(1): 57–67

Judd, L.L., Goldstein, M.J., Rodnick, E.H. and Jackson, N.P. (1970): Premorbid level of adjustment and response to phenothiazine medication in acute schizophrenics. In: Psychopharmacology and the individual patient (Wittenborn, J.R., Goldberg, S.C. and May, P.R.A., eds.), pp. 88–98. New York: Raven Press

Kant, H.S. and Goldstein, M.J. (1970, December): Pornography. Psychology Today 4(7): 50–76

Alkire, A.A., Goldstein, M.J., Rodnick, E.H. and Judd, L.L. (1971): Social influence and counter-influence within families of four types of disturbed adolescents. Journal of Abnormal Psychology 77(1): 32–41

Goldstein, J.J., Kant, H.S., Judd, L.L., Rice, C.J. and Green, R.S. (1971): Experience with pornography: Rapists, pedophiles, homosexuals, transsexuals, and controls. Archives of Sexual Behavior 1: 1–15 reprinted in: Exploring human sexuality (1977), (Byrne, D. and Byrne, L., eds.), pp. 456–468. New York: Thomas Y. Cromwell

Evans, J.R., Rodnick, E.H., Goldstein, M.J. and Judd, L.L. (1972): Premorbid adjustment, phenothiazine treatment and remission in acute schizophrenics. Archives of General Psychiatry 27: 486–490

Goldstein, J.J., Rodnick, E.H., Jackson, N.P., Evans, J.R. and Judd, L.L. (1972): The stability and sensitivity of measures of thought, perception and emotional arousal. Psychopharmacologia 24(1): 107–120

Evans, J.R., Goldstein, M.J. and Rodnick, E.H. (1973): Premorbid adjustment, paranoid diagnosis, and remission in acute schizophrenics treated in a community mental health center. Archives of General Psychiatry 28(5): 666–672

Goldstein, M.J. (1973): Explaining psychopathology: A review of Heilbrun, A. B. Aversive maternal control. Science 181: 1240–1241

Goldstein, M.J. (1973): Exposure to erotic stimuli and sexual deviance. Journal of Social Issues 29(3): 197–219

Goldstein, M.J. (1973): Individual differences in response to stress. American Journal of Community Psychology 1: 113–137

Goldstein, M.J., Kant, H. and Hartman, J.J. (1973): Pornography and sexual deviance: A report of the Legal and Behavioral Institute Beverly Hills. Berkeley, CA: University of California Press [reprinted, in Italian translation 1978]

Goldstein, M.J. and Wilson, W.C. (1973): Introduction. Exposure to erotic stimuli and sexual deviance. Journal of Social Issues 29: 1–5

Judd, L.L., Goldstein, M.J., Rodnick, E.H. and Jackson, N.L. (1973): Phenothiazine effects in good premorbid schizophrenics divided into paranoid-nonparanoid status. Archives of General Psychiatry 29(2): 207–217

McPherson, S.R., Goldstein, M.J. and Rodnick, E.H. (1973): Who listens? Who communicates? How? Styles of interaction among parents and their disturbed adolescent children. Archives of General Psychiatry 28: 393–399

Wilson, W.C. and Goldstein, M.J. (eds.) (1973): Pornography: Attitudes, use and effects. Journal of Social Issues 29

Rodnick, E.H. and Goldstein, M.J. (1974): A research strategy for studying risk for schizophrenia during adolescence and early childhood. In: The child in his family: Children at a psychiatric risk (Anthony, E.J. and Koupernik, C., eds.), Vol. 3, pp. 507–526. New York: Wiley-Interscience

Rodnick, E.H. and Goldstein, M.J. (1974): Premorbid adjustment and the recovery of mothering function in acute schizophrenic women. Journal of Abnormal Psychology 83(6): 623–628

Goldstein, M. J., Rodnick, E.H., Evans, J.R. and May, P.R.A. (1975): Long acting phenothiazine and social therapy in the community treatment of acute schizophrenia. In: Drugs in combination with other therapies: Seminars in psychiatry. (Greenblatt, M., ed.), pp. 63–94. New York: Grune and Stratton

Goldstein, M.J. and Palmer, J.O. (1975): Experience of anxiety: A casebook, 2nd ed. New York: Oxford Press

Goldstein, M.J. and Palmer, J.O. (1975): Experience of anxiety: Teacher's Guide. New York: Oxford Press

Goldstein, M.J. and Rodnick, E.H. (1975): The family's contribution to the etiology of schizophrenia: Current status. Schizophrenic Bulletin 14: 48–63

May, P.R.A., Van Putten, T., Yale, C., Potepan, B.A., Jenden, D.J., Fairchild, M.D., Goldstein, M.J. and Dixon, W.J. (1976): Predicting individual responses to drug treatment in schizophrenia: A test dose model. The Journal of Nervous and Mental Disease 162: 177–183

Diskin, S.D., Grencik, J.M. and Goldstein, M.J. (1977): Coping style of law enforcement officers in response to simulated stress. American Journal of Community Psychology 5(1): 59–73

Goldstein, M.J. (1977): A behavioral scientist looks at obscenity. In: Sales B. (ed.), Perspectives in law and psychology. Vol. 1: The criminal justice system, pp. 1–21. New York: Plenum Publications

Goldstein, M.J. and Jones, J.E. (1977): Adolescent and familial precursors of borderline and schizophrenic conditions. In: Borderline personality: The concept, the syndrome, the patient, (Hartocollis, P., eds.), pp. 213–229. New York: International Universities Press

Jones, J.E., Rodnick, E.H., Goldstein, M.J., McPherson, S.R. and West, K.L. (1977): Parental transactional style deviance in families of disturbed adolescents as an indicator of risk for schizophrenia. Archives of General Psychiatry 34: 71–74

Woodward, J.A. and Goldstein, M.J. (1977): Communication deviance in the families of schizophrenics: A comment on the misuse of analysis of covariance. Science 197(4308): 1096–1097

Goldstein, M.J. (1978): Further data concerning the relationship between premorbid adjustment and paranoid symptomatology. Schizophrenia Bulletin 4(2): 236–243

Goldstein, M.J. (1978): Sex, crime and the law. Review of sex, crime and the law by D.E.J. MacNamara and E. Sagarin, Crime and Delinquency 24: 510–512

Goldstein, M.J. (1978): The study of families of disturbed adolescents at risk for schizophrenia and related conditions. In: The child in his family: Vulnerable children (Anthony, E., Koupernik, C., and Chiland, C., eds.), Vol. 4, pp. 303–312. New York: Wiley

Goldstein, M.J., Rodnick, E.H., Evans, J.R., May, P.R.A. and Steinberg, M. (1978): Drug and family therapy in the aftercare of treatment of acute schizophrenia. Archives of General Psychiatry 35(10): 1169–1177

Goldstein, M.J., Rodnick, E.H., Jones, J.E., McPherson, S.R. and West, K.L. (1978): Familial precursors of schizophrenia spectrum disorders. In: The nature of schizophrenia (Wynne, L.D. Cromwell, R.L. and Matthysse, S., eds.), pp. 487–498. New York: Wiley

King, C.E. and Goldstein, M.J., (1979): Therapist rating of achievement of therapy objectives: An aid to research on psychotherapy with acute schizophrenics. Schizophrenia Bulletin 5(1): 118–129

Goldstein, M.J., Baker, B. and Jamison, K.R. (1980): Abnormal psychology: Experiences, originals and interventions. Boston, MA: Little, Brown & Company

Goldstein, M.J. (1980): The course of schizophrenic psychosis. In: Constancy and change in human development (Brim, O.G. and Kagan, J., eds.), pp. 523–558. Boston, MA: Harvard University Press

Goldstein, M.J. (1980): Family therapy during the aftercare of acute schizophrenia. In: Psychotherapy of schizophrenia: Current status and new directions (Strauss, J.S., Bowers, M., Downey, T.W., Fleck, S., Jackson, S. and Levine, I., eds.), pp. 78–89. New York: Plenum Publishing

Goldstein, M.J. (1980): Environmental factors as stressors in schizophrenia. Report of stress and illness panel in research on stress in health and disease. Washington, DC: National Academy of Sciences, Institute of Medicine.

Baker, B.L. and Goldstein, M.J. (1981): Readings in abnormal psychology. Boston, MA: Little, Brown & Company

Doane, J.A., West, K.L., Goldstein, M.J., Rodnick, E.H. and Jones, J.E. (1981): Parental communication deviance and affective style. Archives of General Psychology 38: 679–685

Doane, J.A., Goldstein, M.J. and Rodnick, E.H. (1981): Cross-situational patterns of parental affective style as a predictor of subsequent schizophrenia-spectrum disorders in vulnerable adolescents. Family Process 20: 337–349

Lewis, J.M., Rodnick, E.H. and Goldstein, M.J. (1981): Intrafamilial interactive behavior, parental communication deviance and risk for schizophrenia. Journal of Abnormal Psychology 90: 448–457

Goldstein, M.J. (1981): Family factors associated with schizophrenia and anorexia nervosa. Journal of Youth and Adolescence 10: 385–405

Goldstein, M.J. (ed.) (1981): New directions for mental health services: New developments in interventions with families of schizophrenics, Vol. 12. San Francisco: Jossey-Bass

Goldstein, M.J. (1981): Editor's notes. In: New directions for mental health services: New developments in interventions with families of schizophrenics, (Goldstein, M.J., ed.), Vol. 12. San Francisco: Jossey-Bass

Goldstein, M.J., (1981): The family. In: Adolescence and stress. Report of an NIMH conference (Moore, C.D., ed.), pp. 59–71. Washington, DC: United States Government Printing Office

Goldstein, M.J. and Kopeikin, H.S. (1981): Short-and long-term effects of combining drug and family therapy. In: New directions for mental health services: New developments in interventions with families of schizophrenics (Goldstein, M.J., ed.), Vol. 12. San Francisco: Jossey-Bass

Lewis, J.M., Rodnick. E.H. and Goldstein, M.J. (1981): Intrafamilial interactive behavior, parental communication deviance, and risk for schizophrenia. Journal of Abnormal Psychology 90(5): 448–457

May, P.R.A., Van Putten, T., Jenden, D.J., Yale, C., Dixon, W.J. and Goldstein, M.J. (1981): Prognosis in schizophrenia: Individual differences in psychological response to a test dose of antipsychotic drugs and their relationship to blood and saliva levels and treatment outcome. Comprehensive Psychiatry 22: 147–152

Asarnow, J.R., Lewis J., Doane, J., Goldstein M. and Rodnick, E. (1982): Family interaction and the course of adolescent psychopathology: An analysis of adolescent and parent effects. Journal of Abnormal Child Psychology 10(3): 427–442

Goldstein, M.J. (ed.) (1982): Preventive intervention in schizophrenia: Are we ready? Washington, DC: United States Government Printing Office

Goldstein, M.J. (1982): What is schizophrenia? Schizophrenia Bulletin 8: 600–601

Goldstein, M.J. and Doane, J.A. (1982): Family factors in the onset, course and treatment of schizophrenia spectrum disorders: An update on current research. Journal of Nervous and Mental Disease 170(11): 692–700

Rodnick, E.H., Goldstein, M.J., Doane, J.A. and Lewis, J.M. (1982): Association between parent-child interactions and risk for schizophrenia: Implications for early intervention. In: Preventative intervention in schizophrenia: Are we ready? (Goldstein, M.J., ed.), Washington, DC: United States Government Printing Office

Snyder, S.H., Kety, S.S. and Goldstein, M.J. (1982): What is schizophrenia? Schizophrenia Bulletin 8(4): 595–602

Doane, J.A. and Goldstein, M.J. (1983): Familial characteristics of adolescents vulnerable to subsequent antisocial disorders. In: Prospective studies of crime and delinquencies (Van Dusen, K.T. and Mednick, S.A., eds.), Boston, MA: Kluwer-Nijhoff Publishing

Goldstein, M.J. (1983): Family interaction: Patterns predictive of the onset and course of schizophrenia. In: Psychosocial intervention in schizophrenia (Stierlin H., Wynne, L.C. and Wirsching, M., eds.). Heidelberg: Springer [reprinted in Goldstein, M.J., Family affect and communication related to schizophrenia. In: Children in families under stress. New directions for child development. (Doyle, A., Gold, G. and Moskowitz, D.S., eds.), Vol. 12, pp. 47–62. San Francisco, CA: Jossey-Bass]

Goldstein, M.J. and Rodnick E.H. (1983): The interaction of drug therapy and family treatment in schizophrenia. In: Psychopharmacology and psychotherapy (Greenhild, M.H. and Gralnick, A., eds.). New York: Free Press

Kopeikin, H.S., Marshall, V. and Goldstein, M.J. (1983): Stages and impact of crisis-oriented family therapy in the aftercare of acute schizophrenia. In: Family therapy in schizophrenia (MacFarlane, W.R., ed.), pp. 690–697. New York: Guilford Press

Miklowitz, D.J., Goldstein, M.J. and Falloon, I.R.H. (1983): Premorbid and symptomatic characteristics of schizophrenics from families with high and low levels of expressed emotion. Journal of Abnormal Psychology 92(3): 359–367

Valone, K., Goldstein, M.J., Norton, J. and Doane, J.A. (1983): Parental expressed emotion and affective style in an adolescent sample at risk for schizophrenia-spectrum disorders. Journal of Abnormal Psychology 92(4): 399–407

Goldstein, M.J. (1984): Family affect and communication related to schizophrenia. New directions for child development. Vol. 24, pp. 47–62. San Francisco, CA: Jossey-Bass

Goldstein, M.J. (1984): Family intervention programs. In: Treatment and care for schizophrenia. (Bellack, A.S., ed.), pp. 281–305. New York: Grune and Stratton

Goldstein, M.J. (1984): Schizophrenia: The interaction of family and neuroleptic therapy. In: Combining psychotherapy and drug therapy in clinical practice (Beitman, B.D. and Klerman, G.L., eds.). New York: Spectrum Publishers

Miklowitz, D.J., Goldstein, M.J., Falloon, I.R.H. and Doane, J.A. (1984): Interactional correlates of expressed emotion in the families of schizophrenics. British Journal of Psychiatry 144: 482–487

Rodnick, E.H., Goldstein, M.J., Lewis, J.M, and Doane, J.A. (1984): Parental communication style, affect and role as precursors of offspring schizophrenia-spectrum disorders. In: Children at risk for schizophrenia (Watt N.F., Anthony, J. et al., eds.). New York: Cambridge University Press

Valone, K., Goldstein, M.J. and Norton, J.P. (1984): Parental expressed emotion and psychophysiological reactivity in an adolescent sample at risk for schizophrenia spectrum disorders. Journal of Abnormal Psychology 93(4): 448–457.

Doane, J.A., Falloon, I.R.H., Goldstein, M.J. and Mintz, J. (1985): Parental affective style and the treatment of schizophrenia. Archives of General Psychiatry 42(1): 34–42

Goldstein, M.J. (1985): Family factors that antedate the onset of schizophrenia and related disorders: The results of a fifteen year prospective longitudinal study. Acta Psychiatrica Scandinavica 71: 7–18

Goldstein, M.J. and Doane, J.A. (1985): Interventions with families and the course of schizophrenia. In: Controversies in schizophrenia: Changes and constancies (Alpert M., ed.), pp. 381–397. New York: Guilford Press

Asarnow, J.R. and Goldstein, M.J. (1986): Schizophrenia during adolescence and early adulthood: A developmental perspective. Clinical Psychology Review 6(3): 211–235

Doane, J.A., Goldstein, M.J., Miklowitz, D.J. and Falloon, I.R.H. (1986): The impact of individual and family treatment on the affective climate of families of schizophrenics. British Journal of Psychiatry 148: 279–287

Goldstein, M.J. (1986): Schizophrenic and affective disorders: Rationale for a biopsychosocial treatment model. Commentary. Integrative Psychiatry 4(3): 180–181

Goldstein, M.J. and Asarnow, J.R. (1986): Prevention of schizophrenia: What do we know? In: Primary prevention: The state of the art (Barter, J.P. and Talbot, S., eds.), pp. 85–116. Washington, DC: American Psychiatric Press

Goldstein, M.J., Baker, B.L. and Jamison, K.R. (eds.) (1986): Abnormal psychology: Experiences, origins, and interventions. Glenview, IL: Scott, Foresman and Co

Goldstein, M.J., Hand, I. and Hahlweg, K. (eds.) (1986): Treatment of schizophrenia: Family assessment and intervention pp. 129–144. Heidelberg: Springer

Goldstein, M.J. and Strachan, A.M. (1986): The impact of family intervention programs on family communication and the short-term course of schizophrenia. In: Treatment of schizophrenia: Family assessment and intervention (Goldstein, M.J. Hand, I. and Hahlweg, K., eds.). Heidelberg: Springer

Magana, A.B., Goldstein, M.J., Karno, M., Miklowitz, D.J., Jenkins, J. and Falloon, I.R.H. (1986): A brief method for assessing expressed emotion in relatives of psychiatric patients. Psychiatry Research 17(3): 203–212

Miklowitz, D.J., Goldstein, M.J., Nuechterlein, K.H., Snyder, K.S. and Doane, J.A. (1986): Expressed emotion, affective style, lithium compliance, and relapse in recent onset mania. Psychopharmacology Bulletin 22(3): 628–632

Miklowitz, D.J., Strachan, A.M., Goldstein, M.J., Doane, J.A., Snyder, K.S., Hogarty, G.E. and Falloon, I.R.H. (1986): Expressed emotion and communication deviance in the families of schizophrenics. Journal of Abnormal Psychology 95(1): 60–66

Strachan, A.M., Leff, J.P., Goldstein, M.J., Doane, J.A. and Burtt, C. (1986): Emotional attitudes and direct communication in the families of schizophrenics: A cross-national replication. British Journal of Psychiatry 149: 279–287

Strachan, A.M., Goldstein, M.J. and Miklowitz, D.J. (1986): Do relatives express expressed emotion? In: Treatment of schizophrenia: Family and intervention (Goldstein, M.J., Hand, I. and Hahlweg, K., eds.), pp. 51–58. Heidelberg: Springer

Wagener, D.K., Hogarty, G.E., Goldstein, M., Asarnow, R.F. and Brown, A. (1986): Information processing and communication deviance in schizophrenic patients and their mothers. Psychiatry Research 18(4): 365–377

Asarnow, J.R., Ben-Meir, S. and Goldstein, M.J. (1987): Family factors in childhood depressive and schizophrenia spectrum disorders. In: Understanding major mental disorder: The contribution of family interaction research (Hahlweg K. and Goldstein, M.J., eds.), pp. 123–138. New York: Family Process Press

Goldstein, M.J. (1987): Family interaction patterns that antedate the onset of schizophrenia and related disorders: A further analysis of data from a longitudinal prospective study. In: Understanding major mental disorder: The contribution of family interaction research (Hahlweg, K. and Goldstein, M.J., eds.), pp. 11–32. New York: Family Process Press

Goldstein, M.J. (1987): Psychosocial issues, special report on schizophrenia. Schizophrenia Bulletin 13(1): 157–171

Goldstein, M.J. (1987): The UCLA High Risk Project. In: High risk studies. Special issue of Schizophrenia Bulletin (Goldstein, M.J. and Tuma, H., eds.), 13(3): 505–514

Goldstein, M.J. and Strachan, A.M. (1987): The family and schizophrenia. In: Family interaction and psychopathology: Theories, methods, and findings, (Jacob, T., ed.), pp. 481–508. New York: Plenum

Goldstein, M.J. and Tuma, H. (eds.) (1987): High risk studies. Schizophrenia Bulletin 13(3)

Hahlweg, K. and Goldstein, M.J. (eds.) (1987): Understanding mental disorders: The contribution of family interaction research. New York: Family Process Press

Hahlweg, K., Nuechterlein, K.H., Goldstein, M.J., Magana, A., Doane, J.A. and Snyder, K.S. (1987): Parental expressed emotion attitudes and intrafamilial communication behavior. In: Understanding mental disorders: The contribution of family interaction research (Hahlweg, K. and Goldstein, M.J., eds.), pp. 156–175. New York: Family Process Press

Miklowitz, D.J., Goldstein, M.J., Nuechterlein, K.H., Snyder, K.S. and Doane, J.A. (1987): The family and the course of recent-onset mania. In: Understanding major mental disorder: The contribution of family interaction research (Hahlweg, K. and Goldstein, M.J., eds.), pp. 195–211. New York: Family Process Press

Mintz, J., Mintz, L. and Goldstein, M.J. (1987): Expressed emotion and relapse in first episodes of schizophrenia: A rejoinder to MacMillian et al. (1986). British Journal of Psychiatry 151: 314–320

Asarnow, J.R., Goldstein, M.J. and Ben-Meir, S. (1988): Parental communication deviance in childhood onset schizophrenia spectrum and depressive disorders. Journal of Child Psychology and Psychiatry 29(6): 825–838

Asarnow, J.R., Goldstein, M.J., Carlson, G.A., Perdue, S., Bates, S. and Keller, J. (1988): Child-onset depressive disorders: A follow-up study of rates of rehospitalization and out-of-home placement among child psychiatric inpatients. Journal of Affective Disorders 15(3): 245–253

Cozolino, L.J., Goldstein, M J., Nuechterlein, K.H., West, K.L. and Snyder, K.S. (1988): The impact of education about schizophrenia on relatives varying in expressed emotion. Schizophrenia Bulletin 14(4): 675–687 [reprinted in Italian Schizofrenia 3(4): 66–77]

Goldstein, M.J. (1988): The family and psychopathology. In: Annual review of psychology (Rosenzwerg, L.W., Porter, M.R. et al., eds.), Vol. 39, pp. 283–299). Palo Alto: Annual Reviews

Goldstein, M.J. (1988): Individual and family therapy of schizophrenia. In: Treatment resistance in schizophrenia (Dencker, S.J., Kulhanek, F., eds.), pp. 65–82. Wiesbaden: Dencker and Kulhanek

Goldstein, M.J. (1988): Patient status, family composition and other structural variables in family therapy research. In: State of the art in family therapy research (Wynne, L.C., ed.), pp. 109–115. New York: Family Process Press

Miklowitz, D.J., Goldstein, M.J., Nuechterlein, K.H., Snyder, K.S. and Mintz, J. (1988): Family factors and the course of bipolar affective disorder. Archives of General Psychiatry 45(3): 225–231

Velligan, D., Christensen, A., Goldstein, M.J. and Margolin, G. (1988): Parental communication deviance: Its relationship to parent, child, and family system variables. Psychiatry Research 26(3): 313–325

Cook, W.L., Strachan, A.M., Goldstein, M.J. and Miklowitz, D.J. (1989): Expressed emotion and reciprocal affective relationships in families of disturbed adolescents. Family Process 28(3): 337–348

Goldstein, M.J. (1989): Intrafamilial communicational patterns observed during adolescence and the subsequent development of schizophrenia in early childhood. In: Psychoses at adolescence (Ladame, F., Gutton, P. and Kalogerakis, M., eds.). Paris: Masson

Goldstein, M.J. (1989): Psychosocial treatment of schizophrenia. In: Schizophrenia: A scientific focus (Schultz, S.C., Tamminga, C.A., eds.), pp. 318–324. New York: Oxford Press

Goldstein, M.J., Miklowitz, D.J., Strachan, A.M., Doane, J.A., Nuechterlein, K.H. and Feingold, D. (1989): Patterns of expressed emotion and patient coping styles that characterize the families of recent onset schizophrenics. British Journal of Psychiatry 155 (Suppl. 5): 107–111

Hahlweg, K., Goldstein, M.J., Nuechterlein, K.H., Magana, A.B., Mintz, J., Doane, J.A., Miklowitz, D.J. and Snyder, K.S. (1989): Expressed emotion and patient-relative interaction in families of recent onset schizophrenics. Journal of Consulting and Clinical Psychology 57(1): 11–18

Miklowitz, D.J., Goldstein, M.J., Doane, J.A., Nuechterlein, K.H., Strachan, A.M., Snyder, K.S. and Magana, A. (1989): Is expressed emotion an index of a transactional process? I. Relative's affective style. Family Process 28(2): 153–167

Mintz, L.I., Nuechterlein, K.H., Goldstein, M.J., Mintz, J. and Snyder, K.S. (1989): The initial onset of schizophrenia and family expressed emotion: Some methodological considerations. British Journal of Psychiatry 154: 212–217

Nuechterlein, K.H., Goldstein, M.J., Ventura, J., Dawson, M.E. and Doane, J.A. (1989): Patient-environment relationships in schizophrenia: Information processing, communication deviance, autonomic arousal, and stressful life events. British Journal of Psychiatry 155 (Suppl. 5): 84–89 [German translation: Schizophrenie als systemische Störung (Böker W. and Brenner H.D., eds.). Bern: Hans Huber]

Strachan, A.M., Feingold, D., Goldstein, M.J., Miklowitz, D.J. and Nuechterlein, K.H. (1989): Is expressed emotion an index of a transactional process? II. Patients' coping style. Family Process 28(2): 169–181

Brenner, H.D., Dencker, S.J., Goldstein, M.J., Hubbard, J.W. et al. (1990): Defining treatment refractoriness in schizophrenia. Schizophrenia Bulletin 16(4): 551–561

Cook, W.L., Asarnow, J.R., Goldstein, M.J., Marshall, V.G. and Weber, E. (1990): Mother-child dynamics in early-onset depression and childhood schizophrenia spectrum disorders. Developmental and Psychopathology 2(1): 71–84

Goldstein, M.J. (1990, Fall): A family-oriented aftercare program for schizophrenia. Transition, pp. 47–51. Mental Health Association Saskatchewan Division

Goldstein, M.J. (1990): Family relations as risk factors for the onset and course of schizophrenia. In: Risk and protective factors in the development of psychopathology (Rolf, J.E., Masten, A., Cicchetti, D., Nuechterlein, K.H., Weintraub, S., eds.), pp. 408–423. New York: Cambridge University Press

Goldstein, M.J. (1990): Psychosocial factors relating to etiology and course of schizophrenia. In: Handbook of schizophrenia (Herz, M.I., ed.). New York: Elsevier Science Publishers

Goldstein, M.J. (1990): Research on family and drug therapy for schizophrenia [in German translation: Kombination therapeutischer Strategien bei schizophrenen Erkrankungen (Hinterhuber, H., Kulhanek, F., Fleischhacker, W., eds.). Braunschweig Wiesbaden: Vieweg]

Goldstein, M.J. (1990): Risk factors and prevention in schizophrenia. In: Recent advances in schizophrenia (Kales, A., Stefanis, C.N., Talbot, J.A., eds.). New York: Springer

Marshall, V.G., Longwell, L., Goldstein, M.J. and Swanson, J.M. (1990): Family factors associated with aggressive symptomatology in boys with attention deficit disorder: A research note. Journal of Child Psychology and Psychiatry 31(4): 629–636

Miklowitz, D.J. and Goldstein, M.J. (1990): Behavioral family treatment for patients with bipolar affective disorder. Behavior Modification 14(4): 457–489

Tompson, M.C., Asarnow, J.R., Goldstein, M.J. and Miklowitz, D.J. (1990): Thought disorder and communication problems in children with schizophrenia spectrum and depressive disorders and their parents. Journal of Clinical Child Psychology 19(2): 159–168

Velligan, D.I., Goldstein, M.J., Nuechterlein, K.H., Miklowitz, D.J. and Ranlett, G. (1990): Can communication deviance be measured in a family problem-solving interaction? Family Process 29(2): 213–226

Cook, W.L., Kenny, D.A., Goldstein, M.J., Feinstein, E. et al. (1991): Parental affective style risk and the family system: A social relations model analysis. Journal of Abnormal Psychology 100(4): 492–501

Goldstein, M.J. (1991): Psychosocial, nonpharmacologic treatments for schizophrenia. In: American Psychiatric Press Review of Psychiatry (Tasman, A, Goldfinger, S.M., eds.), pp. 116–135. Washington, DC: American Psychiatric Press

Goldstein, M.J. (1991): Schizophrenia and family therapy. In: Integrating pharmacotherapy and psychotherapy (Beitman, B.D. Klerman, G.L. et al., eds.), pp. 291–309. Washington, DC: American Psychiatric Press

Goldstein, M.J. (1991): Some thoughts about the possibilities for preventing schizophrenia. In: Psychiatry at the crossroads between social science and biology (Torgerson, S., Abrahamsen, P., Sorensen, T., eds.). Oslo: Norwegian University Press

Goldstein, M.J. (1991): The interaction of drug and family therapy in the prevention of relapse in schizophrenia. In: Guidelines for neuroleptic relapse prevention in schizophrenia (Kissling, W., ed.), Berlin: Springer

Hibbs, E.D., Hamburger, S.D., Lenane, M., Rapoport, J.L., Kruesi, M.J.P., Keysor, C.S. and Goldstein, M.J. (1991): Determinants of expressed emotion in families of disturbed and normal children. Journal of Child Psychology and Psychiatry 32: 757–770

Leeb, B., Hahlweg, K., Goldstein, M.J., Feinstein, E., Mueller, U., Dose, M. and Magana-Amato, A. (1991): The cross national reliability, concurrent validity and stability of a brief method for assessing expressed emotion. Psychiatry Research 39(1): 25–31

Miklowitz, D.J., Velligan, D.I., Goldstein, M.J., Nuechterlein, K.H., Gitlin, M.J., Ranlett, G. and Doane, J.A. (1991): Communication deviance in families of schizophrenic and manic patients. Journal of Abnormal Psychology 100(2): 163–173

Rea, M.M., Strachan, A.M., Goldstein, M.J., Falloon, I.R.H. and Hwang, S. (1991): Changes in patient coping style following individual and family treatment for schizophrenia. British Journal of Psychiatry 158: 642–647

Altman, E., Rea, M., Mintz, J., Miklowitz, D.J., Goldstein, M.J. and Hwang, S. (1992): Prodromal symptoms and signs of bipolar relapse: A report based on prospectively collected data. Psychiatry Research 41: 1–8

Altdorfer, A.A., Goldstein, M.J., Miklowitz, D.J. and Nuechterlein, K.H. (1992): Stress-indicative patterns of non-verbal behaviour: Their role in family interaction. British Journal of Psychiatry 161 (Suppl. 18): 103–113

Goldstein, M.J. (1992): Expressed emotion in depressed patients and their partners. Commentary. Family Process 31(2): 172–174

Goldstein, M.J. (1992): Intrafamilial communication patterns observed during adolescence and the subsequent development of schizophrenia in early adulthood. In: International annals of adolescent psychiatry (Schwartzberg, A.Z., Esman, A.H. et al., eds.), Vol. 2., pp. 47–54. Chicago, IL: The University of Chicago Press

Goldstein, M.J. (1992): Psychosocial strategies for maximizing the effects of psychotropic medications for schizophrenia and mood disorder. Psychopharmacology Bulletin 28(3): 237–240

Goldstein, M.J. (1992): The family and schizophrenia: Some current issues. In: psychotherapy of schizophrenia: Facilitating and obstructive factors (Werbart A., Cullberg, J., eds.). Oslo: Scandinavian University Press

Goldstein, M.J. and Asarnow, J.R. (1992): Prevention in schizophrenia. In: National plan for prevention research. Washington, DC: Government Printing Office

Goldstein, M.J., Talovic, S.A., Nuechterlein, K.H., Fogelson, D.L., Subotnik, K.L. and Asarnow, R.F. (1992): Family interaction versus individual psychopathology: Do they indicate the same processes in the families of schizophrenics? British Journal of Psychiatry 161 (Suppl. 18): 97–102

Nuechterlein, K.H., Dawson, M.E., Gitlin, M., Ventura, J., Goldstein, M.J., Snyder, K.S., Yee, C.M. and Mintz, J. (1992): Developmental Processes in Schizophrenic Disorders: Longitudinal studies of vulnerability and stress. Schizophrenia Bulletin 18: 387–425

Asarnow, J.R., Goldstein, M.J., Tompson, M.C. and Guthrie, D. (1993): One-year outcomes of depressive disorders in child psychiatric inpatients: Evaluation of the prognostic power of a brief measure of expressed emotion. Journal of Child Psychology and Psychiatry 34(2): 129–137

Bergman, R.L. and Goldstein, M.J. (1993): Short-term stability of task-generated interactional patterns in families of schizophrenic patients. Family Process 32(1): 105–116

Cook, W.L. and Goldstein, M.J. (1993): Multiple perspectives on family relationships: A latent variable models. Child Development 64(5): 1377–1388

Friedmann, M.S. and Goldstein, M.J. (1993): Relatives' awareness of their own expressed emotion as measured by a self-report adjective checklist. Family Process 32(4): 459–472

Goldstein, M.J. (1993): A clinician/researcher looks at Andrew and his family. Commentary. Family Process 32(4): 397–404

Goldstein, M.J., Strachan, A.M. and Wynne, L.C. (1993): DSM-IV literature review: Relational problems with high expressed emotion. DSM-IV Sourcebook. Washington, DC: American Psychiatric Press

Miklowitz, D.J. and Goldstein, M.J. (1993): Mapping the intrafamilial environment of the schizophrenic patient. In: Schizophrenia: Origins, processes, treatment, and outcome (Cromwell, R.L., Snyder, C.R. et al., eds.), pp. 313–332. New York: Oxford University Press

Stubbe, D.E., Zahner, G.E., Goldstein, M.J. and Leckman, J.F. (1993): Diagnostic specificity of a brief measure of expressed emotion: A community study of children. Journal of Child Psychology and Psychiatry 34(2): 139–154

Tompson, M.C., Goldstein, M.J., Lebell, M.B., Mintz, L.I. and Marder, S.R. (1993): Relatives' Expressed Emotion (EE) vs. patients' perceptions of EE: Which is a better predictor of course? (Abstract) Schizophrenia Research 9(2,3): 273

Asarnow, J.R., Tompson, M.C. and Goldstein, M.J. (1994): Childhood-onset schizophrenia: A followup study. Schizophrenia Bulletin 20(4): 599–617

Asarnow, J.R., Tompson, M.C., Hamilton, E., Goldstein, M.J. and Guthrie, D (1994): Family expressed emotion, childhood onset-depression, and childhood-onset schizophrenia spectrum disorders: Is expressed emotion a nonspecific correlate of child psychopathology or a specific risk factor for depression? Journal of Abnormal Child Psychology 22(2): 129–146

Castellon, S., Asarnow, R.F., Goldstein, M.J. and Marder, S.R. (1994): Persisting negative symptoms and information-processing deficits in schizophrenia: Implication for subtyping. Psychiatry Research 54: 59–69

Friedmann, M.S. and Goldstein, M.J. (1994): Relatives' perceptions of their interactional behavior with a schizophrenic family member. Family Process 33(4): 377–387

Goldstein, M.J. (1994): Psychoeducational and family therapy in relapse prevention. Acta Psychiatrica Scandinavica 28 (Suppl. 382): 54–57

Goldstein, M.J. and Kern, R. (1994): Psychological factors in schizophrenia. Current Opinion in Psychiatry 7: 61–64

Goldstein, M.J. and Miklowitz, D.J. (1994): Family interventions for persons with bipolar disorder. In: New directions: Interventions with families of the mentally ill (Hatfield, A., et al., eds.), pp. 23–35. San Francisco, CA: Jossey-Bass

Goldstein, M.J., Rosenfarb, I.S., Woo, S. and Nuechterlein, K.H. (1994): Intrafamilial relationships and the course of schizophrenia. Acta Psychiatrica Scandinavica 90 (Suppl. 384): 60–66

Goldstein, M.J. (1995): Psychoeducation and relapse prevention. International Clinical Psychopharmacology 9(6): 59–69

Goldstein, M.J. (1995): Transactional processes associated with relatives' expressed emotion. International Journal of Mental Health 24(2): 76–96

Goldstein, M.J. and Miklowitz, D.J. (1995): The effectiveness of psychoeducational family therapy in the treatment of schizophrenic disorders. Journal of Marital and Family Therapy 21(4): 361–376

Kern, R.S., Green, M.F. and Goldstein, M.J. (1995): Modification of performance on the span of apprehension, a putative marker of the vulnerability to schizophrenia. Journal of Abnormal Psychology 104(2): 385–389

Miklowitz, D.J., Goldstein, M.J. and Nuechterlein, K.H. (1995): Verbal interactions in the families of schizophrenic and bipolar affective patients. Journal of Abnormal Psychology 104(2): 268–276

Rosenfarb, I.S., Goldstein, M.J., Mintz, J. and Nuechterlein, K.H. (1995): Expressed emotion and subclinical psychopathology observable within the transactions between schizophrenic patients and their family members. Journal of Abnormal Psychology 104(2): 259–267

Tompson, M.C., Goldstein, M.J., Lebell, M.B., Mintz, L.I., Marder, S.R. and Mintz, J. (1995): Schizophrenic patients' perceptions of their relatives' attitudes. Psychiatry Research 57(2): 155–167

Davis, J.A., Goldstein, M.J. and Nuechterlein, K.H. (1996): Gender differences in family attitudes about schizophrenia. Psychological Medicine 26: 689–696

Goldstein, M.J. (1996): Treating the person with schizophrenia as a person. Review in Contemporary Psychology 41: 256–258

Goldstein, M.J. (1996): Psychoeducational family programs in the United States. In: Handbook of mental health economics and health policy (Moscarelli, M., Rupp, A., Sartorius, N., eds.), Vol. 1: Schizophrenia, pp. 287–293. Chichester: Wiley

Goldstein, M.J., Rea, M.M. and Miklowitz, D.J. (1996): Family factors related to the course and outcome of bipolar disorder. In: Interpersonal factors in the origin and course of affective disorders (Mundt, C., Goldstein, M.J., Hahlweg, K., Fiedler, P., eds.), pp. 193–203. London: Gaskell Books

Linszen, D., Dingemans, P., Van der Does, J.W., Nugter, A., Scholte, P., Lenior, R. and Goldstein, M.J. (1996): Treatment, expressed emotion and relapse in recent onset schizophrenic disorders. Psychological Medicine 26: 333–342

Mundt, C., Goldstein, M.J., Hahlweg, K., Fiedler, P. (eds.) (1996): Interpersonal factors in the origin and course of affective disorders. London: Gaskell Books

Tompson, M.C., Goldstein, M.J. and Rea, M.M. (1996): Psychoeducational family intervention: Individual differences in response to treatment. In: Advanced prelapse education: Compliance and relapse in practice. Papers presented at a Lundbeck Symposium (Kane, J.M., van den Bosch, R.J., eds.), pp. 21–28. Denmark: Lundbeck Publications

Simoneau, T.L., Miklowitz, D.J., Goldstein, M.J., Nuechterlein, K.H. and Richards, J.A. (1996): Nonverbal interactional behavior in the families of persons with schizophrenic and bipolar disorders. Family Process 35(1): 83–102

Goldstein, M.J., Rosenfarb, I.S., Woo, S. and Nuechterlein, K.H. (1997): Transactional processes which can function as risk or protective factors in the family treatment of schizophrenia. In: Towards a comprehensive therapy for schizophrenia (Brenner, H.D., Böker, W., Genner, R., eds.), pp. 147–157. Göttingen: Hogrefe and Huber Publishers

Miklowitz, D.J. and Goldstein, M.J. (1997): Bipolar disorder: A family-focused treatment approach. New York: Guilford Press

Subotnik, K.L., Nuechterlein, K.H., Asarnow, R.F., Fogelson, D.L., Goldstein, M.J. and Talovic, S.A. (1997): Depressive symptoms in the early course of schizophrenia: Relationship to familial psychiatric illness. American Journal of Psychiatry 154(11): 1551–1556

Tompson, M.C., Asarnow, J.R., Hamilton, E.B., Newell, L.E. and Goldstein, M.J. (1997): Children with schizophrenia-spectrum disorders: Thought disorder and communication problems in a family interactional context. Journal of Child Psychology and Psychiatry 38(4): 421–429

Tompson, M.C., Goldstein, M.J. and Weisman, A. (1997): Do mentally ill patients perceive their family members' expressed emotion? (Abstract) Schizophrenia Research 12: 229

Woo, S.M., Goldstein, M.J. and Nuechterlein, K.H. (1997): Relatives' expressed emotion and non-verbal signs of subclinical psychopathology in schizophrenic patients. British Journal of Psychiatry 170: 58–61

Asarnow, J.R., Tompson, M.C. and Goldstein, M.J. (1998): Psychosocial factors: The social context of child- and adolescent-onset schizophrenia. In: Schizophrenia in children and adolescents: Developmental and clinical perspectives (Remschmidt, H., ed.). Cambridge: Cambridge University Press

Goldstein, M.J. (1998): Adolescent behavioral and intrafamilial precursors of schizophrenia spectrum disorders. International Clinical Psychopharmacology 13 (Suppl. 1): 1

Linszen, D.H., Dingemans, P.M., Lenior, M.E., Scholte, W.F. and Goldstein M.J. (1998): Early family and individual interventions and relapse in recent-onset schizophrenia and related disorders. The Italian Journal of Psychiatry and Behavioural Sciences 2: 77–84

Linszen, D.H., Dingemans, P., Lenior, M.E., Scholte, W.F., de Haan, L. and Goldstein, M.J. (1998): Early detection and intervention in schizophrenia. International Clinical Psychopharmacology 13 (Suppl. 3): 31–34

Linszen, D.H., Dingemans, P.M., Lenior, M.E., Scholte, W.F., de Haan, L. and Goldstein, M.J. (1998): Early intervention, untreated psychotic illness in early recognized schizophrenia. International Clinical Psychopharmacology 15 (Suppl. 3): 45–52

Linszen, D.H., Dingemans, P.M., Scholte, W.F., Lenior, M.E. and Goldstein, M.J. (1998): Early recognition, intensive intervention and other protective and risk factors for psychotic relapse in patients with first psychotic episodes in schizophrenia. International Clinical Psychopharmacology 13 (Suppl. 1): 7–13

Weisman, A.G., Okazaki, S., Gregory, J., Tompson, M.C., Goldstein, M.J., Rea, M.M. and Miklowitz, D.J. (1998): Evaluation of therapist competence and adherence to behavior family management with bipolar patients. Family Process 37(1): 107–121

Weisman, A.G., Nuechterlein, K.H., Goldstein, M.J. and Snyder, K.S. (1998): Expressed Emotion, attributions, and schizophrenia symptom dimensions. Journal of Abnormal Psychology 107(2): 355–359 [reprinted in: Clinician's Research Digest: Briefings in Behavioral Science 16(8), August 1998 edition]

Goldstein, M.J. (1999): Psychosocial treatments for individuals with schizophrenia and related disorders. In: Cost-effectiveness of psychotherapy: A guide for practitioners, researchers, and policy makers (Miller, N.E., Magruder, K.M. et al., eds.), pp. 235–247. New York: Oxford University Press

Goldstein, M.J. (1999): New directions in family intervention programs for psychotic patients: Implications from expressed emotion research. In: Psychotherapy indications and outcomes, Janowsky (D.S. et al., eds.), pp. 323–339. Washington, DC

Rosenfarb, I.S., Ventura, J., Nuechterlein, K.H., Goldstein, M.J., Snyder, K.S. and Hwang, S. (1999): Expressed emotion, appraisal and coping by patients with recent-onset schizophrenia: A pilot investigation. Scandinavian Journal of Behaviour Therapy 28(1): 3–8

Tompson, M.C., Niv, N., Rea, M.M., Miklowitz, D.J. and Goldstein, M.J. (1999): Family-focused treatment for bipolar disorder: Evaluating mechanisms of action. (Abstract). Bipolar Disorders 1 (Suppl. 1): 55

Tompson, M.C., Rea, M.M., Goldstein, M.J., Miklowitz, D.J. and Weisman, A.G. (2000): Difficulty in implementing a family intervention for bipolar disorder: The predictive role of patient and family attributes. Family Process 39: 105–120

Weisman, A.G., Lopez, S.R., Ventura, J., Nuechterlein, K.H., Goldstein, M.J. and Hwang, S. (2000): A comparison of psychiatric symptoms between Anglo-Americans and Mexican-Americans with schizophrenia. Schizophrenia Bulletin 26: 817–824

Weisman, A.G., Nuechterlein, K.H., Goldstein, M.J. and Snyder, K. (2000): Controllability perceptions and reactions to symptoms of schizophrenia: A within family comparison of high-EE and low-EE relatives. Journal of Abnormal Psychology 109(1): 167–171

Rosenfarb, I.S., Miklowitz, D.J., Goldstein, M.J., Harmon, L., Nuechterlein, K.H. and Rea, M.M. (2001): Family transactions and relapse in bipolar disorder. Family Process 40(1): 5–14

Rosenfarb, I.S., Nuechterlein, K.H., Goldstein, M.J. and Subotnik, K.L. (2000): Neurocognitive vulnerability, interpersonal criticism, and the emergence of unusual thinking during family transactions in patients with schizophrenia. Archives of General Psychiatry 57(12): 1174–1179

Weisman, A.G., Lopez, S.R., Ventura, J., Nuechterlein, K.H., Goldstein, M.J. and Hwang, S. (in press): Therapist competency and adherence to family focused therapy as a predictor of outcome in patients with bipolar disorder

Manuscripts in Preparation

Rea, M.M., Tompson, M.C., Miklowitz, D.J., Goldstein, M.J., Hwang, S. and Mintz, J. (in preparation): Family focused treatment vs. individual treatment for bipolar disorder: Results of a randomized clinical trial

Tompson, M.C., Asarnow, J.R., Burney, T., Hamilton, E. and Goldstein, M.J. (in preparation): Communication deviance in the families of children with schizophrenia-spectrum disorders

Presentations (Subset of Presentations, Beginning 1981)

Miklowitz, D.J., Goldstein, M.J. and Falloon, I.R.H. (1981, April): Familial and symptomatic characteristics of schizophrenics living in high and low expressed emotion home environments. Presented at the Annual Western Psychological Association (W. P.A.) Convention, Los Angeles, CA

Cozolino, L.J., Goldstein, M.J., and Nuechterlein, K.H. (1982, May): Family education in the psychosocial treatment of schizophrenia. Presented at NIMH Workshop on Preventive Intervention Programs for Family Units with a Mentally-Ill Relative, La Jolla, CA

Miklowitz, D.J., Goldstein, M.J., Doane, J.A. and Falloon, I.R.H. (1983, April): Cross-situational affective communication in the families of schizophrenics. Presented at the Annual W.P.A. Conference, San Francisco, CA

Asarnow, J.R., Fliegel, S. and Goldstein, M.J. (1985, September): Family factors associated with childhood onset depressive disorders. Paper presented at the Conference on the Impact of Family Interaction Research on our Understanding of Psychopathology, MaxPlanckInstitute for Psychiatry, Munich

Miklowitz, D.J., Goldstein, M.J., Nuechterlein, K.H., Snyder, K.S. and Doane, J.A. (1985, December): Expressed emotion, lithium compliance and relapse in early onset mania. Presented at the Annual Meeting of the American College of Neuropsychopharmacology, Maui, HI

Miklowitz, D.J., Goldstein, M.J. and Nuechterlein, K.H. (1987, March): Patient and family correlates of expressed emotion in schizophrenia. Presented at the International Congress on Schizophrenia Research, Clearwater, FL

Asarnow, J.R. and Goldstein, M.J. (1987, June): A comparative study of childhood onset schizophrenia spectrum and depressive disorders. Poster presented at the Fifth Annual Institute of the MacArthur Foundation Research Network on Risk and Protective Factors in the Major Mental Disorders, San Diego, CA

Asarnow, J.R., Goldstein, M.J., Carlson, G.A., Perdue, S., Bates, S. and Keller, J. (1987, September): Childhood-onset depressive disorders: A follow-up study of rates of rehospitalization and out of home placement among child psychiatric inpatients. Paper presented at the Annual Meeting of the Depression Risk Consortium, Boston, MA

Goldstein, M.J., Miklowitz, D.J., Strachan, A.M., Doane, J.A., Feingold, D. and Nuechterlein, K.H. (1987, September): Family interaction and patient coping style as predictors of the short-term course of schizophrenia. Invited address presented at the International Symposium on Schizophrenia on The Role of Mediating Processes in Understanding and Treating Schizophrenia, Berne

Nuechterlein, K.H., Goldstein, M.J., Ventura, J., Dawson, M.E. and Doane, J.A. (1987, September): Patient-environment relationships in schizophrenia: Attentional functioning, communication deviance, autonomic arousal, and stressful life events. Invited address presented at the International Symposium on Schizophrenia on The Role of Mediating Processes in Understanding and Treating Schizophrenia, Berne

Asarnow, J.R., Goldstein, M.J., and Ben-Meir, S. (1987, November): Parental communication deviance in childhood onset schizophrenia spectrum and depressive disorders. Presentation at the Annual Meeting of the Society for Research in Psychopathology, Atlanta, GA

Miklowitz, D.J., Velligan, D.I., Goldstein, M.J., Nuechterlein, K.H. and Doane, J.A. (1988, November): Communication deviance in parents of schizophrenic and manic patients. Presented at the Society for Research in Psychopathology, Harvard University, Cambridge, MA

Altorfer, A., Goldstein, M.J. and Nuechterlein, K.H. (1989, April): The analysis of verbal and nonverbal communication processes in families of schizophrenic and manic-depressive patients: Connections to "communication deviance" (CD), "affective style" (AS) and "Expressed Emotion" (EE). Presented at the Second International Congress on Schizophrenia Research, San Diego, CA

Goldstein, M.J., Miklowitz, D.J., Strachan, A.M. and Nuechterlein, K.H. (1989, April): Reciprocal interaction patterns in the families of recent onset schizophrenics related to short term course of the disorder. Presented at the Second International Congress on Schizophrenia Research, San Diego, CA

Miklowitz, D.J., Velligan, D.I., Goldstein, M.J., Nuechterlein, K.H. and Gitlin, M.J. (1989, April): Communication deviance in parents of schizophrenic and manic patients. Presented at the Second International Congress on Schizophrenia Research, San Diego, CA

Velligan, D.I., Miklowitz, D.J., Goldstein, M.J. and Nuechterlein, K.H. (1989, April): Can communication deviance be measured in an interactional setting? Presented at the Second International Congress on Schizophrenia Research, San Diego, CA

Miklowitz, D.J., Goldstein, M.J., Nuechterlein, K.H., Strachan, A.M. and Feingold, D. (1989, November): Interactional behavior in families of schizophrenic and manic patients. Presented at Society for Research in Psychopathology, Miami, FL

Goldstein, M.J. and Asarnow, J.R. (1990, June): Prevention in Schizophrenia. Paper commissioned for the National Conference on Prevention Research, National Institute of Mental Health, Rockville, MD

Goldstein, M.J., Talovic, S.A., Nuechterlein, K.H., Fogelson, D.L., Subotnik, K.L. and Asarnow, R.F. (1990, October): Family interaction versus individual psychopathology: Do they indicate the same processes in the families of schizophrenics? Presented at the 3rd International Schizophrenia Symposium, Berne

Goldstein, M.J., Nuechterlein, K.H., Miklowitz, D.J. and Strachan, A.M. (1990, November): The contribution of family interaction to understanding the early course of schizophrenia. Paper presented at Society for Research in Psychopathology, Boulder, CO

Velligan, D.I., Goldstein, M.J. and Miklowitz, D.J. (1990, November): The impact of individual and family treatment on communication deviance in the families of schizophrenic patients. Poster presented at Society for Research in Psychopathology, Boulder, CO

Subotnik, K.L., Nuechterlein, K.H., Asarnow, R.R., Fogelson, D.L., Goldstein, M.J. and Talovic, S.A. (1990, May): Affective and negative symptoms in recent-onset schizophrenia: Relationship to familial psychiatric illness. Presented at the 143rd Annual Meeting of the American Psychiatric Association, New York

Goldstein, M.J. and Asarnow, J.R. (1990, June): Prevention in schizophrenia. Paper commissioned for the National Conference on Prevention Research, National Institute of Mental Health, Rockville, MD

Asarnow, J.R., Goldstein, M.J., Tompson, M.C. and Hornstein, N. (1990, December): Depression in childhood: Factors associated with risk for relapse and/or continuing mood disorder. Paper presented at the 5th Annual Meeting of the Society for Research in Psychopathology, Boulder, CO

Goldstein, M.J., Talovic, S.A., and Nuechterlein, K.H. (1991, April): Family interactions vs. individual psychopathology. Presented at the 3rd International Congress on Research in Schizophrenia, Tucson, AZ

Miklowitz, D.J., Goldstein, M.J. and Nuechterlein, K.H. (1991, April): The predictive utility of schizophrenic symptoms in patients with a recent episode of mania. Presented at the 3rd International Congress on Research in Schizophrenia, Tucson, AZ

Asarnow, J.R., Goldstein, M.T., Tompson, M.C. and Hornstein, N. (1991, April): A comparative study of children with depressive disorders and schizophrenia spectrum disorder: Short-term outcome. Paper presented at the Meeting for the Society for Research in Child Development

Tompson, M.C., Goldstein, M.J., Lebell, M.B., Marder, S.R. and Mintz, L. (1991, April): Schizophrenic patients' perceptions of their relatives' attitudes. Poster presented at the International Conference on Schizophrenia Research, Tucson, AZ

Asarnow, J.R., Bates, S., Tompson, M.C, Goldstein, M.J. and Hornstein, N. (1991, October): Depressive and schizophrenia spectrum disorders in childhood: A follow-up study. Paper presented at the Annual Meeting of the American Academy of Child and Adolescent Psychiatry

Rea, M.M., Goldstein, M.J. and Miklowitz, D.J. (1992, November): Patterns of family interaction as they relate to the course of bipolar disorder. Society for Research in Psychopathology, Palm Springs, CA

Subotnik, K.L., Goldstein, M.J., Nuechterlein, K.H., Mintz, J. and Talovic, S.A. (1992, November): The relationship between family interaction attributes and family history of psychiatric disorders in parents of recent-onset schizophrenic patients. Presented at the 7th Annual Meeting of the Society for Research in Psychopathology, Palm Springs, CA

Asarnow, J.R., Hamilton, E., Tompson, M.C. and Goldstein, M.J. (1993, February): Childhood-onset depression: Examination of patterns of affective expression among depressed children and their parents. Paper presented at the Annual Meeting of the Society for Research in Child and Adolescent Psychopathology, Santa Fe, NM

Altorfer, A., Goldstein, M.J., Nuechterlein, K.H. and Miklowitz, D.J. (1993, April): The patient's nonverbal behaviour in family interactions. Presented at the Fourth International Congress on Schizophrenia Research, Colorado Springs, CO

Miklowitz, D.J., Goldstein, M.J. and Nuechterlein, K.H. (1993, April): A comparison of verbal interactional styles among families of schizophrenic and bipolar patients. Presented at the 4th International Congress on Schizophrenia Research, Colorado Springs, CO

Rosenfarb, I.S., Goldstein, M.J., Mintz, J. and Nuechterlein, K.H. (1993, April): Expressed emotion and subclinical psychopathology observable within the transactions between recent-onset schizophrenics and their families. Presented at the Fourth International Congress on Schizophrenia Research, Colorado Springs, CO

Simoneau, T.L., Stackman, D.K., Miklowitz, D.J., Goldstein, M.J. and Nuechterlein, K.H. (1993, April): Nonverbal interactional behaviour in the parents of schizophrenic and bipolar patients. Presented at the 4th International Congress on Schizophrenia Research, Colorado Springs, CO

Tompson, M.C., Goldstein, M.J., Lebell, M.B., Mintz, L.I. and Marder, S.R. (1993, April): Relatives' Expressed Emotion (EE) vs. patients' perceptions of EE: Which is a better predictor of course? Poster presented at the 4th International Congress on Schizophrenia Research, Colorado Springs, CO

Woo, S.M., Goldstein, M.J. and Nuechterlein, K.H. (1993, April): Manifestations of subclinical psychopathology in schizophrenics from high and low EE families. Presented at the Fourth International Congress on Schizophrenia Research, Colorado Springs, CO

Rosenfarb, I.S., Miklowitz, D.J., Goldstein, M.J., Harmon, L. and Nuechterlein, K.H. (1993, October): Family transactions and relapse in bipolar disorder. Society for Research in Psychopathology, Chicago, IL

Tompson, M.C., Goldstein, M.J. and Rea, M.M. (1996, August): Psychoeducational family therapy with bipolar patients: Predicting treatment difficulty. Poster presented at the 104th American Psychological Association Convention, Toronto, Canada

Goldstein, M.J. and Tompson, M.C. (1996, September): Coping with psychosis: Patients, relatives, assessments. Paper presented at the 9th Congress of the European College of Neuropsychopharmacology, Amsterdam, Holland

Weisman, A.G., Nuechterlein, K.H. and Goldstein, M.J. (1996, August): Expressed emotion, attributions, and schizophrenia symptom dimensions. Poster presented at the American Psychological Association, Toronto, Canada

Goldstein, M.J. (1998, November): Adolescent behavioral and intrafamilial precursors of schizophrenia spectrum disorders. Congress on First Psychotic Episode in Schizophrenia, Amsterdam

Linszen, D.H., Dingemans, P.M., Lenior, M.E., Scholte, W.F., de Haan, L., and Goldstein, M.J. (1997, March): Early detection and intervention in schizophrenia, Lundbeck Symposium, Rome

Tompson, M.C., Goldstein, M.J. and Weisman, A.G. (1997, April): Do mentally ill patients perceive their family members' expressed emotion? Paper presented at the Biennial International Congress on Schizophrenia Research, Colorado Springs, CO

Subotnik, K.L., Nuechterlein, K.H., Asarnow, R.F., Fogelson, D.L., Goldstein, M.J. and Mintz, J. (1997, May): Depressive symptoms in recent-onset schizophrenia patients are associated with a family history of depression. Presented at the Annual Meeting of the American Psychiatric Association, San Diego, CA

Weisman, A.G., Ventura, J., Nuechterlein, K.H., López, S.R., Goldstein, M.J. and Hwang, S. (1997, August): Manifestations of psychopathology in Anglo-American and Mexican-American patients with schizophrenia. Paper presented at the Regional Congress of Psychology for Professionals in the Americas, Mexico City, Mexico

Niv, N., Rea, M.M., Tompson, M.C., Goldstein, M.J. and Miklowitz, D.J. (1997, October): Axis II comorbidity in bipolar patients. Poster presented at the meeting of the Society for Research in Psychopathology, Palm Springs, CA

Rea, M.M., Niv, N., Miklowitz, D.J., Tompson, M.C. and Goldstein, M.J. (1997, October): Axis II comorbidity in bipolar disorder. Poster presented at the Society for Research in Psychopathology, 10th Annual Meeting, Palm Springs, CA

Rea, M.M., Tompson, M.C., Miklowitz, D.J. and Goldstein, M.J. (1997, October): The UCLA Bipolar/Family Treatment Project: Preliminary efficacy results. Paper presented at the Society for Research in Psychopathology, 10th Annual Meeting, Palm Springs, CA

Weisman, A.G., Okazaki, S., Gregory, J., Tompson, M.C., Rea, M.M. and Goldstein, M.J. (1997, November): Therapist competence and adherence to behavioral family management in a bipolar sample. Paper presented at the Annual Conference of the Association for the Advancement of Behavior Therapy, Miami, FL

Weisman, A.G., Okazaki, S., Gregory, J., Goldstein, M.J., Tompson, M.C., Rea, M.M. and Miklowitz, D.J. (1998, May): Evaluation of therapist competence and adherence to behavioral family management with bipolar patients. Annual Meeting of the American Psychological Society, Washington, DC

Rea, M.M., Goldstein, M.J., Tompson, M.C. and Miklowitz, D.J. (1998, May): Family and individual therapy in bipolar disorders: Outline and first results of the study. World Association for Psychiatric Rehabilitation, Hamburg, Germany

Rosenfarb, I.S., Goldstein, M.J., Miklowitz, D.J., Harmon, L., Nuechterlein, K.H. and Rea, M.M. (1998, November): Patient subclinical psychopathology during family transactions in schizophrenia and bipolar disorder. Poster presented at the Society for Research in Psychopathology, 13th Annual Meeting, Boston, MA

Subotnik, K.L., Nuechterlein, K.H., Asarnow, R.F., Goldstein, M.J., Fogelson, D.L. and Torquato, R.D. (1999, April): Communication deviance is associated with putative genetic vulnerability indicators in recent-onset schizophrenia. Presented at the Biennial Meeting of the International Congress on Schizophrenia Research, Santa Fe, NM

Tompson, M.C., Niv, N., Rea, M.M., Miklowitz, D.J. and Goldstein, M.J. (1999, June): Family-focused treatment for bipolar disorder: Evaluating mechanisms of action. Poster presented at the 3rd International Conference on Bipolar Disorder, Pittsburgh, PA

Niv, N., Rea, M.M., Miklowitz, D.J., Tompson, M.C. and Goldstein, M.J. (1999, August): Comorbid Bipolar Disorder and Personality Disorders. Poster presented at the American Psychological Association Annual Convention, Boston, MA

Weisman, A.G., Nuechterlein, K.H., Goldstein, M.J. and Snyder, K.S. (1999, August): Controllability perceptions and reactions to symptoms of schizophrenia: A within family comparison of high-EE and low-EE relatives. Poster presented at the American Psychological Association, Boston, MA

Miklowitz, D.J. and Goldstein, M.J. (1999, November): The relationship between expressed emotion and individual psychopathology among relatives of bipolar patients. 14th Annual Society for Research in Psychopathology meeting, Montreal, Quebec, Canada

Weisman, A.G., Okazaki, S. Gregory, J., Tompson, M.C., Goldstein, M.J., Rea, M.M. and Miklowitz, D.J. (2000, November): Therapist competency and adherence to family focused therapy as a predictor of outcome in patients with bipolar disorder. Poster presented at the Association for the Advancement of Behavioral Therapy, New Orleans, LA

Part II

High Expressed Emotion and Associated Research in Schizophrenia and in Borderline Personality

3
Early Psychosis, Schizophrenia and the Family

Don H. Linszen and Peter M. Dingemans

Schizophrenia remains the most severe psychotic disorder and a source of intense distress for the family. With the typical onset of the first psychotic episode of schizophrenia in adolescence or early adulthood the productive years of young people are interrupted. When parents generally expect their children to become adult and independent, deterioration of functioning starts, even before the first psychotic episode (Jones et al., 1993; Häfner et al., 1995). Precisely in this period the severity of schizophrenia will be established, i.e. in the early phase 5 years after the first psychotic episode (Bleuler, 1978; McGlashan, 1996). Eighty percent of people with first episode schizophrenia or related disorders relapse at least once or more within five years (Sheperd et al., 1989; Robinson et al., 1999). There is a decline in social contacts with the peer group, especially in young men with an earlier age of onset than females (mean difference: 5 years, Angermeyer and Kühn, 1988). The early phase of psychosis and schizophrenia can thus be seen as a 'critical period' with major implications for the prevention of disease and psychosocial deterioration (Birchwood et al., 1998). Early recognition and intervention may thus lead to a better outcome. Evidence for that idea is based on the following findings:

(1) the early onset and the varying symptomatic and functional course of schizophrenia (Bleuler, 1978),

(2) poorer outcome associated with delay in adequate intervention (Crow, 1986; Loebel et al., 1992), and

(3) the rapid deterioration in the two years, after the first psychotic episode (Birchwood and MacMillan, 1993).

In the critical period the severity of psychosis will be established, and the role of the family in the first episode is a crucial one. Two concepts of schizophrenia have exerted their influence in focussing on the role of the family and their attitudes. In the first concept the family is seen from the medical point of view: schizophrenia is a disease and the family is generating genetic risk factors for schizophrenia. The other point of view has been represented by the emphasis on psychosocial factors. Goldstein et al. (1978) integrated both medical and psychosocial views in a seminal intervention study, combining drug and psychosocial interventions, with a sample of young psychotic patients and their families. This study was characterized by 1) a family oriented preventive approach to psychosis and schizophrenia, 2) a community-based approach, and 3) attention for the burden of psychosis on the family.

In this chapter, the views on the family and schizophrenia will be discussed, followed by an overview of different family intervention models of patients with a first psychotic episode or with mixed patient groups. Finally, Goldstein's model will be applied and extended in a preventive study model with families in the recognition and intervention of first episode psychosis during the critical period in an attempt of altering the natural course of schizophrenia.

Concepts on Family and Schizophrenia

The interest in the family of patients with schizophrenia has fluctuated between two basic concepts and can be traced back to the start of last century. Kraepelin (1919) unified a number of psychiatric conditions (hebephrenia, catatonia and paranoia) in one disease: "dementia praecox". The disease had its onset in adolescence and young adulthood and was initially thought to lead inevitably to intellectual deterioration, from which patients inevitably failed to discover. Later Kraepelin recognised that a small group of hebephrenic and catatonic patients recovered fully. One should realise that Kraepelin's emphasis was on negative symptoms and early deterioration, and not so much on psychotic episodes in actual terminology. The family carried genetic factors, that caused metabolic changes; "autotoxins", independent from the family environment, were thought to cause this early dementia type. With severe forms of schizophrenia the patient was often institutionalised and the family felt only the burden of stigma and not of the daily care.

The disease concept of schizophrenia was influential in studies of the last two decades. In this concept the emotional reactions of the family to the disease are emphasised; they will be the same or even worse – because of the young age of the patient – as those of any other family with a more or less genetically determined chronic disease. Their reaction will be one of loss: mourning, denial, despair and anger, being frightened because of the genetic risk and feeling burdened in the case of inadequate care.

Bleuler (1911) introduced the second concept with the term schizophrenia instead of dementia praecox. He noticed that the slow progression to a demented state was only true in a subset of the patients with the symptoms of dementia praecox. Also the age of onset was not always precocious. According to his view schizophrenia should be seen as a group of disorders, differing in (also genetic) causes, clinical picture and outcome. With Jung, he pointed out the psychological and social aspects, including family life factors, influencing the course of schizophrenia. His ideas may be interpreted as the forerunner of the vulnerability/stress models (Zubin and Spring, 1977; Goldstein, 1978; Nuechterlein and Dawson, 1984). A non-genetic family theory was developed in the late 1940s and the 1950s. Bateson et al. (1956) improvised on the theme of ambivalence in relationships, expanded the concept of the schizophrenogenic mother of Melanie Klein to a family level and developed the "double bind" theory. The basic idea of this theory was that there were conflicting overt verbal and a more abstract nonverbal communication patterns of parents towards their child. The child was not able to distinguish the conflicts in message correctly and could not withdraw from the situation. The thought and communication disorders of adolescents and young adults with schizophrenia were thought to arise from this situation. Lidz and his colleagues (1957) used the term "marital schism" (overt conflicts between the parents) and "marital skew" (in which the disturbed functioning of one parent was compensated by distorted communication of the other) as the underlying condition of schizophrenia. Wynne et al. (1958) described "communication deviance", "pseudomutuality" and "pseudohostility" as the characteristically disordered communication patterns and emotional relation of parents of patients with schizophrenia. One must realize that in those days the adaptational aspect of symptoms was in the centre of interest, and that the effect of antipsychotic medication had not been tested yet.

Based on these theories many family therapies for schizo-phrenic patients were developed and applied to families with young first episode patients (Lidz, 1973; Selvini-Palazzoli et al., 1978). The goal of the etiologically oriented family therapy was to alter the described pathological family, thus improving the course of schizo-phrenia or even curing the disease. At the same time acute and maintenance antipsychotic medication appeared to be effective against psychotic signs and symptoms and as prevention against relapse. The etiologically oriented family therapists tended to see medical interventions such as the use of antipsychotic medication as inflicting the "sick role" on the schizophrenic family member. However, despite their attractiveness for many professionals the results of these family therapy approaches turned out to be disap-pointing, mainly because of a lack of empirical evidence. Moreover, Terkelsen (1983), and Lefley (1992) have also convincingly argued that families and patients experienced negative "side" effects from this type of family intervention. Relatives felt they were scapegoated or the cause of the illness and experienced therapy sessions as a burden. This alienated families from professionals and hindered a useful co-operation, a development that was detrimental especially with young patients.

Families and the Course of Schizophrenia: The Empirical Past and Present

The interest for the families of patients with schizophrenia changed again during the 1970s to the role of the family and the course instead of the cause of the disease. During the sixties families were treated as adversaries in the therapeutic process; later on they were considered to be allies. This reorientation can be traced back to the influence of three important interacting factors: (1) deinstitutiona-lisation and increase of extramural care; (2) the relative importance of pharmacotherapy, and (3) "Expressed Emotion" (EE) research and the family burden.

Deinstitutionalisation

The deinstitutionalisation in the United States and Italy and the corresponding shift from intramural to extramural care reunited many patients with schizophrenia on the spot where their illness had started: the nuclear family. In the United States two-thirds of these patients returned to their homes. This return often meant a burden for the family. Family members were handicapped by a lack of knowledge of coping with such a severe disorder. This also turned out to be true for many professionals: they also suffered from a lack of knowledge and interest in the slow and difficult process of motivating the patient for their treatment.

The Relative Importance of Pharmacotherapy

Antipsychotic medication has proven to be effective in the treatment of schizophrenia, has been successfully applied in the acute and maintenance treatment of all forms of schizophrenia and related disorders and has become the mainstay of intervention (Kane, 1989). Compliance with antipsychotic medication has been found the major predictor of a favourable outcome over a 5 year follow-up period (Robinson et al., 1999). Untreated non-affective psychoses with a duration longer than one year found to predict more severe forms of schizophrenia, e.g. more psychotic relapses (Crow et al., 1986) and delay in psychotic symptom remission, representing the feature of deterioration (Loebel et al., 1992). Both psychotherapists and system therapists have underestimated the importance of this finding. Depot-antipsychotic medication offered the best insight in the effect on relapse of the antipsychotic drugs. The relapse rate with depots fluctuated from 40% with recent discharged patients (Hogarty et al., 1979) to 8% (Rifkin et al., 1977). Antipsychotic drugs are of a considerable value, but are not conclusively effective against relapse in the treatment of schizophrenia. An important reason for the addition of family intervention to antipsychotic medication was the incomplete protection of antipsychotic maintenance medication against psychotic relapse (Vaughn and Leff, 1976). Low EE (absence of family stress) was considered to be as valuable clinically as maintenance medication, as EE and medication each accounted for about a 30% of the relapse rate (Bebbington and Kuipers, 1994). These findings gave an impetus of combining the pharmacotherapy of psychosis with other treatments, i.e. family intervention.

The Family and Expressed Emotion (EE): A Shift to Need of Support

The original EE finding dated back to the fifties (Brown et al., 1958), showed the same interest for ambivalent emotions as the family theorists from that time and was replicated in 1972 (Brown et al., 1972). Patients with schizophrenia who returned from the hospital and who lived with relatives expressing themselves in a critical, hostile or emotionally over-involved way about the patient and his/her disease or behavior in a standardized interview (high EE) experienced psychotic relapses more often than patients who lived on their own or with relatives who expressed themselves less or not emotionally (low EE). Since then numerous studies supported the value of high EE in predicting substantially higher rates of psychotic relapses and thus the severity of schizophrenia (Kavanagh, 1992). Low EE was clinically as valuable as maintenance medication, as EE and medication each accounted for about a 30% of the relapse rate (Bebbington and Kuipers, 1994). The classical interpretation of the EE finding has been that a high EE was an indicator of stressful family interactions. As stressful life events and high EE attitudes of relatives were thought to contribute to a high level of environmental stress, which then interacted with the biological vulnerability factors, and increased the likelihood of relapse, thus influencing the severity and course of schizophrenia.

In two first episode studies parental high EE had prognostic value and predicted psychotic relapse within a year. The Los Angeles group interpreted their finding as underlining the importance of the vulnerability stress model (Nuechterlein and Dawson, 1984). Again they assumed an interaction between a biological (genetic and neuropsychological) vulnerability and environmental stressors (EE) in precipitating a psychotic relapse during the short-term course of first episode schizophrenia. Alternatively, in a separate analysis the authors found that severity of illness could have elicited high EE, an early onset and living at home. In a study in Amsterdam (Linszen et al., 1996) high EE in families with young patients was found to be a predictor as well as in a one-year family intervention trial. In this cohort the short-term course was not confounded by repeated admissions or by more than one year duration of untreated psychosis. The high EE of the parents of these adolescent and young adult patients in the early phase of their disease was interpreted as an acute emotional reaction (a state factor) to the crisis elicited by the recent onset episode of the disease and admission and a strong need for support. Pathological reactions could then arise as a response to the stress of coping with a disturbed adolescent.

In other studies with young patients with a first psychotic episode of schizophrenia or related disorders the results of EE research have been more controversial. In some studies of first episode patients EE was not found to be a predictor at 12 months follow up (Barrelet et al., 1990; Stirling et al., 1991; Rund et al., 1994). Interesting findings of these non-replicating first episode studies were the high occurrence of emotional overinvolvement (EOI) compared with criticism and hostility expressed by the parents with a tendency of EOI to turn into criticism (Stirling et al., 1991). In the last double-blind placebo controlled study with first psychotic episode patients EE turned out to be a significant, but spurious predictor. In the last double-blind placebo controlled antipsychotic medication study – with first episode psychotic patients – they found a significant but marginal difference in psychotic relapse rate: 40% and 60% relapse after two years in the active versus placebo medication group respectively (Mac Millan et al., 1986). Untreated duration of psychosis more than a year and medication use appeared to be the better predictor of poor outcome compared with high EE.

A strong indicator for the need of support was the founding of organisations of family members of patients with chronic schizophrenia, in the USA ("the National Alliance of Mentally Ill – NAMI"), in England ("the National Schizophrenia Fellowship") and in the Netherlands ("Ypsilon"). For the family deinstitutionalisation resulted in an increase in contacts with their schizophrenic family member. They felt a need for information about coping with the illness and for support. They experienced a lack of services; because they felt dissatisfied with the mental services, they created self-help groups and organisations for issues of support and information.

Family Interventions

Family Intervention Programs with Patients with Chronic Schizophrenia

The EE family intervention programs, which were superimposed on maintenance antipsychotic drug treatment, were developed to change the critical, hostile or overinvolved climate of the family of the patient with schizophrenia, thus reducing stress and the risk of a psychotic relapse. There were four family intervention programmes, all tested against maintenance pharmacotherapy, and all with high EE families, that succeeded in their goal of relapse reduction over 1 to 2 year period (Leff et al., 1982; Falloon et al., 1982; Hogarty et al., 1986; Tarrier et al., 1988). They reduced the level of negative family interaction (Falloon et al., 1985), high EE (Lam, 1991), in particular the high emotional involvement (Mari and Streiner, 1994).

In the London intervention (Leff and Vaughn, 1981; Leff et al., 1982) 24 patients with a PSE diagnosis of schizophrenia were included and received antipsychotic medication. Their high EE families were randomized over a experimental family intervention (educational multiple family groups and individual family intervention) and a standard condition. The results showed a 9% relapse rate after 9 months and a 33% relapse rate after two years in the experimental condition against 33% and 75% consecutively in the control condition. The USCAL model (Falloon, 1982; Falloon, 1984) included 36 patients with PSE diagnoses of schizophrenia. The majority came from high EE families. One third of the cohort of 36 patients were admitted for the first time. All patients were on oral antipsychotic medication; when they appeared to be non-compliant (measured by blood levels), they received depot anti-psychotic medication. The family intervention was home-based with the patient and consisted of psycho-education, communication training and problem solving. Crisis-intervention was possible. The results showed a 6% and 17% relapse rate for the family intervention at 9 and 24 months follow-up against a 44% and 83% relapse rate for the individual intervention.

In the Pittsburgh study (Hogarty et al., 1986) 103 patients came from high EE families. Patients were randomised over 4 conditions: family intervention, social skills training, a combination of both and antipsychotic medication. The family intervention was characterized by (1) creation of a working alliance, (2) the "survival-skills"-workshop, (3) application, and (4) continuity of treatment (Anderson et al., 1986).

Relapse rates after one year follow-up showed 41% in the medication group; in the family intervention group 19% of the patients relapsed, as 20% of them did in the social skills training group. 0% of the patients relapsed in the family intervention plus social skills training group. These results are the same as in the Amsterdam study with similar results (Linszen et al., 1996).

Most of the high EE and intervention studies used psycho-educational and behavioral models and studied older patients with relapsing, non-remitting and chronic outcomes of schizophrenia. Authors emphasised that EE as a predictor in the epidemiological sense could also be interpreted as expression of burden of the family by a severe mental disease. The group of Jackson examined the relation between EE and family burden. High levels of criticism corresponded with the burden felt by disease and patient charac-teristics (Jackson et al., 1990). The Amsterdam group found the same relation in a new first psychotic episode study (Wolthaus et al., in press).

Family Intervention in First Episode Psychosis

The classical family intervention studies used a select sample of patients with different ages and in different phases of schizophrenia, namely those from families rated as high expressed emotions (high EE) and with a mixed sample of first episode and more chronic patients.

Recently a new shift took place in the interest in first episode schizophrenia and the family, this in time with a preventive approach, since early recognition and intervention might lead to a better outcome. Only in three intervention trials young patients with first psychotic episodes and their families have been evaluated.

Goldstein et al. (1978) at the UCLA in California did the first and seminal study. They emphasised the crisis of psychosis in the 96 adolescent patients and their family and used crisis intervention techniques in their family intervention program in combination with a mean and low dosage of antipsychotic medication in a randomized design. "Expressed Emotion" was not measured. The ingredients of the family intervention were information about the characteristics of the illness, inventarisation of stressors, expressing feelings about the psychotic episode and the development of strategies to cope actively with stressors now and in the future. Family members had to learn to make realistic estimations about the social functioning of their child and to decrease high expectations. The last phase consisted of anticipation on stressors, the early recognition and active management of prodromal signs and compli-ance issues. Other problems that were discussed often were work, making friends and housing. After 6 months of follow-up no patients (0%) relapsed in the mean dosage/family intervention group, 14% in the mean dosage/no family intervention group, 21% in the low dosage/family intervention group and 48% in the low dosage/no family intervention group. The weakness of the Goldstein study was obviously the short duration.

Rund et al. (1994) studied 24 young patients and their families in Norway in a controlled study. Family intervention was composed of creating a working alliance, training in problem solving skills, and maintenance sessions. The control condition consisted of standard services. There was a significant lower relapse rate in the family intervention condition.

In a Chinese study (Zhang et al., 1994) family group therapy or individual family therapy, all with patients, was applied during 18 months in a flexible way and contrasted with a 'standard care' control group. The experimental group had a significant lower readmission rate than the control group, a shorter hospital stay and a better overall level of functioning. Education and stress reduction were the main ingredients of both family interventions with the aim prevention of chronicity of the patients and reduction of the burden on the family. There was a strong effect of compliance to antipsychotic medication. A weakness was the ill-defined outcome criteria, i.e. hospitalisation.

The Amsterdam Study

The Amsterdam first episode study (Linszen et al., 1996) did not attempt to merely replicate the strong evidence supporting family psychoeducation as in Goldstein's intervention. The study compared different family intervention strategies and compared family psychoeducation with more sophisticated individual therapy than previously available. The study applicated the Goldstein model over a 15 month period. The duration of untreated psychotic illness of the young patients (mean age 20.6) turned out to be short, compared with the Northwick Park Study (Crow et al., 1986). 71 of the patients appeared to have untreated psychotic symptoms between 0 and 6 months (74%), 14 between 7 and 12 months (14%) and 12 of the patients more than 12 months (12%). Duration of untreated psychotic illness as a risk factor, categorised in less and more than 12 months, appeared not to be predictive of psychotic relapse either. Moreover, in the first two studies EE was not reported (Goldstein et al., 1978; Zhang et al., 1994); in the Amsterdam study a full sample of high and low EE families was used (Linszen et al., 1996).

Patients were stratified by levels of EE before condition assignment. In all the empirical family intervention approaches, whether psycho-educational or behavioral, with first episode or with more chronic patients, the families were considered to be allies in the treatment and rehabilitation of patients with schizophrenia. The approaches gave support when relatives experienced burden and educated the family about the illness (i.e., the genetic role in schizophrenia). An attempt was made to avoid making scapegoats of the relatives of patients, but the question remained whether the therapists succeeded in their effort avoiding stress – and guilt indication. In Falloon's family behavioral therapy (1982) and in the Amsterdam study (Linszen et al., 1996), training and problem solving skills followed psychoeducation. An unresolved issue regarding these family programs was how much of the efficacy was due to the provision of support and education and how much to the specific behavioral interventions. This question turned out to be relevant for the results of the Amsterdam controlled clinical trial. The experimental behavioral family intervention of that study (including two supportive and education sessions) did not influence the relapse rate (16%) when contrasted with the standard treatment condition (15%). This result turned out to be the first failure of finding an effect of family intervention in the high EE condition. The finding was interpreted as follows: the inpatient treatment, including the two family education sessions and the continuity of care, provided such a "high" baseline that family intervention could not manage to show an additional increment in effectiveness. Some additional remarks can be made when the results of our study are compared with the methods and findings of similar studies in the UK and the United States. The inpatient phase of the treatment program continued relatively long (3 months), while in the United States insurance policies typically necessitate discharging the patients after 2–3 weeks. Compared with the United States, the inpatient treatment program with both the patients and the families appeared to be close to optimal. Furthermore, an active family-oriented treatment program had already taken place during inpatient care before the start of the trial. This made the program different from the cited EE-family intervention studies in which only incidental family treatment was undertaken during the inpatient phase. One can assume that the inpatient program influenced the outpatient results for the entire sample. Although it is speculative, one may hypothesise that the inpatient programs with a few supportive and education sessions was all the help that the low-EE families needed. Cozolino et al. (1988) found that a brief psycho-educational module, along the line as developed by Anderson et al. (1986), did produce a number of positive effects on family sense of support of the treatment team. Also interesting was the slightly higher incidence of relapses in the low EE/standard plus family treatment group. The follow-up behavioral family intervention phase may have put pressure on the low-EE families to look for and produce clinical changes in the patient, thus increasing the relapse rate. Post hoc analysis revealed that the behavioral family interventions may have interfered with the "grief process" and that there may have been other "adverse" labelling effects in what may be an essentially "good prognosis population". This is a criticism increasingly frequently levelled at EE interventions that may have some validity. There may be a danger of using EE as a criterion for family intervention, rather than a "needsled" family approach (Smith and Birchwood, 1990). In a further study of a smaller sample the Amsterdam group found that with 27% of the families remaining low in expressed emotion and 25% remaining high and with 40% moving in either direction, unstable expressed emotion was linked to relapse in this young sample (Nugter et al., 1997). Expressed emotion as measured by the Five Minutes Speech Sample (Magana et al., 1986) could then be seen as a characteristic of a process of adjustment to psychosis, perhaps at its zenith in this early critical phase (Birchwood et al., 1998). However, one should be cautious with this interpretation, since only two patients relapsed in the low EE/family plus standard intervention contrasted with no relapses in the low EE/ standard treatment group. As mentioned earlier standard treatment patients received psycho-educational components regarding their illness, their prodromal signs, coping strategies, three months of post-hospital day treatment, assistance with employment, education and finances, a well organised medication protocol and home visits when the patients appeared to be non complying. Compliance with anti-psychotic medication was deemed high throughout the study. This therapeutic package may have had an effect on the low relapse rate of the entire sample. Additional family intervention sessions could then not conceivably add anything to the standard treatment. Predictors of psychotic relapse turned out to be heavy cannabis abuse (Linszen et al., 1994) and high EE and cannabis use (Linszen et al., 1997), suggesting that much of the critical remarks and over involvement of the parents was directed towards behavior attributed to cannabis use.

A crucial question was whether the favourable effects lasted after the end of the intensive 15-month intervention program with this young population with a short duration of untreated psychosis (Linszen et al., 1998). Therefore data were gathered from these patients, who were carefully transferred to other agencies and whose follow up period was varying form 17 to 55 months. Psychotic relapses and exacerbations could be rated for 63 patients during the follow up period after the 15-month transmural intervention. The median survival time turned out to be 19 months. 40 Patients (63.5%) suffered from at least one psychotic relapse or exacerbation, despite the short duration of illness in the sample. 21% of the patients suffered from one relapse only; the other patients became chronic. In a similar first episode study from the Hillside more than 80% of the patients suffered from at least one relapse within 5 years of recovery from a first psychotic episode of schizophrenia or schizo-affective disorder. Maintenance antipsychotic medication was found to be best predictor of the relapse rate (Robinson et al., 1999).

The Patient, the Family and the Professional: An Integrative model in the "Critical Period" of Schizophrenia

The first psychotic episode of schizophrenia or a related disorder of an adolescent or young adult patient heralds a "critical period" with a high risk of psychotic relapse or psychosocial decline (Birchwood, 1998). Recognition and active intervention at the earliest possible stage of florid psychosis has been shown to contribute to early symptom remission, delay of psychotic relapse and prevention of suicide and psychosocial deterioration over a one year period (Linszen et al., 1996; Power et al., 1998). Important ingredients of this initial success were based on Goldstein's model. Family members, most of them parents, were approached as actively as their psychotic child, whose psychotic episode revealed itself in the period where other children, including in their own family, were in the process of becoming independent (Goldstein et al., 1978).

The only way to prevent poor outcomes is to continue medication and stress management for a period up to 5 years, which approaches the "critical period", as articulated by Birchwood et al. (1998). The basic attitude of professionals is to approach the parents of first episode patients as allies in the fight against a severe but treatable mental disease. Professionals are aware that every well meant activity can be considered as stigmatising. They also are aware of the need of the family including the patient for genuine support and empathy, avoided blaming.

Support, relief of burden, facilitation of mourning and psycho-education during in-patient or community based treatment during the acute phase followed by an outpatient educational, medication and stress-management treatment during the maintenance phase with a continued relationship with the treatment staff are other effective ingredients. The effectiveness of the program was reflected in the excellent drug compliance during the intervention. This may not have been the case in the period after the intervention program. One may presume that the favourable effect of the intervention program would last after the intensive 15-month treatment program. The results of the follow-up study were in sharp contrast with that expectation. The relapse findings at follow-up underscore McGlashan's (1996) remark, that interventions in schizophrenia are effective as long as they are active, both for families and patients. After the intervention study all patients were referred to other mental health facilities, such as community mental health centres or rehabilitation centres. The favourable effects of the family intervention on relapse and a possible effect of the relatively short duration of untreated psychosis disappear rapidly, underlining that early age of onset of schizophrenia is associated with a poor symptomatic and functional outcome (Häfner et al., 1995; Kessler et al., 1995). The only way to prevent relapse and psychosocial decline after the symptom remission and relapse delay after the first psychotic episode of schizophrenia seems to be (1) continuation of medication compliance, and (2) individual treatment with the effective ingredients disease management, medication management and stress management. This short-term effective intervention should last for a minimum period of five years, a period that approaches the critical period (Birchwood et al., 1993). In that period professionals have to create a good relation with the patient and the family and support, educate and inform them continuously. They can help the family understand and respond to stigma and they may stimulate contacts with self-help and support groups.

Finally, the family research on the coping skills of the family with the patient's disorder patient should be developed further during the critical period. Targets are for instance lack of insight or medication compliance or the patient's drug misuse, the emotional adjustment to the disorder and their effort in supporting the psychological adjustment and rehabilitation of the patients. Results of these studies can be indicators for an optimal approach towards the vulnerable patient during the critical period. Autonomy and dependence needs in relation to that vulnerability can be operationalized in a working alliance between parents, patient and professional with a working plan with clear strategies of disease management, and psychosocial rehabilitation.

Acknowledgments

The authors want to thank Marion van Bruggen, Hugo van Engelsdorp, Lieuwe de Haan, Marijke Krikke, Jules Lavalaye, Marie Lenior, Dorien Nieman, Pim Scholte, André te Winkel and Jiska Wolthaus for their review of this chapter.

References

Anderson, C.M., Reiss, D.J., and Hogarty, G.E. (1986): Schizophrenia and the family. New York London: Guilford Press

Angermeyer, M., and Kühn, L. (1988): Gender differences in age of onset of schizophrenia. An overview. European Archives of Psychiatry and Neurology Science 237: 351–365

Barrelet, L., Ferrero, F., Szigethy, L., Giddey, C., and Pellizer, G. (1990): Expressed emotion and first-admission schizophrenia, nine-month follow-up in a French cultural environment. British Journal of Psychiatry 156: 357–362

Bateson, G., Jackson, D.D., Haley, J., and Weakland, J. (1956): Toward a theory of schizophrenia. Behavioral Science 1: 251–264

Bebbington, P., and Kuipers, L. (1994): The predictive utility of expressed emotion in schizophrenia: an aggregate analysis. Psychological Medicine 24: 707–718

Birchwood, M., and MacMillan, J.F. (1993). Early intervention in schizophrenia. Australian and New Zealand Journal of Psychiatry 27: 374–378

Birchwood, M., Todd, P., and Jackson, C. (1998): Early intervention in psychosis. The critical period hypothesis. British Journal of Psychiatry 172 (Suppl. 33): 53–59

Bleuler, E. (1911): Dementia Praecox or the Group of Schizophrenias. Translated by Zinkin, J. (1950). New York: International Universities Press

Bleuler, M. (1978): The schizophrenic disorders: long term patient and family studies. Translated by S. Clements. New Haven: Yale University Press

Brown, G.W., Carstairs, G.M., and Topping, G.G. (1958): Post-hospital adjustment of chronic mental patients. Lancet 2: 685–689

Brown, G.W., Birley, J.L.T., and Wing, J.K. (1972): Influence of family life on the course of schizophrenics disorders: A replication. British Journal of Psychiatry 121: 241–258

Cozolino, L.J., Goldstein, M.J., Nuechterlein, K.H., West, K.L., and Snyder, K.S. (1988): The impact of education about schizophrenia on relatives vyraing in expressed emotion. Schizophrenia Bulletin 14: 675–687

Crow,T.J., MacMillan, J.F., and Johnson, A.L. (1986): A randomized controlled trial of prophylactic neuroleptic treatment. British Journal of Psychiatry 148: 120–127

Falloon, I.R.H., Boyd, J., McGill, C.W., et al. (1982): Family management in the prevention of exacerbations of schizophrenia - a controlled study. New England Journal of Medicine 306: 1437–1440

Falloon, I.R.H., Boyd, J.L., and McGill, C.W. (1984): Family care of schizophrenia. New York London: Guilford Press

Falloon, I.R., Boyd, J.L., McGill, C.W., Williamson, M., Razani, J., Moss, H.B., Gildeman, A.M., and Siomson, G.M. (1985): Family management in the prevention of morbidity of schizophrenia. Clinical outcome of a two-year longitudinal study. Archives of General Psychiatry 42: 887–896

Goldstein, M.J., Elliot, H., Evans, J.R., May, P.R.A., and Steinberg, M.R. (1978): Drug and family therapy in the aftercare of acute schizophrenics. Archives of General Psychiatry 35: 1169–1177

Goldstein, M.J. Rodnick E.H., Evans J.R., May, P.R., and Steinberg, M.R. (1978) Drug and family therapy in the aftercare of acute schizophrenia. Archives of General Psychiatry 35: 1169–1177

Häfner, H., Maurer, K., Löffler, W., Bustamante, S., van der Heiden, W., Riechler-Rössler, A., and Nowotny, B. (1995): Onset and early course of schizophrenia. In: The Search for the Causes of Schizophrenia. H.H. Häfner, and W.F. Gattaz, (eds.), Vol III, pp. 43–66, Berlin: Springer

Hogarty, G.E., Schooler, N.R., Ulrich, R.F., Mussare, F., Ferro, P., and Herron, E. (1979): Fluphenazine and social therapy in the aftercare of schizophrenic patients: Relapse analyses of a two-year controlled trial. Archives of General Psychiatry 36: 1283–1294

Hogarty, G.E., Anderson, C.M., Reiss, D.J., Kornblith, S.J., Greenwald, D.P., Javna, C.D., Madonia, M.J. (1986): Family psychoeducation, social skills training and maintenance chemotherapy in the aftercare of schizophrenia: I. One year effects of a controlled study on relapse and expressed emotion. Archives of General Psychiatry 43

Jackson, H.J., Smith, N., and McGorry, P. (1990): Relationship between expressed emotion and family burden in psychotic disorders: an exploratory study. Acta Psychiatrica Scandinavica 82: 243–249

Jones, P.B., Bebbington, P., Foerster, A., Lewis, S.W., Murray, R.M., Russel, A., Sham, P.C., Tone, B.K., and Wilkins, S. (1993): Premorbid social underachievement in schizophrenia: results from the Camberwell Collaborative Psychosis Study. British Journal of Psychiatry 162: 65–71

Kane, J.M. (1989): The current status of neuroleptic therapy. J Clin Psychiatry 50: 322–328

Kavanagh D.J. (1992): Recent developments in expressed emotion and schizophrenia. British Journal of Psychiatry 160: 601–620

Kessler, R.C., Foster, C.L., Saunders, W.B., and Stang, P.E. (1995): Social consequences of psychiatric disorders, I: Educational attainment. American Journal of Psychiatry 152: 1026–1031

Kraepelin, E. (1919): Dementio praecox and paraphrenia. Translated by Barclay, R.M. and Livingstone, S. Edingburgh. Reprinted in 1971 by Huntington. New York: Krieger Publishing Co

Lam, D.H. (1991): Psychosocial family intervention in schizophrenia: a review of empirical studies. Psychological Medicine 21: 423–441

Lefley, H.P. (1992): Expressed emotion: conceptual, clinical, and social policy issues. Hospital Community and Psychiatry 43: 591–598

Leff, J., Kuipers, L, Berkowitz, R., Eberlein-Vries, R. and Sturgeon, D. (1982): A controlled trial of social interaction in the families of schizophrenic patients. British Journal of Psychiatry 141: 121–134

Leff, J., and Vaughn, C. (1981): The role of maintenance therapy and relatives' expressed emotion in relapse of schizophrenia: a two-year follow-up. British Journal of Psychiatry 139: 102–104

Lidz, T., Cornelison, A.R., Fleck, S., and Terry, D. (1957): The intrafamilial environment of schizophrenic patients: II. Marital schism and marital skew. American Journal of Psychiatry 114: 241–248

Lidz, T. (1973): The origin and treatment of schizophrenic disorders. New York: Basic Books.

Linszen, D.H., Dingemans, P.M., and Lenior, M.E. (1994): Cannabis abuse and the course of recent-onset schizophrenic disorders. Archives of General Psychiatry 51: 273–279

Linszen, D.H., Dingemans, P.M., Scholte, W.F., Van der Does, J.W., Nugter, M.A. Lenior, M.E., and Goldstein, M.J. (1996): Treatment, expressed emotion and relapse in recent onset schizophrenic disorders. Psychological Medicine 26: 333–342

Linszen, D.H., Dingemans, P.M., Nugter, M.A., Van der Does, J.W., Scholte, W.F., and Lenior, M.E. (1997): Patient attributes and expressed emotion (EE) as risk factors for psychotic relapse. Schizophrenia Bulletin 23: 119–130

Linszen, D.H., Lenior, M., Haan L. de, and Dingemans, P. (1998): Early intervention, untreated psychosis and the course of recent-onset schizophrenia. British Journal of Psychiatry 172 (suppl. 33): 83–88

Loebel, A.D., Lieberman, J.A., Alvir, J.M.J., Mayerhoff, D.I., Geisler, S.H., and Szymanski, S.R. (1992): Duration of psychosis and outcome in first-episode schizophrenia. American Journal of Psychiatry 149: 1183–1188

Mari, J.D., and Steiner, D.L. (1994): An overview of family interventions and relapse on schizophrenia. Meta-analysis of recent findings. Psychological Medicine 24: 565–578

MacMillan, J.F., Crow, T.J., Johnson, A.L., and Johnstone, E.C. (1986): Expressed emotion and relapse. British Journal of Psychiatry 148: 133–143

Magana, A.B., Goldstein, J.M., Karno, M., Miklowitz, D.J., Jenkins, J., and Falloon, I.R. (1986): A brief method for assessing expressed emotion in relatives of psychiatric patients. Psychiatry Research 17: 203–212

McGlashan, T.H. (1996): Early detection and intervention in schizophrenia. Schizophrenia Bulletin 22: 197–200

Nuechterlein, K.H., and Dawson, M.E. (1984): A heuristic vulnerability/stress model of schizophernic episodes. Schizophrenia Bulletin 10: 300–312

Nugter, M.A., Dingemans, P.M., Van der Does, A.J., Linszen, D.H., and Berthold, G. (1997): Family treatment, expressed emotion and relapse in recent onset schizophrenia. Psychiatry Research 72: 23–31

Power, P., Elkins, K., Adlard, S., Curry, C., McGorry, P., and Harringan, S. (1998): Analysis of the initial treatment phase in first-episode psychosis. British Journal of Psychiatry, 33 (suppl. 172): 71–76

Robinson, D., Woerner, M., Alvir, J.A., et al. (1999): Predictors of relapse following response from a first psychotic episode of schizophrenia or schizoaffective disorder. Archives of General Psychiatry 56: 241–247

Rund, B.R., Moe, L., Sollien, T., Fjell, A., Borchgrevink, T., Hallert, M., and Naess, P.O. (1994): The psychosis project: outcome and cost-effectiveness of a psycho-educational program for schizophrenic adolescents. Acta Psychiatrica Scandinavica 89: 211–218

Selvini-Palazzoli, M., Cecchin, A., Prata, G., and Boscolo, L. (1978): Paradox and couterparadox. New York: Jason Aronson

Sheperd, M., Watt, D., Falloon, I., et al. (1989). The natural history of schizophrenia: a five year follow-up in a representative sample of schizo-phrenics. Psychological Medicine, Monograph (suppl. 15).

Smith, J., and Birchwood, M. (1990): Relatives and parents as partners in the management of schizophrenia. The development of a service model. British Journal of Psychiatry 156: 654–660

Stirling, J., Tantam, D., Thomas, P., Newby D., Montague, L., Ring, N., and Rowe, S. (1991): Expressed emotion and early onset schizophrenia: a one year follow-up. Psychological Medicine 21: 675–685

Tarrier, N., Barrowclough, C., Proceddu, K., Watts, S., and Freeman, H. (1988): The community management of schizophrenia. A controlled trial of a behavioral intervention with families to reduce relapse. British Journal of Psychiatry 153: 532–542

Terkelsen, K.G. (1983): Schizophrenia and the family: II. Adverse effects of family therapy. Family Process 22: 191–200

Vaughn, C.E., and Leff, J.P. (1976): The measurement of expressed emotion in the families of psychiatric patients. British Journal of Social Psychology 15: 157–165

Wolthaus, J.E., Dingemans, P.M., Linszen, D.H., et al. (submitted) Caregiver burden, personality traits and symptoms in recent-onset schizophrenia

Wynne, L.C., Ryckoff, I., Day, J., and Hirsch, S. (1958): Pseudo-mutuality in the family relations of schizophrenics. Psychiatry 21: 205–220

Zhang, M., Wang, M., Li, J. and Phillip, M.R. (1994): Randomised control trial of family intervention for 78 first-episode male schizophrenic patients. British Journal of Psychiatry 165 (suppl.): 96–102

Zubin, J., and Spring, B. (1977): Vulnerability: a new view of schizophrenia. Journal of Abnormal Psychology 86: 103–126

4

Examining Patients' Perceptions of their Relatives' Expressed Emotion

Martha C. Tompson and Amy G. Weisman

Introduction

Numerous studies have demonstrated that critical or emotionally overinvolved attitudes on the part of family members can be a significant stressor for mentally ill patients (for review, see Butzlaff and Hooley, 1998). High levels of these attitudes, referred to as Expressed Emotion (EE), have been shown to predict both the development of schizophrenia (Goldstein, 1987) and a poorer course of illness in a variety of psychiatric disorders, including schizophrenia (Brown, Birley and Wing, 1972; Vaughn and Leff, 1976a; Vaughn, Snyder and Jones et al., 1984), bipolar disorders (Miklowitz et al., 1988), substance abuse (O' Farrell, Hooley, Fals-Stewart, and Cutter, 1998), unipolar depression (Hooley, Orley and Teasdale, 1986; Vaughn and Leff, 1976a), and eating disorders (LeGrange, Eisler, Dare, and Hodes, 1992; Van Furth et al., 1996). While relatives' attitudes may be viewed as a potential stressor for patients with psychiatric illnesses, the mechanism by which they exert their influence is still unclear. Measures of EE have traditionally been made by counting the number of criticisms and making ratings of emotional overinvolvement (EOI) based on the Camberwell Family Interview (Vaughn and Leff, 1976b), or more recently, by the Five Minute Speech Sample (Magana et al., 1986). EE has been reliably assessed using the CFI (Hooley, 1998) and the FMSS (Asarnow et al., 1994; Tompson et al., 1995) and is associated with psychiatric outcome using both the CFI (Butzlaff and Hooley, 1998) and the FMSS (Asarnow et al., 1993). It is important to note that these assessments are conducted individually with the relative by an interviewer and not in the presence of the patient. Thus, while an examiner interviewing the relative and making ratings of EE may view him or her as critical or emotionally overinvolved, it is not clear that the patient's perception is similar. Family interaction studies indicate that high EE relatives express more criticism and perhaps are more intrusive than low EE relatives during laboratory based family discussion tasks (Miklowitz, Goldstein, Falloon, and Doane, 1984; Strachan, Leff, Goldstein, Doane, and Burtt, 1986), and physiological data suggest that patients react with higher levels of arousal to the presence of high versus low EE relatives (Sturgeon et al., 1981; Tarrier et al., 1979; Tarrier et al., 1988). Thus, there is some evidence that patients react to these negative attitudes at least to some degree.

Several studies have also examined the congruence between patients' views of their family climates and their relatives' views. These studies demonstrate only modest associations between patients' and relatives' perceptions (Lebell et al., 1993; Scott, Fagin and Winter, 1993). In addition several studies indicate that the patients' perceptions also have an impact on their illness course, with more negative perceptions being associated with a more symptomatic course (Lebell et al., 1993; Scott, Fagin and Winter, 1993; Warner and Atkinson, 1988). Yet measures of patients' perceptions have often been indirect, measuring the overall family environment using the Family Environment Scale (Moos and Moos, 1981) or some perception of the early parent-child relationship using the Parental Bonding Instrument (Parker, Tupling and Brown, 1979). Tompson and colleagues (1995) have addressed this issue more directly by administering a detailed interview to patients' about their family relationships, specifically asking them about their interactions with their relatives, those aspects they liked and those they wished to change. Questions were included about critical behavior, nagging, worrying, and over-protective behavior on the part of their relatives. The interview was carefully coded for examples of perceived criticism, nagging, and emotional overinvolvement. Results indicated a significant association between ratings of relatives' EE and patients' perceptions of relatives' behavior, with high EE/Critical relatives perceived as more critical than low EE/Critical relatives but they were not perceived as more nagging or emotionally overinvolved. The small number of relatives rated as high EOI made it difficult to separately examine patients with high EOI relatives. Interestingly, while EE did not predict outcome in this sample, patients' perceptions of criticism were highly predictive of relapse during the one-year follow-up period.

Psychiatric patients demonstrate a number of interpersonal distortions. Schizophrenic patients have been found to be poor judges of others' emotional states when compared to normal controls; this may be particularly true when there is some ambiguity in the situation (Cramer, Weegman and O'Neil, 1989). In affective disorders, depressed mood is also believed to be associated with distorted cognitive processes, illogical pessimistic attitudes (Beck, 1979), and perceptions of rejection from others (Dobson, 1989). Thus there may be elements of patients' psychiatric symptoms that alter their perceptions of their relatives. In other words, patients' perceptions of their family members may correlate with symptoms of their psychiatric disturbance. This issue of the validity of patients' perceptions is examined as part of the present study.

In general, past research has indicated that patients living in high EE families do not appear to differ from those living in low EE families in their premorbid functioning or in their overall level of psychiatric symptoms at the time that EE is assessed (Hooley, 1998; Kavanagh, 1992). However, Glynn and colleagues (1990) examined a full range of psychiatric symptoms on the Brief Psychiatric Rating Scale (BPRS) and the Scale for the Assessment of Negative Symptoms (SANS) among patients with schizophrenia. They found that patients from high EE families had significantly higher ratings of positive symptoms, anxious depression, and overall psychopathology, but not negative symptoms. Thus, specific types of patient symptoms and negative behaviors may contribute to ongoing negative family transactions. By further examining the relationship between patients' symptoms and EE, we may better understand how patients contribute to the family interactional processes associated with the EE construct.

The current study explored the relationship between family members expressed emotion and both patients' perceptions of their family members attitudes and their psychiatric symptoms. Assessments of family members' expressed emotion were made using the Five Minute Speech Sample. While highly critical and emotionally overinvolved (EOI) relatives are both designated as high EE, we combined EOI and low EE groups in these analyses. This is because the types of behaviors and attitudes resulting in the high EOI designation (e.g., overprotective behavior) are quite different then those resulting in the high EE/critical designation (e.g., critical comments about the patient), and because the beliefs and attributions made by high EE/EOI relatives are thought to be more similar

to those made by low EE relatives than those of other high EE
(critical and hostile) family members (Hooley, 1987). Patients were
administered an interview designed to assess their perceptions of
their relatives' attitudes and their family environments (Tompson
et al., 1995). The following three questions were addressed: (1) Do
patients perceive their relatives' EE? Given earlier finding demonstrating an association between high EE/critical attitudes and
patients' perceptions of critical behavior (Tompson et al., 1995), we
anticipated replicating these results. (2) Are patients' perceptions of
their family relationships associated with the content and/or severity
of their psychiatric symptoms? Given the literature reviewed above
suggesting that psychiatric patients demonstrate a number of interpersonal distortions (Beck, 1979; Dobson, 1989; Cramer et al., 1989),
we anticipated that patients' perceptions of their relatives' attitudes
may be associated with their level of psychiatric disturbance. (3) What
is the relationship between residual psychiatric symptoms and relatives' EE? In other words, what role might specific psychiatric
symptoms play in the ongoing transactions indexed by the Expressed
Emotion construct? Given the findings of Glynn and colleagues
(1990), we anticipated that high EE might be associated with certain
types of patient symptoms, such as anxious depression and positive
symptoms.

Method

Participants

Family members of patients with chronic and persistent mental
illness were recruited through a grass-roots organization which
offers support and advocacy for family members of individuals with
various mental illnesses. At local support group meetings interested
family members signed up and agreed to be contacted by the
primary investigator. These family members were screened for
inclusion criteria over the telephone and, if they met criteria and
agreed to participate, subsequently interviewed individually in their
homes. Criteria for inclusion in the study were:
(a) availability of a close family member who both was diagnosed
with schizophrenia or major affective disorder and agreed to be
contacted by the primary investigator,

and (b) ability of both family members to give informed consent. Potential participants were excluded from the study if the mentally ill family member had a primary diagnosis of substance abuse or dependence, was residing in a locked residential facility, or lived out of the area.

A total of 35 family members were interviewed. Of these family members 10 had mentally ill relatives who subsequently refused to participate. Thus, complete data (from both family member and mentally ill relative) were available for 25 families. These family members were on average 60 years of age (range = 39–75) and had 13.4 (range 4–18) years of education. The sample was composed primarily of mothers of mentally ill patients (18; 72%), but four fathers, one sibling, and one spouse also participated.

The family members had a total of 21 mentally ill relatives who participated in the study. Although formal diagnostic assessments were not conducted, patients clinical diagnoses were recorded based on information from both patients and relatives. Of these ten (48%) had diagnoses of schizophrenia, seven (33%) had schizoaffective diagnoses, and four (19%) had diagnoses of bipolar disorder. The 15 men and 6 women ranged from 21 to 46 years of age (mean age = 33.8), and had on average 13.3 years of education. Seventeen (81%) were single, and four (19%) were married, separated or divorced. Their ages of onset ranged from 13 to 28 years (mean = 20), and they had on average a history of 6.2 psychiatric hospitalizations for an average of 15.5 months total time hospitalized. Sixty-two percent were Caucasian, and the remainder were Latino.

Procedure

Family members were interviewed in a session lasting approximately one and one half hours. This session included administration of the Five Minute Speech Sample (FMSS), a coping questionnaire, and a demographic questionnaire. Their mentally ill relatives participated in a one-hour individual interview. During this session they were administered the FMSS about their relative, the Patients' Interview for Assessing Patient Perceptions of Family Relationships, the Brief Psychiatric Rating Scale, and a demographic questionnaire.

Measures

Five Minute Speech Sample

All participants were administered the FMSS, which is a brief measure of Expressed Emotion (Magana et al., 1986). During the FMSS the examinee speaks for five minutes about his/her relative, discussing what kind of person he/she is and how they get along together. (For additional information on the administration of the FMSS see Magana et al., 1986). All FMSS protocols were audiotaped for coding purposes.

The FMSS ratings of EE were made using criteria developed by Magana et al. (1986). As with the Camberwell Family Interview, a relative is given a high EE rating on the basis of criticism or emotional overinvolvement. **High EE/Critical** – the criteria for a rating of high EE based on criticism are any of the following:
(a) a negative initial statement,
(b) on overall negative rating for the patient-relatives relationship,
or (c) one or more critical comments about the patient.
High EE/Emotionally overinvolved – the criterion for a rating of high EE based on emotional overinvolvement (EOI) include any of the following:
(a) a report of self-sacrificing/overprotective behavior,
(b) an emotional display during the interview,
or (c) a combination of two of the following: excessive detail about the past, one or more statements of positive attitude, and excessive praise (five or more positive remarks).
An individual can be rated as high EE for both criticism and EOI. All FMSS ratings were completed by a trained rater. Ten protocols, not included in the present analyses, were taken from a related study to examine interrater reliability. The kappa statistics reflected complete agreement between raters for overall FMSS-EE ($k = 1.00$, $p < 0.01$) FMSS-EE/critical ($k = 1.00$, $p < 0.01$), and FMSS-EE/EOI ($k = 1.00$, $p < 0.01$).

The Patients' Interview for Assessing Patient Perceptions of Family Relationships (PPI; Tompson et al., 1995)

This interview was designed to elicit psychiatric patients' perceptions of their family members' emotional attitudes towards them and how they cope with family stress when it occurs. The PPI consists of questions about the relationship in nine areas and focuses on eliciting descriptions of the patients' perceptions about the behavior of their relatives. The nine areas include four groups of questions about the relatives' criticism, four about EOI, and one group about how much the relative nags the patient. Each time patients endorse a problem area, they are queried as to how they coped with the situation (for additional information on the content of the interview, see Tompson et al., 1995).

The Manual for Coding Patients' Perceptions of their Relatives' EE was used to assess the amount of criticism, EOI, and nagging that patients perceive and their coping strategies for dealing with stressful family situations (for further information on coding see Tompson et al., 1995). There are three perceptions categories, each reflecting the number of statements the patient made in that category. The three perception categories included (a) perceived Criticism, (b) perceived Nagging and (c) perceived Emotional Overinvolvement. Twenty-one of the interviews were coded by an additional rater and Pearson correlation coefficients between the raters reflected adequate reliability for perceived criticism ($r = 0.88$), perceived nagging ($r = 0.96$), and perceived emotional overinvolvement ($r = 0.87$). Patients' perceptions of criticism were further categorized into five content groups which reflected the topic of the criticism. These included harsh or generalized criticisms, criticisms of personal goals, criticisms of day to day habits, criticisms about medication and treatment management, and criticisms about symptoms and illness related issues. Raters demonstrated complete agreement on the content codes.

Brief Psychiatric Rating Scale

The Brief Psychiatric Rating Scale (BPRS; Lukoff, Nuechterlein, and Ventura, 1986) was administered to all patients to assess psychiatric symptomatology. Based on the BPRS items, four conceptually-defined cluster scores were calculated:

(a) anxiety/depression – anxiety, guilt, and depressed mood,

(b) paranoia – hostility, suspiciousness, and uncooperativeness,

(c) schizophrenia – conceptual disorganization, unusual thought content, and hallucinatory behavior, and

(d) residual symptoms – emotional withdrawal, blunted affect, and motor retardation.

A total BPRS score was also obtained by summing patients' scores on all items. An interclass correlation coefficient for the BPRS ratings calculated based on 9 interviews demonstrated high reliability (ICC = 0.93).

Results

The first question addressed in this study was: Do patients with psychiatric disorders perceive their relatives' Expressed Emotion? Three t-tests were conducted to compare patients with high EE/ critical relatives to those with low EE or high EOI (combined) relatives on perceived criticism, perceived EOI and perceived nagging. The findings, which are displayed in Table 1, replicated previous research (Tompson et al., 1995) in demonstrating that patients with high EE/critical relatives perceived these relatives as more critical than patients with low EE or high EOI relatives ($t = 4.37$, $p < 0.05$). However, patients whose relatives were high EE/critical did not differ from patients with low EE or high EOI relatives in their perceptions of emotionally overinvolved behavior or nagging. To further examine differences in the content of patients' perceptions we conducted five chi-square tests on the association between relatives criticism (from the EE ratings) and patients perceptions of critical content, including criticisms about personal goals, daily living issues, medication and treatment management issues, symptoms, and global/harsh criticisms. Interestingly, patients with high EE/critical relatives did not differ from patients with low EE or high EOI relatives on any of these content categories, except harsh criticisms. Indeed, 80% of patients with high EE/Critical relatives reported at least one harsh criticism; whereas only 12% of patients

Table 1. Relatives' expressed emotion and patients' perceptions of criticism, emotional overinvolvement and nagging

	Relatives' expressed emotion	
	Low EE/EOI ($n = 16$)	High EE/critical ($n = 5$)
Perceived criticism[a]	1.37 (1.15)	3.00 (2.45)
Perceived emotional overinvolvement	1.81 (1.51)	2.40 (2.19)
Perceived nagging	2.69 (1.81)	4.60 (3.05)

[a]$p < 0.05$

Table 2. Relatives' EE and patients' symptoms ($n = 21$)

	Relatives' expressed emotion	
	Low EE/High EOI ($n = 16$)	High EE/Critical ($n = 5$)
Total BPRS	41.50 (11.67)	52.80 (8.23)
Anxiety/Depression	7.18 (2.71)	7.60 (3.78)
Paranoia[a]	4.81 (2.07)	8.40 (2.88)
Schizophrenia	5.63 (3.81)	6.80 (3.11)
Residual	4.75 (2.79)	6.60 (3.91)

[a] $p < 0.05$

with low EE or high EOI relatives reported a harsh criticism ($X^2 = 8.51$, $p < 0.01$).

The second question addressed in the study was: Are patients' perceptions of their relatives' criticism a reflection of their psychiatric symptoms? Our results indicated no significant association between patients' reports of criticism by their relatives and their overall BPRS score ($r = 0.16$) or their scores on the thinking disturbance ($r = 0.11$), hostility/suspiciousness ($r = -0.04$), anxiety/depression ($r = 0.15$) or residual symptoms ($r = -0.28$) clusters of the BPRS. Thus, patients who perceived high levels of criticism did not appear to be more symptomatic than those who reported low levels.

The third question addressed in the study was: What is the relationship between current psychiatric symptoms and relatives Criticism on the EE measures? Analyses revealed a trend for patients with high EE/Critical relatives to have slightly higher total BPRS scores than patients with low EE or high EOI relatives ($t = 3.99$, $p < 0.06$). A closer examination of the BPRS data revealed that patients with high EE/critical relatives did not differ from patients with low EE/high EOI relatives on anxiety/depression, thinking disturbance and residual symptoms scores. However, patients with high EE relatives had significantly higher scores on hostility/suspiciousness than did patients with low EE or high EOI relatives ($t = 9.54$, $p < 0.01$).

Discussion

This small study revealed that (1) patients' with highly critical relatives (compared with those with low EE or EOI relatives) perceived more criticisms on the part of their family members, particularly harsh, generalized criticisms; (2) these perceptions are unrelated to patients' levels of current psychopathology; and (3) patients' with high EE relatives may be more symptomatic, particularly demonstrating hostility and suspiciousness.

These findings replicate previous work (Tompson et al., 1995) indicating that relatives who are rated high in criticism on measures of Expressed Emotion are perceived by patients as more critical than relatives who are rated low in criticism. These results are consistent with studies indicating that in laboratory-based family discussion tasks, high EE/critical family members make more critical comments than family members who are either high EOI or low EE (Miklowitz, Goldstein, Falloon, and Doane, 1984; Strachan, Leff, Goldstein, Doane and Burtt, 1986). Interestingly, patients with high EE relatives perceived more generalized/harsh types of criticisms than patients with low EE relatives, but there were no differences in perceptions of other types of criticisms. Perhaps these global types of criticism represent particularly destructive forms of interpersonal communication which are quiet salient to those patients who experience them and are indices of more disturbed family relationships.

Second, in this study patients' perceptions of the amount of criticism, nagging and emotionally overinvolved behavior which their family members directed toward them were not associated with their psychiatric symptoms. This finding supports the validity of examining patients' perceptions of their family environments. However, it should be noted that the patients in this study had clinical diagnoses within the psychotic-spectrum and demonstrated relatively low levels of residual symptomatology. Thus, these findings may not generalize to patients in other diagnostic groups or those experiencing high levels of symptoms. Indeed, the stability and the validity of patients' perceptions may be somewhat dependent on current clinical state, with patients in relative symptom remission able to provide valid information on their typical reactions to their family members.

In this study we found no overall differences in psychiatric symptoms between patients in high versus low EE families; however, one cluster of symptoms, specifically hostility/suspiciousness, did distinguish between the two groups. Patients with high EE relatives displayed significantly higher scores on these symptoms than did patients with low EE relatives. Although not within the clinical range of severity,[1] certain subclinical symptoms or other nonsymptomatic behaviors may elicit high EE attitudes, as well as result from them. These results may be viewed as supporting a family transactional model and appear consistent with the findings of Rosenfarb and colleagues (1995). In the Rosenfarb study (Rosenfarb et al., 1995) investigators found that during a laboratory-based family interaction task schizophrenic patients with high EE relatives demonstrated more subtle "subclinical" manifestations of odd and disruptive behavior; in these families the appearance of these subclinical behaviors was predictive of subsequent critical comments by relatives; and relatives' criticisms increased the probability of additional "subclinical" odd/disruptive behaviors. In a parallel study Woo (1997) examined patients' *nonverbal* behavior during the family interaction task and its relationship to family member EE. Results indicated that odd or hostile nonverbal behaviors were more common in the interactional behavior of patients with high EE relatives than those with low EE relatives. It should be noted that in both of these studies, as well as in the present study, the measures of patient symptoms/behavior are clearly "subclinical" and may represent nonsymptomatic behaviors or personality characteristics. Our findings in conjunction with Rosenfarb (1995) and Woo and colleagues (1997) support a transactional model in which odd and/ or hostile patient behaviors may lead to negative familial attitudes (or EE), which are perceived by patients and might lead to negative/ hostile patient behaviors toward family members, and in turn increase negative familial attitudes and behaviors (Goldstein, Rosenfarb, Woo, and Nuechterlein, 1997). This escalating cycle may elevate levels of stress for both patients and family members, leading to symptom exacerbation and increased family burden.

The current study was limited by the small sample size, the lack of diagnostic verification, and the combination of patients with various psychiatric disorders. However, the results underscore the need to examine both the role of patients' perceptions and behaviors in family transactions and their relationship to Expressed Emotion measures. By understanding the patient's role in such transactions, we can further identify the contributions of all involved, examine strategies for disrupting these patterns and specify family

---

[1]Scores of 4 or above on individual items on the BPRS are considered clinically meaningful (Ventura, Green, Shaner, and Liberman, 1993).

treatment strategies which will be more effective for helping high EE families.

Acknowledgements

This chapter is dedicated to the memory of Michael J. Goldstein, Ph.D., those work has improved understanding of both family processes and family treatment for individuals with serious mental disorders.

References

Asarnow, J.R., Goldstein, M.J., Tompson, M.C., and Guthrie, D. (1993): One-year outcomes of depressive disorders in child psychiatric inpatients: Evaluation of the prognostic power of a brief measure of expressed emotion. Journal of Child Psychology and Psychiatry 34(2): 129–137

Asarnow, J.R., Tompson, M.C., Hamilton, E., Goldstein, M.J., and Guthrie, D (1994): Family expressed emotion, childhood onset-depression, and child-hood-onset schizophrenia spectrum disorders: Is expressed emotion a nonspecific correlate of child psychopathology or a specific risk factor for depression? Journal of Abnormal Child Psychology 22(2): 129–146

Beck, A.T., Rush, A.J., Shaw, B.F., and Emery, G. (1979): Cognitive therapy of depression. New York: Guilford Press

Brown, G.W., Birley, J.L.T., and Wing, J.K. (1972): Influence of family life on the course of schizophrenic disorders: A replication. British Journal of Psychiatry 121: 241–258

Butzlaff, R.L. and Hooley, J.M. (1998): Expressed emotion and psychiatric relapse. Archives of General Psychiatry 55(6): 547–552

Cramer, P., Weegman, M., and O'Neil, M. (1989): Schizophrenia and the perception of emotions: How accurately do schizophrenics judge the emotional states of others? British Journal of Psychiatry 155: 225–228

Dobson, K.S. (1989): Real and perceived interpersonal responses to subclini-cally anxious and depressed targets. Cognitive Therapy and Research 13(1): 37–47

Glynn, S.M., Randolph, E.T., Eth, S., Paz, G.G., Leong, G.B., Shaner, A.L., and Strachan, A. (1990): Patient psychopathology and expressed emotion in schizophrenia. British Journal of Psychiatry 157: 877–880

Goldstein, M.J. (1987): Family interaction patterns that antedate the onset of schizophrenia and related disorders: A further analysis of data from a longitudinal prospective study; In: Understanding major mental disorders: The contribution of family interaction research (Halweg, K. and Goldstein, M.J., eds.). New York: Family Process Press

Goldstein, M.J., Rosenfarb, I., Woo, S., and Nuechterlein, K. (1997): Transac-tional processes which can function as risk or protective factors in the family treatment of schizophrenia. In: Towards a comprehensive therapy for schizophrenia (Brenner, H.D., Boeker, W., and Genner, R., eds.), pp. 147–157. Göttingen: Hogrefe and Huber Publishers

Hooley, J.M. (1998): Expressed emotion and psychiatric illness: From empirical data to clinical practice. Behavior Therapy 29: 631–646

Hooley, J.M. (1987): The nature and origins of expressed emotion. In: Understanding Major Mental Disorder: The Contribution of Family Interaction Research (Hahlweg, K. and Goldstein, M., eds.), pp. 176–194. New York: Family Process.

Hooley, J.J.M., Orley, J., and Teasdale, J.D. (1986): Levels of expressed emotion and relapse in depressed patients. British Journal of Psychiatry 148: 642–647

Kavanagh, D.J. (1992): Recent developments in expressed emotion and schizophrenia. British Journal of Psychiatry 160: 601–620

Lebell, M.B., Marder, S.R., Mintz, J., Mintz, L.I., Tompson, M.C., Wirshing, W., Johnston-Cronk, K., and McKenzie, J. (1993): Patients' perceptions of family emotional climate and outcome in schizophrenia. British Journal of Psychiatry 162: 751–754

LeGrange, D., Eisler, I., Dare, C., and Hodes, M. (1992): Family criticism and self-starvation: A study of expressed emotion. Journal of Family Therapy 14(2): 177–192

Lukoff, D., Nuechterleih, K.H., and Ventura, J. (1986): Manual for the Expanded Brief Psychiatric Rating Scale. Schizophrenia Bulletin 12: 594–602

Magana, A.B., Goldstein, M.J., Karno, M., Miklowitz, D.J., Jenkins, J., and Falloon, I.R.H. (1986): A brief method for assessing expressed emotion in relatives of psychiatric patients. Psychiatry Research 17: 203–212

Miklowitz, D.J., Goldstein, M.J., Falloon, I.R.H., and Doane, J.A. (1984): Interactional correlates of expressed emotion in the families of schizophrenics. British Journal of Psychiatry 144: 482–487

Miklowitz, D.J., Goldstein, M.J., Nuechterlein, K.H., Snyder, K.S., and Mintz, J. (1988): Family factors and the course of bipolar affective disorder. Archives of General Psychiatry 45: 225–231

Moos, R.H., and Moos, B.S. (1981): Family Environment Scale Manual. Palo Alto, CA: Consulting Psychologist's Press

O'Farrell, T.J., Hooley, J., Fals-Stewart, W., and Cutter, H.S.G. (1998): Expressed emotion and relapse in alcoholic patients. Journal of Consulting and Clinical Psychology 66: 744–752

Parker, G., Tupling, H., and Brown, L.B. (1979): A parental bonding instrument. British Journal of Medical Psychology 52: 1–10

Rosenfarb, I.S., Goldstein, M.J., Mintz, J., and Nuechterlein, K.H. (1995): Expressed emotion and subclinical psychopathology observable within the transactions between schizophrenic patients and their family members. Journal of Abnormal Psychology 104(2): 259–267

Scott, R.D., Fagin, L., and Winter, D. (1993): The importance of the role of the patient in the outcome of schizophrenia. British Journal of Psychiatry 163: 62–68

Strachan, A.M., Leff, J.P., Goldstein, M.J., Doane, J.A., and Burtt, C. (1986): Emotional attitudes and direct communication in the families of schizophrenics: A cross-national replication. British Journal of Psychiatry 149: 279–287

Sturgeon, D., Kuipers, L., Berkowitz, R., Turpin, G., and Leff, J.P (1981): Psychophysiological responses of schizophrenic patients to high and low expressed emotion relatives. British Journal of Psychiatry 138: 40–45

Tarrier, N., Barrowclough, C., Porceddu, K., and Watts, S. (1988): The assessment of psychophysiological reactivity to the expressed emotion of the relatives of schizophrenic patients. British Journal of Psychiatry 152: 618–624

Tarrier, N., Vaughn, C., Lader, M.H., and Leff, J.P. (1979): Bodily reactions to people and events in schizophrenics. Archives of General Psychiatry 36: 311–315

Tompson, M.C., Goldstein, M.J., Lebell, M.B., Mintz, L.I., Marder, S.R., and Mintz, J. (1995): Schizophrenic patients' perceptions of their relatives' attitudes. Psychiatry Research 57: 155–167

Vaughn, C.E., and Leff, J.P. (1976a): The influence of family and social factors on the course of psychiatric illness: A comparison of schizophrenic and depressed neurotic patients. British Journal of Psychiatry 129: 125–137

Vaughn, C., and Leff, J. (1976b): The measurement of expressed emotion in the families of psychiatric patients. British Journal of Social Psychology 15: 157–165

Vaughn, C.E., Snyder, K., Jones, S.J., Freeman, W.B., and Falloon, I.R.H. (1984): Family factors in schizophrenic relapse. Archives of General Psychiatry 41: 1169–1177

Van Furth, E.F., Van Strien, D.C., Martina, L.M.L., Van Son, M.J.M., Hendricks, J.J.P., and Van Engeland, H. (1996): Expressed emotion and the prediction of outcome in adolescent eating disorders. International Journal of Eating Disorders 20(1): 19–31

Ventura, J., Green, M.F. Shaner, A., and Liberman, R. (1993): Training and quality assurance with the brief psychiatric rating scale 'The drift busters.' International Journal of Methods in Psychiatric Research 3: 221–244

Warner, R. and Atkinson, M. (1988): The relationship between schizophrenic patients' perceptions of their parents and the course of their illness. British Journal of Psychiatry 153: 344–353

Woo, S.M., Goldstein, M.J. and Nuechterlein, K.H. (1997): Relatives' expressed emotion and non-verbal signs of subclinical psychopathology in schizo-phrenic patients. British Journal of Psychiatry 170: 58–61

5

Patient Psychopathology and Parental Expressed Emotion in Schizophrenia Revisited

Peter M. Dingemans, Don H. Linszen and Maria E. Lenior

Psychopathology and Expressed Emotion

Research with Expressed Emotion (EE) showed a high profile score to be associated with psychiatric disturbance. Kavanagh (1992) found 21 percent of patients from low EE families and 48 percent from high EE families to experience a psychotic relapse within a year after discharge. Up to now the meaning that should be attributed to the relation between psychotic relapse and EE (Hooley et al., 1987) is still unclear. Some think the parental EE score to reflect the patient's severity of pathology (Glynn et al., 1990; MacMillan et al., 1987; Parker et al., 1988), but Miklowitz et al. (1983) could not substantiate this hypothesis. Goldstein et al. (1994) found patients from high EE homes to show significantly more odd and disruptive behaviors than those from low EE families. The latter ones were more anxious and fearful. This hypothesis was supported by research of Rosenfarb et al. (1995). In this research it was also suggested that there is some reciprocity in behaviors of high EE parents and their psychotic offspring: being exposed to higher levels of odd and disruptive behaviors of their offspring elicits higher levels of criticism and/or overinvolvement.

Barrowclough et al. (1994) have employed an attributional theory to explain high parental EE scores. In their opinion parents assume that children are and should be in control of at least part of their behavior. This should apply more to negative than to positive symptoms. Negative symptoms like e.g., anhedonia, lack of concentration, flat affect should therefore be evaluated more as a sign of unwillingness than positive symptoms like delusions, hallucinations. The latter will be more interpreted as signs of illness, and thus powerlessness. Consequently, negative symptoms and a high EE profile should co-occur more often than positive symptoms and a high EE parental profile. We wanted to test Goldstein's (1994) and Barrowclough's (1994) hypotheses in this project.

Method

Patients

Inclusion criteria for clinically admitted adolescents were: clinical schizophrenia or schizophrenia spectrum diagnosis (schizophreniform and schizoaffective), which needed antipsychotic medication in patients within the age range of 15 and 26 years, and close contact with their parents before clinical admission. Patients with primary alcohol and/or drug dependence in need of detoxification, or patients with a brief reactive psychosis were excluded. Of the 98 consecutively admitted patients, who gave informed consent, 85 parents were available for interviewing. Of the 85 patients 2 refused psychopathology interviewing, and so 83 patient remained for analyses.

Instruments

Psychopathology was assessed by the expanded version of the BPRS (BPRS-E; Lukoff et al., 1986). Interrater reliability (ICC) with a reference group at UCLA was: .81.

BPRS-E analyses (Dingemans et al., 1995) employed a four component model: positive symptoms, negative symptoms, depression and mania. The component scales had an internal reliability of 0.74, 0.75, 0.76 and 0.64, respectively (Cronbach's alpha). The total scale scores were used for analyses.

Expressed Emotion was assessed 11 days on average (s.d. 9.5) after admission of the patient with the Camberwell Family Interview (CFI; Vaughn and Leff, 1976). Assessment took place for separate parents (mother and father) if possible (when both parents wanted to participate regardless of separation and/or divorce). Criteria for scoring were conform with the literature (Linszen et al.,

1994): if one or both parents met the criteria for high EE or low EE respectively a high or low profile score were given for the family. Of the high EE-profiles 41 families were found to be critical whereas 20 were found to be high emotionally overinvolved. The remainder of the high EE profiles had a mixture of criticism and overinvolvement.

Training for the CFI took place in London with L. Berkowitz and reliability was checked repeatedly with the UCLA reference group (profile percentage reliability > 0.80).

Procedure

After informed consent was given the clinical assessment with the BPRS-E of the patient and the interviewing with the separate parent(s) was planned as soon as possible. Interviews of patients and parents were carried out separately and independently.

Results

The patient group has been described elsewhere (Linszen et al., 1994), and therefore the demographics will be summarized here (Table 1):

It appears from Table 1 that the participating group (as opposed to the non-participating group) was clinically in a somewhat better condition.

Patients were divided with regard to their parental EE-scores (high and low), and compared with regard to their premorbid functioning (Goldstein, in: Kokes et al., 1977), prognosis (Strauss and Carpenter, in Kokes et al., 1977), mean item scores on the BPRS-E (Lukoff et al., 1986), and sumscores of the BPRS-E component scales. The significant results are summarized in Table 2:

It may be noted from Table 2 that patients from high EE homes show better premorbid functioning.

The second column of Table 2 shows patients from the different parental EE-groups (high versus low) neither to be different on individual items nor on symptom component scales (positive, negative, mania and depression).

When the profile scores (high versus low) are decomposed in "criticism" and "emotional overinvolvement" it is noticed that the patients can be differentiated on their parental emotional

Table 1. Demographic and psychiatric characteristics of the sample

	Participants (N=83)	Low EE (N=31)	High EE (N=52)	Test for difference (p)
Demographic				
Age at admission (mean, sd)	20.7 (2.4)	20.7 (2.4)	20.7 (2.4)	U 796 (0.92)
Sex, n (%)				
female	25 (30)	7 (23)	18 (35)	CHI 1.34 (0.25)
male	28 (70)	24 (77)	34 (65)	
Education, n (%)				
<highschool	16 (19)	6 (19)	10 (19)	CHI 0.01 (0.99)
≥highschool	67 (81)	25 (81)	42 (81)	
SES, n (%)[2]				
low (1–2)	64 (77)	23 (74)	41 (79)	CHI 0.24 (0.63)
high (3–5)	19 (23)	8 (26)	11 (21)	
Premorbid functioning[3], mean (sd)	62.3 (11.2)	60.4 (10.6)	63.4 (11.4)	U 667 (0.19)
Psychiatric				
Age schiz. started mean (sd)	19.4 (2.4)	19.2 (2.6)	19.5 (2.2)	U 763 (0.68)
Months psychotic mean (sd)	9.5 (9.6)	11.5 (11.4)	8.3 (8.22)	U 612 (0.09)
Discharge diagnosis schizophrenia (DSM-III-R), n (%)				
no	38 (46)	14 (45)	24 (46)	CHI 0.01 (0.93)
yes	45 (54)	17 (55)	28 (54)	
Sumscore pos. and neg. symptoms discharge[4], mean (sd)	14.9 (14.9)	14.6 (5.1)	15.1 (4.8)	U 752 (0.61)
Drugs				
Alcohol abuse, n (%)				
no	75 (92)	28 (90)	47 (92)	CHI 0.08 (0.77)
yes	7 (8)	3 (10)	4 (8)	
Cannabis abuse, n (%)				
no	62 (75)	23 (74)	39 (75)	CHI 0.08 (0.93)
yes	11 (25)	8 (26)	13 (25)	
Use hard drugs, n (%)				
no	80 (98)	30 (97)	50 (98)	CHI 0.13 (0.72)
yes	2 (2)	1 (3)	1 (2)	

Table 1. Continued

Medication compliance[5] mean (sd)	3.8 (0.5)	3.7 (0.44)	3.8 (0.6)	U 696 (0.22)
Antipsychotic medication[6] Mean (sd)	3.5 (1.2)	3.5 (1.2)	3.5 (1.1)	U 779 (0.99)

[1] For categorical variables Chi^2 tests were used (df = 1); for interval variables Mann-Whitney tests (U) were employed.
[2] Hollingshead Redlich Index (Hollingshead and Redlich, 1958).
[3] Strauss and Carpenter (in: Kokes et al., 1977).
[4] Positive symptoms: unusual thought contents, hallucinations, conceptual disorganization and excitement. Negative symptoms: motor retardation, flat affect, autism. (Breier et al., 1991).
[5] Mean medication compliance in clinical and ambulatory care. Medication compliance was rated from 1 (no compliance: 0%) to 5 (100% compliance, depot included).
[6] Mean haloperidol equivalents during clinical and ambulatory care. Dose was scored from 1 (none) to 6 (>15 haloperidol equivalents).

Table 2. Analysis (P) of scale scores (BPRS) and Expressed emotion (profile CFI EE, subscales Criticism and Emotional Overinvolvement (N=83)

	EE-profile	p-value	p-value Criticism	p-value EOI
Premorbid functioning [1]	L < H [2]	**0.005** [3]	0.11	**0.0004**
Prognostistic scale [3]	L < H	0.24	0.76	**0.005**
BPRS-E-items				
Elated mood	L < H	0.35	0.19	**0.01**
Suicidality	H < L	0.13	0.24	0.06
Guilt	H < L	0.12	0.55	0.07
BPRS-E Factors				
Factor 2 (depression)	H < L	0.19	0.23	0.09
Factor 4 (mania)	L < H	0.91	0.30	0.06

[1] Goldstein (in: Kokes et al., 1977).
[2] First column depicts patient group differences (L < H: patients from parents with low EE-profile had a lower score on this variable than patients from parents with a high EE-profile scores. The p-value of this test in column 1 is depicted in column 2. In column 3 and 4 differences on EE-subscales are tested.
[3] Strauss and Carpenter (in: Kokes et al., 1977).

overinvolvement scores (column 4) but not on the criticism scale (column 3). In column 4, we see that parental emotional overinvolvement has more relationship with a low prognostic score and grandiosity of the patient than other items. Column 4 also shows that there is a statistical trend in the relation between parental emotional overinvolvement and patient psychopathology.

Discussion

This research did not support the hypothesis that patient's (subtle) psychopathology can be differentiated on the basis of their parental EE-profile (high versus low). This finding is in line with Vaughn's et al. (1984).

We did not find experimental support for the idea that patients from high EE milieus are more challenging or disruptive when compared with patients from low EE families who are hypothesized to be more anxious and fearsome. Therefore Goldstein's et al. (1994) hypothesis and Rosenfarb's et al. (1995) findings are therefore not corroborated by the findings of this study.

Like Glynn et al. (1990) we also did not find a relationship between negative symptoms and parental EE-score. The results of this study therefore do not support Barraclough's (1994) hypothesis either. The findings of this study are also not in line with those of Hibbs et al. (1991) who found patient depression and hostility to be related to parental EE-score.

When patients were categorized on their parental EE profile they could be distinguished with regard to their premorbid functioning. Miklowitz et al. (1983) found high parental EE to be related to low premorbid functioning of patient. In this study the opposite was found. When looking at the patient samples from both studies we note that in Miklowitz's study the patients were more chronic (had more psychotic relapses), and were from a more multicultural and multiracial background than in this study (first or second break psychosis; mainly caucasian). Various studies (for review: Dingemans and Linszen, 1988) have shown these factors (chronicity, age, culture) to be related to EE.

An interesting finding in this study was that a high parental EE score was more often given because of high emotional overinvolvement than because of high criticism. This findings is in line with Mavreas' et al. (1992) research.

This finding suggests the possibility that when schizophrenia is in it's early phase parents tend to react to this with emotional overinvolvement; particularly so when the patient had a good premorbid functioning. This suggestion should further be explored of course, but when this is found to be true, this finding will have two important implications. The one implication is that EE level is not a parental trait marker, but dependent on the psychotic process within the patient (state dependent). When this is found to be true it will explain part of the sometimes contradictory findings with regard to the stability of parental EE-level (Nugter, 1997).

The second implication is that psycho-educational programs may currently be too rigid in their approach (trying to get parental EE-levels down as soon as possible) and should focus instead more on the accommodation of parental needs (in this view criticism is perceived as different from emotional overinvolvement) in handling the schizophrenia breakdown of their offspring. On a more speculative level it may be possible that parental EE-level is related to parental personality, and therefore also to patient personality factors. In this way Mike Goldstein's hypotheses may be purposely further refined and investigated with regard to patient and parent personality variables in the future.

References

Barrowclough, C., Johnston, M., and Tarrier, N. (1994): Attributions, expressed emotion, and patient relapse: An attributional model of relatives' response to schizophrenic illness. Behavior Therapy 25: 67–88

Breier, A., Schreiber, J.L., Dyer, J., and Pickar, D. (1991): National institute of Mental Health Longitudinal study of chronic schizophrenia Prognosis and predictors of outcome. Archives of General Psychiatry 48: 239–246

Camberwell Family Interview (CFI): MRC Social Psychiatry Research Unit, Maudsley Hospital, London SE 5

Dingemans, P., Linszen, D.H., Lenior, M.E., et al. (1995): Component structure of the Expanded Brief Psychiatric Rating Scale (BPRS-E). Psychopharmacology 122: 263–267

Dingemans, P., and Linszen, D.H. (1988): Communicatie deviatie, expressed emotion en affectieve stijl in relatie tot het symptomatische beloop van schizofrene psychosen. In: Schizofrenie. Recente ontwikkelingen in onderzoek en behandeling (van den Bosch R.J., van Meer C.R., Dingemans P.M.A.J., eds.), pp. 204–229. Deventer: Van Loghum Slaterus

Goldstein, M.J., Rosenfarb, I., Woo, S., et al. (1994): Intrafamilial relationships and the course of schizophrenia. Acta Psychiatrica Scandinavica (Suppl. 90/384:) 60–66

Glynn, S. M., Randolph, E.T., Eth, S., et al. (1990): Patient psychopathology and expressed emotion in schizophrennia. British Journal of Psychiatry 157: 877–880

Hibbs, E.D., Hamburger, S.D., Lenane, M., et al. (1991): Determinants of Expressed Emotion in families of disturbed and normal children. Journal of Child Psychology and Psychiatry 32: 757–770

Hollingshead, A.B., and Redlich, F.C. (1958): Social class and mental illness. New York: Wiley

Hooley, J.M., Richters, J.E., Weintraub, S., et al. (1987): Psychopathology and marital distress: The positive side of positive symptoms. Journal of Abnormal Psychology 96: 27–33

Kavanagh, D.J. (1992): Recent developments in expressed emotion and schizophrenia. British Journal of Psychiatry 160: 601–620

Kokes, R.F., Strauss, J.S., and Klorman, R. (1977): Part II. Measuring premorbid adjustment: the instruments and their development. Schizophrenia Bulletin 2: 212–213

Linszen, D.H., Dingemans, P.M.A.J., Scholte, W.F., et al. (1994): Expressed emotion en patientgebonden kenmerken als risicofactoren voor psychose-recidief bij schizofrene stoornissen. Tijdschrift voor Psychiatrie 36: 495–508

Lukoff, D., Nuechterlein, K.H., and Ventura, J. (1986): Manual for the expanded BPRS. Schizophrenia Bulletin 12: 594–602

Mavreas, V.G., Tomaras, V., Karydi, V., et al. (1992): Expressed emotion in families of chronic schizophrenics and its association with clinical measures. Social Psychiatry and Psychiatric Epidemiology 27: 4–9

Macmillan, J.F., Crow, T.J., Johnson, A.L., et al. (1987): Expressed emotion and relapse in first episodes of schizophrenia. British Journal of Psychiatry 151: 320–323

Miklowitz, D.J., Goldstein, M.J., and Falloon, I.R.H. (1983): Premorbid and symptomatic characteristics of schizophrenics from families with high and low levels of expressed emotion. Journal of Abnormal Psychology 92: 359–367

Nugter, A. (1997): Family factors and interventions in recent onset schizophrenia. Amsterdam: University of Amsterdam Dissertation

Parker, G., Johnston, P., and Hayward, L. (1988): Parental 'expressed emotion' as a predictor of schizophrenic relapse. Archives of General Psychiatry 45: 806–813

Rosenfarb, I.S., Goldstein, M.J., Mintz, J., and Nuechterlein, K.H. (1995): Expressed emotion and subclinical psychopathology observable within transactions between schizophrenic patients and their family members. Journal of Abnormal Psychology 104(2): 259–267

Vaughn, C., and Leff, J. (1976): The measurement of expressed emotion in the families of psychiatric patients. British Journal of Social and Clinical Psychology 15: 157–165

Vaughn, C.E., Snyder, K.S., Jones, S., Freeman, W.B., and Falloon, J.R. (1984): Family factors in schizophrenic relapse. Replication in California of British research on expressed emotion. Archives of General Psychiatry 41: 1169–1177

6
Psychophysiological Evaluation of Verbal Interaction during Conversations between Psychotic Patients and their Relatives

Andreas Altorfer and Marie-Louise Käsermann

Introduction

In the context of a vulnerability stress model of schizophrenic episodes (e.g., Zubin and Spring, 1977), behavioral events in communication such as negative attitudes in high Expressed Emotion (EE, Leff and Vaughn, 1985), negative Affective Style (AS, Doane et al., 1981) and high Communication Deviance (CD, Doane et al., 1982; Interactional Measure of CD, Velligan et al., 1990) are conceived of as specific stressors which interfere with the patients' ability to adapt to life outside the confines of the hospital. Numerous studies e.g. from the "Family Research Group" at University of California in Los Angeles (UCLA) have demonstrated this important relation between specific events during family communication and increased risk of relapse (see reviews by Goldstein, 1987; 1988; 1991).

However, these studies only produce scarce evidence of an actual or even a remote effect of communicative stressors on the level of physiological arousal (Tarrier and Turpin, 1992; Sturgeon et al., 1984). Furthermore, the question of whether a given stress response may be modified by an individual's communicative reactions to it (in the sense of active coping with stressors) or by modifications of the course of the communicative exchange e.g., introduced elusively by both interactants, is not addressed at all. This lack of pertinent substantial evidence with regard to both the question concerning the immediate physiological effect of stressors, and the related question concerning individual- or interaction-dependent physiological modifications of stress responses mainly seems to be due to two methodological limitations. On the one hand, well established physiological measures of arousal processes are not subtle enough to depict relevant changes occurring during short time (Altorfer et al., 1998). On the other hand, although the target of research cited above is communication, ongoing processes of communicative exchange are not directly investigated. For instance, the coding systems applied to quantify stressors during conversations are established by referring mainly to large passages in discourse of the relatives (e.g., up to six lines of uninterrupted speech) which are rated according to defined categories (Leff and Vaughn, 1985; Doane et al., 1981; Velligan et al., 1990). Therefore, rather than specifically assigning a score to each statement made by participants, codes are applied within a critical incident model by tabulating phases during the interactional course meeting at least one of the criteria. That is, ongoing communicative interaction consisting of minimally two or three functionally related turns of two interactants (e.g., question-answer pairs [P1-X1] and subsequent qualification of answer [P2]) are not considered as the critical unit of analysis. Furthermore, these coding systems do not provide categories for the identification of events **without** any stressor, though this would form an irrevocable prerequisite for the identification of pertinent **baseline data against which events carrying a stressor might be statistically compared** (cf. Altorfer et al., 1998). Thus, from a microanalytical point of view, construing communicative stressors in such a nonspecific manner can only provide a very rough picture of the occurrence and nature of concomitant physiological stress because (1) there is no way to coordinate changes of arousal with relevant communicative acts on an exact, time-locked basis, and (2) there do not exist any methodological procedures which try to investigate the relations between communicative events with and without stressors.

Nevertheless, studies concerning familial stressors yield substantially important evidence with regard to an effect of social psychological factors on the incidence and the course of psychiatric illnesses. However, they do not treat variables of communicative stressors and concomitant autonomous stress responses in a way that is conducive to the examination of ongoing social interactions. Therefore, the impact of communicative events is inferred and the collection of data on concomitant stress responses is either neglected or is carried out using methods (e.g., ratings of arousal) which tap the stress response, i.e. underlying processes of arousal, in a rather crude manner. In contrast, a specific methodology (Käsermann et al., 2000; Jossen et al., 2000) yields pertinent results. **First**, it can be shown that relevant changes in arousal are systematically associated with a defined set of communicative stressors. That is, "emotionally-loaded" (i.e., "invasive") and "emotionally-neutral" events that take place during a conversation between parents and their schizophrenic (Käsermann and Altorfer, 1989) or healthy son (Altorfer et al. 1991), respectively, as well as "disturbing" (interruptions, misinterpretations of verbal content and unjustified pauses made by a person instructed to do so) and "neutral" situations in the course of conversations between five pairs of healthy adults (Käsermann and Altorfer, 1991) consistently display this effect. Thus, specific events, which may be conceived of **as violations of conversational maxims** (Grice, 1975), are correlated with specific changes in the period of the pulse volume curve (a sudden or continuous decrease in period length, i.e., increase of heart rate) in the case of both schizophrenic and healthy individuals. Based on the comparison with neutral situations, these changes in cardiovascular functioning may be interpreted as stress reactions. **Second**, by tackling questions about the instrumentality of communicative behavior in modifying a given level of arousal, it can be shown that equivalent stressors are accompanied by stress reactions which are more pronounced in schizophrenic interactants than in healthy ones, although both groups react to equivalent stressors with equivalent communicative coping behavior (Käsermann and Altorfer, 1994). This result demonstrates that the potential effect of an objectively defined stressor (e.g., intrusiveness of P1) is mediated by a subjective interpretation or appraisal (e.g. Lazarus and Folkman, 1984) made by the index person.

This process of interpretation and its potential effect on arousal can be revealed only if one looks at communicative units consisting of at least two turns. Therefore, as in previous studies the **sections of verbal communication** investigated in what follows are derived from a functional model of communicative exchange (see Käsermann, 1983; 1986; 1987). It defines a sequence unit consisting of three subsequent statements by two (or three) different speakers – relative (P1)→patient (X1)→relative (P2). The inclusion of the third statement makes it possible to monitor the effect of given patterns of communicative exchange on the course of activation in the index person. Within this theoretical framework, the present study aims at advancing our understanding about the interplay between interactional communicative stressors and physiological stress response, and the power of verbal interaction in modifying a given stress response. Specifically, it will be shown

(1) whether and to what extent P1s containing a potential stressor (compared with neutral P1s) are correlated with physiological stress reactions of index persons;
(2) whether and to what extent states of arousal are systematically changed by the way index persons in X1s communicatively react to P1s; and
(3) whether and to what extent states of arousal are systematically changed by characteristic features of the course of the subsequent communicative exchange (P2s).

Patients and Methods

Patients

Thirteen dyadic and triadic conversations between relatives and their schizophrenic or bipolar manic offspring, spouse or sibling are examined. During their hospital stay, all patients underwent a clinical interview (Present State Examination, PSE, Wing et al., 1974) which was crucial for establishing a diagnosis according to DSM-III-R criteria (American Psychiatric Association, 1987). Shortly before discharge, the patients and their relatives were invited to participate in a family conversation session. They were advised to discuss a problem which had to be solved in the near future (e.g., planning a vacation, looking for an apartment, etc.). Data about the patients are summarized in Table 1.

Categories of verbal communication

With regard to communicative exchange, a defined section (sequence) of the interactional course is selected consisting of the aforementioned three consecutive statements – relative (P1)→patient (X1)→relative (P2). Since the main interest is on changes in psychophysiological arousal in the course of communicative interaction (cf. questions 2. and 3.), it is necessary not only to categorize

Table 1. Characteristics of patients

Con- versat- ion	Family members involved in con- versation	Age of patient	Sex	Diag- nosis DSM- III-R	Duration of index- hospitali- zation (days)	Pulse (overall mean)	Pulse (overall SD)
#1	Dyad**	21	male	295.31	49	92.79	12.36
#2	Triad*	28	female	295.70	60	76.61	6.56
#3	Dyad****	42	female	295.40	21	57.09	6.60
#4	Triad*	24	male	295.33	148	66.89	6.46
#5	Dyad**	29	male	295.33	106	68.44	5.99
#6	Dyad**	27	male	295.70	53	92.32	11.00
#7	Triad*	26	male	295.33	176	67.11	5.39
#8	Triad*	29	female	295.33	73	91.26	12.48
#9	Dyad***	28	female	298.80	25	78.01	6.45
#10	Dyad***	32	female	295.70	47	70.39	8.27
#11	Triad*	17	male	295.40	46	71.19	6.43
#12	Dyad**	29	female	295.13	96	74.08	8.74
#13	Dyad***	26	female	295.70	74	91.43	12.05

*Patient and parents **Patient and mother ***Patient and spouse ****Patient and sister

295.13... Schizophrenia, disorganized type, subchronic, with acute exacerba- tion
295.31 ... Schizophrenia, paranoid type, subchronic
295.33... Schizophrenia, paranoid type, subchronic with acute exacerbation
295.40... Schizophreniform disorder
295.70... Schizoaffective disorder
295.80... Brief reactive psychosis

statements as such (e.g., P1s), but also to consider the functional relation between consecutive statements (Fig. 1).

(1) The starting-point of coding are the relatives' (parents', spouses' or siblings') P1 statements which are coded as either containing a "**stressor**" (B) or being "**neutral**" (N) (see category descriptions for P1 statements in Table 2).

(2) The sequences P1-X1-P2 are categorized according to the relation between X1 respectively P2 to the opening statement P1. A "**cooperative-affiliative**" sequence is characterized by a coherent connection between X1 and P1 – the patient in X1 either verbally responds to the content (e.g. discussing the criticized behavior, answering a given question, etc.) or to the "stressful" or "neutral" connotation of the statement made in P1 (e.g., discussing the

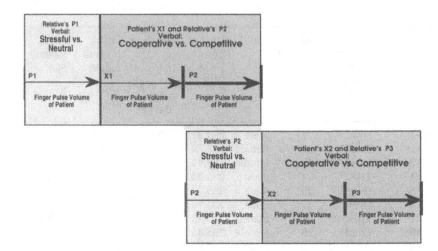

Fig. 1. Course of verbal interaction, relative's P1 neutral vs. stressful statements and cooperative vs. competitive sequences (P1-X1-P2/P2-X2-P3/P3-X3-P4...)

relative's attitude). Non-overlapping adjacency pairs (Sacks et al., 1974) are coded by passing a moving "time window" throughout the conversation (P1-X1, P2-X2, etc.). Additionally, a reference between the content of P2 and P1 is found, in other words, coding is required which indicates a repetition of the content of the P1 statement. The relative's statements P1-...-P2 are coded throughout the conversation by tallying overlapping pairs (P1-...-P2, P2-...-P3, etc.). Maximally deviating from this communicative exchange is a "**competitive-agonistic**" course of interaction where P1 addresses topic 1, X1 changes to topic 2 (incoherent connection to P1), and P2 changes again to topic 1. "**Mixed**" sequences are courses of interaction in which either X or P behave competitively/cooperatively and vice versa (see category descriptions for sequences P1-[X1-P2] in Table 2).

Interaction transcripts were coded by two trained raters who were blind to each patient's symptomatology data. Coder training requires about five hours; with trained coders, it takes about three times the original interaction time to code transcribed interactions. Interrater reliabilities, calculated for each code of the relative's statement P1, were found to yield levels ranging from 0.79 (reflexive impediments) to 0.93 (criticism, prospective impediments) (Cohen's kappa, $p<0.001$; Cohen, 1960). Interrater reliability calculated across

Table 2. Coding of verbal stressors during P1 statements of relatives (A) and coding of "competitive" vs. "cooperative" sequences (P1-X1-P2)

Category	Description
(A) P1 Statements	
(A1) Criticism	Benign criticism which is directed toward specific incidents or sets of behavior; personal criticism which has qualities of unnecessary or overly harsh modifiers, reference to broad classes of behavior, or reference to the patient's character or nature
(A2) Guilt induction	Behavior which conveys that the patient is to blame or at fault for a negative event and that the relative has been distressed or upset by the event
(A3) Obstruction of participation in conversation	
(A3.1) Reflexive impediments	Referring to some aspects of the patients's utterance but neglecting the important ones; misinterpreting, ignoring or not taking a previous statement of the patient seriously
(A3.2) Prospective impediments	Obligation to respond to a certain topic with emotional component; questions with obstructive tendency by anticipating an emotionally negative quality
(A4) Intrusiveness	Relative is taking responsibility for the patient's affairs and advising him/her without respecting personal distance; relative implies knowledge of the patient's thoughts, feelings, conditions or motives when in fact there is no apparent basis for such knowledge
(B) Sequences P1-[X1-P2]	
	X1 and P2 rejudged in relation to the sequence-opening statement P1:
(B1) cooperative-affiliative sequence	In statement X1 coherent verbal response to content or connotation of statement P1 and in statement P2 referring to statement P1 (by implication referring also to statement X1)
(B2) competitive-agonistic sequence	In statement X1 in coherent verbal response to content or connotation of statement P1, however, in statement P2 referring to statement P1

Table 2. (Continued)

Category	Description
(B3) mixed sequence	In statement X1 coherent verbal response to content or connotation of statement P1, however, in statement P2 no reference to statement P1
	In statement X1 in coherent verbal response to content or connotation of statement P1 and in statement P2 reference to statement P1

the relational categories and summarized for all possible courses of interaction (neutral/stressor × coherent/incoherent × reiteration/no reiteration) was 0.94 (Cohen's kappa, $p<0.001$; Cohen, 1960).

Psychophysiological Measurement

For each statement of a sequence in the interactional course, the psychophysiological concomitants are registered by continuously measuring the cardiovascular activity of the patient using a photoplethysmographic recording of the finger pulse volume (FPV). As a result of a highly accurate quantification of the photometric signal and a time-exact representation of the cardiovascular measures (Altorfer et al., 1990; Jossen et al., 2000), it is possible to coordinate them to the ongoing conversation. In this respect, temporal coordination of physiological and communicative data allows for a qualitative and quantitative description of psychophysiological effects immediately at the point of occurence. We use six physiological indices to quantify experienced stress during the different statements of conversations:

(1–2) In line with traditional parameters, **mean** and **standard deviation of the vessel volume changes** is calculated for each statement of the conversation.

(3–5) Based on the individual overall mean and standard deviation (calculated in each subject for the whole conversation), for each statement we count the **number of values** which exceed the sum of the overall mean and one standard deviation, **the number of series** which meet these criteria and the **duration of these series**.

(6–7) Additionally, **integrals** of sections of vessel volume changes are computed for each statement.

With regard to changes of physiological activity in the course of interaction, we first address the question whether sequences with an objectively defined **communicative stressor** in a relative's utterance P1 are accompanied by a stress response in the index person, secondly, we compare the course of physiological activation during **cooperative-affiliative** sequences with the respective course of physiological activation during **competitive-agonistic** sequences. This analytical step is critical with regard to the question whether and how the quality of communicative exchange (as opposed to an individual's specific communicative moves) may affect arousal in a psychotic patient.

Data Analysis

The physiological analysis of the communicative sequences is conducted by means of analysis of variance designs (ANOVA). The number of cases is determined by the number of family conversations and the existence of the verbal codes for communicative events. The frequency that verbal categories occur is determined in each family conversation. In order to guarantee the assessment of an adequate number of distinct verbal situations, the means of the physiological variables are computed based exclusively on verbal categories which on the one hand occur at various points throughout the conversation and which on the other hand occur at least 5 times in each conversation. The fact that 8 different courses of communicative exchange are coded for each conversation respectively (4 for stressful and 4 for neutral sequences based on P1 codings) yields a maximum of 8 means of the physiological variable. Within 13 families this results in a maximum of 104 cases. The criterion "more than 5 situations per category" does, however, reduce the number of cases included in this study by 14 to 90. Concerning sequential dependencies and sampling of cases, note that categories of verbal stressors reduced to the dichotomy between **"stressful"** and **"neutral"** situations as well as coding adjacency pairs as **"coherent"** and **"incoherent"** reactions of the patients to relatives' statements are regarded as independent samples of cases. Based on investigations of Bakeman (1991) and Marascuilo and Serlin (1988), categorical data satisfy claims of sampling independence as a procedural matter if sufficiently trained coders assign codes "only to events at hand and are not influenced by their coding of the previous event" (Bakeman, 1991, p. 264). Even if tallying overlapping sequences by analyzing "**cooperative**", "**competitive**" and "**mixed**" sequences including three statements (P1-...-P2, P2-...-P3, etc.) appears objectionable on formal grounds (lack of sampling independence), it turns out to be empirically inconsequential because subsequent codings are not affected by previous ones (Bakeman, 1991). Subsequent statements demand that the physiological measures are considered as repeated measure throughout verbal interaction (whole sequences three levels). For all univariate ANOVAs involving more than two levels of the repeated measure, reported *p*-values are based on the Greenhouse-Geisser correction (Jennings and Wood, 1976) and adjusted df, truncated to the nearest integer, are reported.

Results

Psychophysiological Comparisons of Neutral and Stressful Statements

Table 3 shows the relationship between "**stressful**" or "**neutral**" statements P1 of the relatives and the psychotic patients' psychophysiological indices. A univariate 1-way analysis of variance (ANOVA) is conducted separately for each proposed indicator of stress. Thirteen families were included into this analysis which result in a total number (N) of 26 independent situations (for each family two situations, i.e. a "stressful" and "neutral" one). The variables which quantify sequences of increased pulse volume (number and duration of stress values/series) or the local shape of the pulse volume curve (integral) show highly significant correlations to the verbal coding of P1 statements. With explained variances (w^2) ranging from 15 to 68 percent, these psychophysiological variables indicate **higher arousal during** "stressful" P1s than during "neutral" P1s.

Cooperative vs. Competitive Sequences

The question of features of communicative interaction (as opposed to an individual's communicative moves) being factors of a systematic modification of arousal is tackled by comparing the three types of courses defined above (**cooperative, competitive**, and **mixed**

Table 3. Neutral vs. stressful statements in P1, physiological correlates: 13 families which include 13 "neutral" and 13 "stressful" cases (N=26) (1-way ANOVA)

Indicator of stress	Verbal coding of P1	Mean	SD	F(df J-1,N-J)	p-level	ω^2 (Strength of statistical relation)
Mean heart rate during statement	Neutral	75.91	11.65	0.17 (df 1.24)	<0.6860	0.0069
	Stressful	77.73	10.97			
SD heart rate during statement	Neutral	4.41	1.78	2.86 (df 1.24)	<0.1040	0.1063
	Stressful	5.78	2.31			
Number of stress values	Neutral	4.46	3.46	11.87 (df 1.24)	<0.0021	0.3308
	Stressful	11.90	6.98			
Number of stress series	Neutral	0.67	0.25	51.49 (df 1.24)	<0.00001	0.6820
	Stressful	1.65	0.42			
Duration of stress series	Neutral	0.56	0.51	14.53 (df 1.24)	<0.0008	0.3770
	Stressful	1.98	1.24			
Integral statement	Neutral	7.19	2.75	4.44 (df 1.24)	<0.0456	0.1563
	Stressful	10.87	5.64			

sequences) and by specifically contrasting the two extreme types of courses. That is, the **cooperative-affiliative** course as default value of a totally coherent communicative situation is compared with the **competitive-agonistic** course.

A first analysis of all courses (total N of cases = 90) shows that there is a significant main effect of type of change within courses (2-way ANOVA, three level repeated measure; course P1-X1-P2: F [2, 165] = 3.394, $p = 0.036$) and a significant interaction between type of courses (cooperative vs. competitive vs. mixed) and type of change within courses (F [4, 165] = 2.711, p = 0.032; Rao R [4, 172] = 2.44, $p = 0.049$). Note with regard to the **mixed** courses that the level of arousal is relatively high throughout the sequences, and that there are no significant changes in arousal (Duncan's multiple range tests; P1 = 8.56, X1 = 9.46, $p = 0.634$; X1 = 9.46, P2 = 8.68, $p = 0.667$). This result is in line with the evidence cited above (Tarrier and Turpin, 1992; Sturgeon et al., 1984) that arousing effects of communicative stressors cannot be found within a communicatively unspecific frame of reference. However, except for **mixed** courses, our analysis **does not replicate** the Tarrier and Turpin (1992) and Sturgeon et al. (1981) results.

A subsequent comparison (2-way ANOVA, three level repeated measure) between **cooperative** and **competitive** courses (total N of cases = 42) yields a significant main effect of the type of change (F [2, 78] = 8.48, $p = 0.000$) and a significant interaction between type of sequences and type of change (F [2, 78] = 2.99, $p = 0.056$; Rao R [2, 39] = 3.49, $p = 0.040$). The main differences between **cooperative** and **competitive** courses are the following ones: (1) Starting from an almost equally high arousal during P1s, the decrease in arousal seen during answers of the patients (X1) is more pronounced in **competitive** sequences (Duncan's multiple rang tests: P1 = 7.66, X1 = 2.63, $p = 0.002$) than in **cooperative** sequences (Duncan's multiple rang tests: P1 = 8.05, X1 = 5.68, $p = 0.149$). Additionally, the difference between the levels reached in answers of the patients (X1) are significantly different for **cooperative** and **competitive** sequences (Duncan's multiple rang tests: X1: cooperative = 5.68, X1: competitive = 2.63, $p = 0.044$). (2) **Competitive** sequences which are comprised of **incoherent** answers of the patients (X1) and reiterations of the P1-topic in P2 lead to a significant increase in arousal during relatives' P2s (Duncan's multiple rang tests: X1 = 2.63, P2 = 8.98, $p = 0.000$) while the equivalent rise in **cooperative** sequences is not significant (Duncan's multiple rang tests: X1 = 5.68, P2 = 6.89, $p = 0.415$). That is, an effect of features of communication on specific changes in arousal may be detected as soon as the analysis concentrates on events which can be interpreted in a communicatively meaningful way: Index persons' being coherent in X1s and inducing cooperativeness in their partners (in P2) attenuate overall tension, while being evasive without inducing the partners to accept that evasion leads to extreme reactions of relief in X1s to subsequent reinforcement of tension during P2s.

The same pattern of arousal modification can be observed when **cooperative** and **competitive** sequences are distinguished as to **whether their P1s contain a stressor or not** (2-way ANOVA, three level repeated measure, "stressful" P1, total N of cases = 21, Fig. 2 and "neutral" P1, total N of cases = 21, Fig. 3): There is a significant main effect of the type of course in "**stressful**" (Fig. 2; F [2, 36] = 14.54, $p = 0.000$) as well as in "**neutral**" sequences (Fig. 3; F [2, 34] = 3.50, $p = 0.42$). The most important difference between **cooperative** and **competitive** courses is again due to a significant increase in arousal in relatives' P2s after incoherent answers of the patients (X1) in both situations with (Duncan's multiple range tests; X1 = 2.56, P2 = 9.74, $p = 0.002$) **and** without P1-stressors (Duncan's multiple rang tests: X1 = 2.70, P2 = 8.22, $p = 0.013$). That is, regardless of the differential amount of stress in P1s, the pattern of modification by subsequently **cooperative** or **competitive** interaction remains the same. Thus, the given results show that the occurrence of stressor-

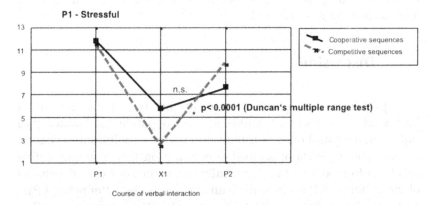

Fig. 2. Course of verbal interaction (three level repeated measure), course of arousal in cooperative and competitive sequences P1-X1-P2, in "stressful" situations, total N of cases = 21 (2-way interaction: F(2,36)=1.81; $p<0.178$)

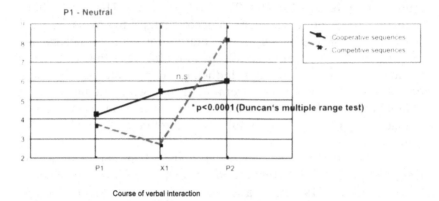

Course of verbal interaction

Fig. 3. Course of verbal interaction (three level repeated measure), course of arousal in cooperative and competitive sequences P1-X1-P2, in "neutral" situations, total N of cases = 21 (2-way interaction: $F(2,34)=1.72$; $p<0.195$)

dependent experience of stress may **determine** a given level of arousal, but its subsequent modification seems to be **entirely dependent on the quality of a given communicative exchange** (as opposed to the meaning or content of an individual communicative move). Specifically, the **default courses of cooperation** between index persons and relatives are a little bit more demanding on the patients' part but on the whole lead to a more stable level of arousal if the psychotic patients **succeed in inducing cooperation in the relatives**. On the other hand, although being incoherent is communicatively less demanding, the patients' failure to induce the relatives to drop a disagreeable topic leads to quite an extreme level of instability in arousal.

Discussion

The preceding paragraphs demonstrated that patients exhibit increased arousal when relatives express negative emotional topics rather than neutral ones. Furthermore, there is a differential change in the patients' level of arousal depending on their communicative reactions to relatives' P1s. Especially incoherent or evasive answers of the patients (X1) seem to have an arousing effect after neutral P1s, and a tension-reducing effect after stressful P1s. However, whether individuals' evasive utterances have to be conceived of as a successful coping strategy remains ambiguous, because ANOVA-treatment of the given material does not provide the basis to decide whether this verbal behavior is an antecedent or a consequence of a given change in arousal. Instead, it seems to be the quality of communicative interaction following "neutral" or "stressful" P1s which is important for the modification of arousal: Interactive cooperativeness within sequences is associated with a relatively **stable reduction**, while interactive competitiveness is accompanied by **both extremely reduced and increased** arousal levels. The results suggest that there is a close relationship between communicative and physiological aspects of behavior, and that linguistic and content-related qualities of single utterances determine significant changes in arousal to a lesser extent than features of the ongoing communicative exchange. This would ask for modifications of traditional concepts of coping as called for by e.g. Nuechterlein and Dawson (1984). The notion that schizophrenic patients are likely to have fewer and less flexible personal resources to cope with stressful events than most people should be expanded by introducing **a systemic level which covers violations of** "interactive kindness" (e.g., cooperativeness) by relatives as well.

Obtaining these results requires using a methodology which comprises a highly resolving physiological measurement on the one hand and a minimal model of the process of communicative exchange which allows for an exact coordination of communicatively relevant events with their respective physiological concomitants on the other. The functional relation of consecutive statements which is the basic feature of communicative exchange is used to investigate different types of ongoing verbal interaction. A contrastive analysis of different communicative situations in defined local contexts is a necessary prerequisite to comparing accompanying quantifications of physiological variables. This methodological claim is strongly supported (ex negativo) by the results of the analysis of communicatively mixed courses which parallel the results reported by other authors (see Tarrier and Turpin, 1992).

The presented results may be viewed as further evidence for the relevance of stressful verbal events of relatives during family conversation. In this respect, the relationship between verbal stressors and physiological arousal supports the notion of the stressful impact of behavioral elements in family communication on the patients' experience of stress. Additionally, subsequent verbal communicative moves of patients and relatives are important determinants for regulating given levels of physiological arousal.

Further research should amplify this global relationship by introducing a single-case level of analysis which quantifies the individual's monitoring of stressor and stress. In-depth analyses are needed to attain greater understanding of the complex processes of regulational systems during conversation. Future results should clarify questions about the stressful impact of specific verbal and nonverbal moves of patients during conversation. In this framework, therapeutic applications of coping training programs turn out to be significant only if validation of the individual patients' coping behavior during conversation can be realized. In this respect, the presented methodological procedure is a powerful instrument to gain insight into processes of stress and their modifications by means of communicative factors. It may be applied as an important prerequisite for developing individual therapeutic interventions which aim to reduce the patient's autonomic responses by means of providing successful communicative strategies.

Acknowledgement

This research was supported by grants from the Swiss National Science Foundation (grant number: 32-26488.89) and the Sandoz Research Foundation.

References

Altorfer, A., Hirsbrunner, H.P., and Käsermann, M.L. (1990): Messung psychophysiologischer Variablen während Gesprächen: Die Quantifizierung des Pulsvolumengeschehens. Zeitschrift für Psychologie 198: 293–308

Altorfer, A., Käsermann, M.L., and Hirsbrunner, H.P. (1998): Arousal and communication I. Relationship between nonverbal behavioral and physiological indices of the stress response. Journal of Psychophysiology 12: 40–59

Altorfer, A., Käsermann, M.L., and Hirsbrunner, H.P. (1991): Erhebung und Analyse des Fingerpulsvolumens auf der Basis einer quasi-kontinuierlichen Messung von Periode und Amplitude. Zeitschrift für Differentielle und Diagnostische Psychologie 12: 33–41

American Psychiatric Association (1987): DSM-III-R: Diagnostic and statistical manual of mental disorders, 3rd revised ed. Washington, DC: American Psychiatric Association

Bakeman, R. (1991): Analyzing categorical data. In: Studying interpersonal interaction (Montgomery, B.M. and Duck, S., eds.), pp. 255–274. New York: Guilford Press

Doane, J.A., Jones, J.E., Fisher, L., Ritzler, B., Singer, M.T., and Wynne, L.C. (1982): Parental communication deviance as a predictor of competence in children at risk for adult psychiatric disorder. Family Process 21: 211–223

Doane, J.A., West, K.L., Goldstein, M.J., Rodnick, E.H., and Jones, J.E. (1981): Parental communication deviance and affective style: Predictors of subsequent schizophrenia spectrum disorders in vulnerable adolescents. Archives of General Psychiatry 38: 679–685

Goldstein, M.J. (1991): Psychosocial nonpharmacological treatments for schizophrenia. In: American Psychiatric Press Review of Psychiatry. (Tasman, A., and Goldfinger, M., eds.), Vol. 10, pp. 116–135. Washington, DC: American Psychiatric Press

Goldstein, M.J. (1988): The family and psychopathology. Annual Review of Psychology 39: 283–299

Goldstein, M.J. (1987): The UCLA high-risk project. Schizophrenia Bulletin 13: 505–514

Grice, H.P. (1975): Logic and conversation. In: Syntax and semantics (Cole, P., and Morgan, J.L., eds.), Vol. 3: Speech acts, pp. 41–58. New York: Academic Press

Jennings, J.R., and Wood, C.C. (1976): The e-adjustment procedure for repeated-measures analyses of variance. Psychophysiology 13: 277–278

Jossen, S., Käsermann, M.L., Altorfer, A., Foppa, K., and Zimmermann, H. (2000). Pheripheral blood flow as an indicatior of activation. Behavior Research Methods, Instruments, and Computers 32: 47–55

Käsermann, M.L. (1987): The analysis of dialogues with a schizophrenic patient. In: Neurotic and psychotic language behavior (van de Craen, P., and Wodak, R., eds.), pp. 277–303. Clevedon: Multilingual Matters

Käsermann, M.L. (1986): Das Phänomen der sprachlichen Inkohärenz in Dialogen mit einem Schizophrenen. Sprache und Kognition 3: 111–126

Käsermann, M.L. (1983): Form und Funktion schizophrener Sprachstörungen. Sprache und Kognition 3: 132–147

Käsermann, M.L., Altorfer, A., Foppa, K., Jossen, S., and Zimmermann, H. (2000). Measuring emotionalization in everyday face-to-face communicative interaction. Behavior Research Methods, Instruments, and Computers 32: 33–46

Käsermann, M.L., and Altorfer, A. (1994): Communicative stress and coping in schizophrenic and healthy persons. In: Past, present and future of Psychiatry, IX World Congress of Psychiatry (Beigel, A., Lopez Ibor, J.J., and Costa e Silva, J.A., eds.), pp. 451–455. Singapore: World Scientific Publishing

Käsermann, M.L., and Altorfer, A. (1991): Was uns in Gesprächen aufregt. Störendes kommunikatives Verhalten und seine Wirkung auf den Gesprächspartner. In: Über die richtige Art, Psychologie zu betreiben (Grawe, K. Hänni, R. Semmer, N., and Tschan, F., eds.), pp. 343–356. Göttingen: Hogrefe

Käsermann, M.L., and Altorfer, A. (1989): Family discourse: Situations differing in degree of stress and their physiological correlates. British Journal of Psychiatry 155(Suppl. 5): 136–143

Lazarus, R.S., and Folkman, S. (1984): Stress, appraisal, and coping. New York: Springer

Leff, J., and Vaughn, C.E. (1985): Expressed emotion in families. New York: Guilford Press

Nuechterlein, K.H., and Dawson, M.E. (1984): A heuristic vulnerability/stress model of Schizophrenic episodes. Schizophrenia Bulletin 10: 300–312

Sacks, H., Schegloff, E.A., and Jefferson, G.A. (1974): A simplest systematics for the organization of turn-talking for conversation. Language 50: 696–735

Sturgeon, D., Turpin, G., Kuipers, L. Berkowitz, R., and Leff, J. (1984): Psychophysiological responses of schizophrenic patients to high and low expressed emotion relatives: A follow-up study. British Journal of Psychiatry 145: 62–69

Tarrier, N., and Turpin, G. (1992): Psychosocial factors, arousal and schizophrenic relapse, the psychophysiological data. British Journal of Psychiatry 161: 3–11

Velligan, D.I., Goldstein, M.J., Nuechterlein, K.H., Miklowitz, D.J., and Ranlett, G. (1990): Can communication deviance be measured in a family problem-solving interaction? Family Process 29: 213–226

Wing, J.K., Cooper, J.E., and Sartorius, N. (1974): The measurement and classification of psychiatric symptoms: An instruction manual for the PSE and CATEGO program. Cambridge: Cambridge University Press

Zubin, J., and Spring, B. (1977): Vulnerability: A new view of schizophrenia. Journal of Abnormal Psychology 86: 103–126

7
Predictors of Relapse in Recent-Onset Schizophrenia

Kenneth L. Subotnik, Keith H. Nuechterlein, Joseph Ventura

Introduction

The course of schizophrenic disorders is likely to be a product of a number of different influences that can be broadly separated into vulnerability, stressor, and protective factors. In this chapter we will discuss recent evidence from a longitudinal study of the impact of stressors on the early course of schizophrenia.

Vulnerability or liability factors for schizophrenia are conceptualized as being present before illness onset and enduring throughout both psychotic episodes and periods of clinical remission (Zubin and Spring, 1977; Nuechterlein and Dawson, 1984). The psychobiological vulnerability factors leading to a liability for the development of schizophrenia may not necessarily be the same factors that influence the course of the disorder once manifested. Genetic influences are likely to contribute to both liability factors for the development of schizophrenia as well as to factors associated with differential course. The evidence from family, twin, and adoption studies support the view that 60–80% of the liability to schizophrenia can be attributed to genetic factors (Kendler and Diehl, 1993; Cannon et al., 1998). Other contributors to psychobiological liability to schizophrenia may be environmental in nature, such as exposure to influenza virus during the second trimester of fetal development or the impact of obstetric complications (Lewis and Murray, 1987; Mednick et al., 1988). These nongenetic contributors to vulnerability to schizophrenia may either potentiate the genetic predisposition or create brain dysfunctions that parallel those that develop from genetic factors (Murray et al., 1992; Parnas and Mednick, 1991).

In addition to psychobiological factors which influence the course of schizophrenia, several lines of evidence suggest that the reemergence of psychosis may also be influenced by proximal environmental stress factors such as life events and a stressful emotional social environment. Much of the earlier work demonstrating a relationship between stressful life events and return of psychosis relied on retrospective reporting of life events after the relapse occurred, thus introducing a potential memory bias (Brown and Birley, 1968; Day et al., 1987). The first well-designed study that did not rely on retrospective reporting showed that negative symptoms, but not positive symptoms, were significantly increased following independent life events (Hardesty et al., 1985). This finding of an increase in negative symptoms suggests that not all patients respond to stressors in similar ways. The earlier report from our UCLA longitudinal project (Ventura et al., 1989), which will be reviewed later in this chapter, was the first study to show a significant link between stressful independent life events and psychotic exacerbation in schizophrenia using prospective data gathering methods. Another prospective study has since also supported a link between the occurrence of stressful life events and a return of positive symptoms of schizophrenia (Malla et al., 1990).

Another source of psychosocial stress that is associated with illness course is an immediate social environment wherein significant others in the patient's life are characterized by lack of acceptance of the illness and lack of social support, and hold highly critical, hostile, or emotionally overinvolved attitudes toward the ill individual. This attitudinal construct has been termed "high expressed emotion" (Leff, 1987), although this term should not be taken to mean that these significant others are simply "highly emotional." High expressed emotion (EE) has been found to predict higher relapse rates (Kavanagh, 1992; Miklowitz, 1994) with a meta-analytic effect size of $r = 0.31$ across 27 studies (Butzlaff and Hooley, 1998). An effect size of this magnitude roughly translates into a high-versus low-EE relapse rate of 65% versus 35%. The association between high EE and psychotic relapse has also been observed in longer follow-up studies (McCreadie, Robertson, Hall, and Berry, 1993; Huguelet et al., 1995; Schulze et al., 1997).

Although these attitudes were originally examined in research with the family members of schizophrenic patients, critical, hostile, or emotionally overinvolved attitudes towards others are certainly present in many social environments and are not specific to relatives of schizophrenia patients. Similarly, the relationship between EE and course of illness is not specific to schizophrenic disorders (Miklowitz et al., 1988; Hooley et al., 1986). The presence of high-EE attitudes among relatives is viewed as an indicator that there are strains in the relationship between the patient and the relatives that lead to a stressful social environment. The origins of these attitudes and the direction of any effects of these attitudes remain continuing issues in this literature.

We and others have conceptualized both discrete stressful life events and a high-EE family environment as being components of an overstimulating social environment; the impact of the two is usually assumed to be additive (Brown et al., 1972; Leff, 1987; Nuechterlein and Dawson, 1984). The examination of the impact of these socio-environmental factors on schizophrenia has been studied primarily among individuals who are already affected with the disorder. Thus, their role, if any, in the initial development of schizophrenia is still unknown.

In the prospective longitudinal project, Developmental Processes in Schizophrenic Disorders, that we have conducted at UCLA, a set of summary variables was selected a priori for a multivariate predictive model of relapse, work outcome, and social functioning in the early course of schizophrenia (Nuechterlein et al., 1992). Some variables represented indicators of hypothesized vulnerability factors (familial history of schizophrenia spectrum disorder, certain neurocognitive deficits, and autonomic hyperactivation and hyperreactivity), others were stressors (expressed emotion and stressful life events), and two others represented baseline indices of variables to be examined as outcomes (symptomatic level and premorbid adjustment level) (see Fig. 1).

Method

Subjects

The participants in the schizophrenia group in the Developmental Processes in Schizophrenic Disorders project were required to have had a first onset of psychotic symptoms within two years of project contact (Nuechterlein et al., 1992). Of the 104 participants, 76% were in the midst of a first psychotic episode at initial project contact.

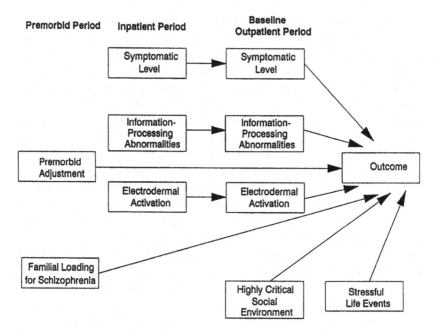

Fig. 1. An a priori multivariate model for predictors of relapse and early course in schizophrenia, which combines selected prominent variables from the scientific literature. Reprinted from Nuechterlein et al., 1992

Thus, many potential effects of chronic illness where minimized in this sample of recent-onset and first-episode patients.

A confirmed diagnosis of schizophrenia or schizoaffective disorder, mainly schizophrenic, by Research Diagnostic Criteria and age at entry between 18 and 45 years were required for study entry. Additional exclusion criteria required participants to have no evidence of a known neurological disorder, recent significant and habitual substance abuse, or premorbid mental retardation (see Nuechterlein et al., 1992 for full inclusion and exclusion criteria). Demographic data for 104 schizophrenic participants are presented in Table 1.

Procedures

To provide a relatively standardized approach to the outpatient psychopharmacologic and psychotherapeutic treatment, all schizophrenia participants were provided treatment at the UCLA Aftercare Program following hospital discharge. Medication was prescribed by two clinic psychiatrists. After an initial period of clinical stabilization averaging two to three months, patients who were judged to be

Table 1. Descriptive data for the 104 schizophrenic participants in longitudinal study

	Age	Gender	Ethnicity/Race	Education
Mean (SD)	23.3 (4.3) years	85 male 19 female	90 Caucasian 7 Hispanic 3 Asian 4 Other	12.4 (2.1) years

appropriate for the standardized starting maintenance dosage of 12.5 mg fluphenazine (Prolixin) decanoate every two weeks were moved to that dosage. This dosage was selected as one that was likely to balance the prophylactic effect and the adverse side effects of this medication (Burnett et al., 1993; Marder et al., 1984). If patients found the antipsychotic medication side effects to be intolerable (10% of cases), dosages as low as 6.25 mg every two weeks were used. The dosage of antipsychotic medication was increased if a psychotic exacerbation, relapse, or other significant increase in symptoms occurred or if a medication increase was otherwise judged clinically indicated. Patients were not entered into this protocol if they had not shown sufficient clinical stability for use of the standard maintenance dose. The psychotherapeutic orientation used at the Aftercare Program was supportive and behaviorally-oriented, with an emphasis on group training in social skills, symptom recognition, and medication usage. Family education was offered to the patients' family members and significant others.

A subsequent phase of this project was designed to identify patients with a short history of illness who do well without continuous antipsychotic medication. Following the one-year period of outpatient treatment with depot antipsychotic medication, schizophrenic participants who were judged to show sufficient remission of psychotic symptoms were invited to participate in a 24-week double-blind placebo-controlled crossover study. Participants who completed the 24 week phase without recurrence of significant psychotic symptoms were invited to try a non-blind period without antipsychotic medication. Patients were urged to resume continuous antipsychotic medication if clinically significant symptoms returned at any time during the crossover or open drug-free periods.

Outcome criteria for significant psychotic exacerbation and psychotic relapse for the initial medicated period were based on the Expanded Brief Psychiatric Rating Scale, as discussed by Nuechter-

lein et al. (1992). Exacerbation and relapse categories were combined into a single class for these analyses, which we refer to as
"relapse" for simplicity. Similar criteria, but with a lower threshold,
were used for the drug crossover and withdrawal period.

Results

Analyses of the relationships of individual predictor variables to
psychotic relapse are summarized here. During this initial 12-month
period in which continuous antipsychotic medication is ensured
through the use of an injectable form of fluphenazine, it is
noteworthy that, among all of our planned univariate course
predictors, only measures of environmental stressors significantly
predict relapse. In other preliminary univariate analyses, the
hypothesized vulnerability factors in the neurocognitive and autonomic domains do predict which patients are able to return to work
or school, but do not significantly predict psychotic relapse (Dawson
et al., 1992; Nuechterlein et al., 1992). Thus, for the purposes of this
chapter on predictors of relapse, we will focus on the results
regarding stressful life events and expressed emotion.

During the period of regular depot antipsychotic medication,
the frequency of stressful life events in the month preceding psychotic
relapse was found to be significantly higher than in comparable
comparison months (Ventura et al., 1989). This was the case even
when only those events that were independent of the patient's control
and not secondary to symptoms were examined (see Fig. 2). Although
causality cannot be proven by this statistical association, the use of
prospective gathering of life events data and a relatively standardized
treatment program allows strong inferences to be drawn in support of
the hypothesis that such independent life events serve as contributing factors or triggers for return of psychotic symptoms.

Unpublished analyses that involve data from some of these
same participants at a later point in time suggest why schizophrenia
patients are so vulnerable to the impact of negative interpersonal life
events (e.g., an argument with a friend). Coping styles, such as the
use of active and avoidant strategies were assessed with the Coping
Responses Inventory (Moos, 1986). Schizophrenic participants failed
to use active problem-focused coping strategies as often as normal
control participants (Ventura et al., 1998). In particular, schizophrenic patients were much less likely to use cognitively oriented problem

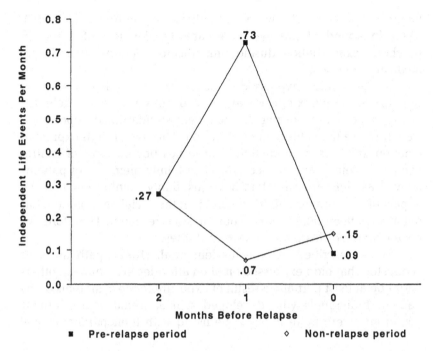

Fig. 2. Mean number of independent life events per month for 11 medicated patients during the months before a psychotic relapse as compared to months that did not precede a relapse. Reprinted with permission from Ventura et al., 1989. Copyright ©American Psychological Association, 1989

solving approaches (e.g., "Making a plan of action and following it") than were normal participants. Furthermore, this failure to use active coping strategies, such as "Logical Analysis" and "Positive Reappraisal" was associated with poorer neurocognitive performance on an early perceptual processing task (Ventura et al., 1998). Thus, a neurocognitive deficit thought to be associated with a vulnerability to schizophrenia may leave patients less able to cope actively with interpersonal life events, and thus make them more likely to be negatively impacted by them.

The findings from schizophrenic participants who had a psychotic exacerbation during the trial without antipsychotic medication provide a powerful comparison to the findings for regularly medicated participants, albeit counterintuitive at first blush. As shown in Fig. 3, patients who had a return of psychotic symptoms while drug-free had significantly fewer independent life events in the month before psychotic exacerbation than during a parallel

month for patients who were on medication (Ventura et al., 1992).
Thus, independent life events apparently play less of a role in
psychotic exacerbation during unmedicated periods than during
medicated periods.

The level of expressed emotion among significant others at
the time of the index episode also significantly predicted likelihood
of psychotic relapse during the one-year standardized depot medication phase (Nuechterlein et al., 1992). The role of high expressed
emotion attitudes in predicting relapse has been a topic of contro-
versy in recent years, particularly since family members of patients
as well as some investigators have justifiably pointed out that the
impact of a severe psychiatric disorder on the social environment has
not always been taken into account in such research. Therefore, we
have examined this issue in several studies.

As described in Nuechterlein et al. (1992), path analyses
suggested that high expressed emotion attitudes in significant others
might be at least partially a result of exposure to the symptoms of the
patient. Individuals who developed schizophrenia at a relatively
young age were more likely to be living with their parents at that

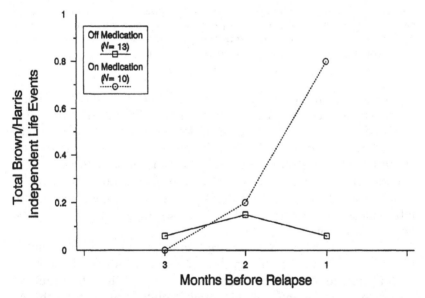

Fig. 3. Mean number of independent life events in the three months preceding
on-medication ($n = 10$) and off-medication ($n = 13$) psychotic relapses. Reprinted with permission from Ventura et al., 1992. Copyright © The Royal College of
Psychiatrists, 1992

point, and these parents were more likely to have high-EE attitudes toward these ill family members. High-EE attitudes, in turn, increased the likelihood of psychotic relapse during the subsequent period on antipsychotic medication (see Fig. 4). Thus, direct exposure to the developing illness was associated with critical or emotionally overinvolved attitudes, which might then function as nonspecific stressors in a vulnerability/stress conception of psychotic relapse.

Our content analysis of the types of behaviors and symptoms most frequently criticized by family members regarding patient behaviors in sample 1 may help to clarify the dynamic relationship between the family's exposure to the ill relatives and the development of high EE attitudes. We found that some of the critical reactions to patients' behavioral deficits were linked to beliefs by family members that the behaviors were intentional as opposed to being part of a psychiatric disorder that was not under the patient's control (Weisman et al., 1998).

In order to understand better the relationship between high EE and the recurrence of psychotic symptoms, in collaboration with our friend and colleague Michael J. Goldstein, microanalyses of 20-

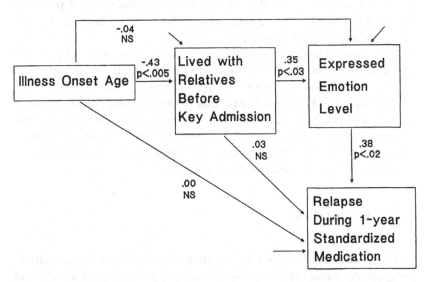

Fig. 4. Path analysis of chain of effects from age of onset of patient's illness through patient's residence before key hospital admission and expressed emotion level to likelihood of psychotic relapse. Reprinted with permission from Nuechterlein et al., 1992. Copyright © The Royal College of Psychiatrists, 1992

minute family interactions were completed for these same families. High EE-critical relatives were characterized by a more negative interactional style and showed a pattern of negative escalation of nonverbal behavior during these interactions (Hahlweg et al., 1989). In results of a separate microanalysis of patient behaviors related to subclinical psychopathology during these family interactions, patient's odd and disruptive verbal behavior appeared to elicit criticism from their high-EE family members, which in turn was followed by more unusual and disruptive behavior (Rosenfarb et al., 1995). These findings support the conceptualization of EE as a bidirectional or transactual process. Convergent evidence comes from the microanalyses of the nonverbal and parlinguistic behaviors during these interactions, which revealed more hostile and unusual behavior in the patients from high-EE families than patients living in low-EE environments (Woo et al., 1997). Further analysis of the subclinical psychopathology ratings in patients revealed that the unusual behavior following criticism was present mainly for patients with working memory deficits (Rosenfarb et al., 2000). This finding illustrates how an interpersonal stressor may interact with a neurocognitive vulnerability factor to contribute to increased psychopathology.

In order to conclude that high-EE attitudes contribute to a stressful environment and is not in itself an indication of personal psychiatric illness or a genetic vulnerability to schizophrenia, the independence of EE from these other factors needs to be demonstrated. We found that EE level is generally independent of parental psychiatric illness, except in the rare case in which the parent has a very severe mental disorder (Goldstein et al., 1992). We have also demonstrated that high EE attitudes do not correspond to a family history of psychiatric disorders in the parents' own families of origin (Subotnik et al., 2001). Thus, the presence of high-EE attitudes does not appear to be an indirect indicator of personal psychopathology or of a genetic susceptibility to schizophrenia.

Discussion

Our research group at UCLA has conducted a series of longitudinal, prospective studies of psychobiological and psychosocial factors that contribute to the initial course of schizophrenia (Nuechterlein et al., 1992), some of which involved a collaboration with our late friend and colleague Michael J. Goldstein, Ph.D. In this chapter we emphasize results concerning psychosocial stressors, which were found to be significant predictors of the reemergence of psychosis during a one-year follow-through period on depot maintenance antipsychotic medication. Although neurocognitive and psychophysiological factors were significantly related to important aspects of functional outcome, these factors did not by themselves predict psychotic relapse.

As described by Ventura et al. (1989), the use of monthly, prospective assessments of stressful life events made it possible to avoid recall biases that often occur when a patient who has already relapsed is asked to report the events that occurred in the weeks just prior to the relapse. We also focused on those life events that could not logically be under that patient's control or a result of the patient's illness. Under these rigorous methodological conditions, our finding that the number of stressful life events in the month preceding psychotic relapse was significantly higher than in comparison months allows us to more confidently infer that the life events contributed to triggering the return of psychosis (Ventura et al., 1989). Two studies reported subsequent to our initial 1989 report of these findings have supported the evidence for increased rates of independent life events in the six months prior to the exacerbation of psychosis (Bebbington et al., 1993; Hirsch et al., 1996). Neither of these subsequent studies have replicated, however, the specific timing of a marked increase in the frequency of life events in the month prior to exacerbation or relapse. Our own subsequent analyses using survival analyses with the entire initial schizophrenia sample from this project (Ventura et al., 2000) also suggests that the period of increased risk of exacerbation after an independent life event extends through at least the subsequent three months. Other prospective research has shown that life events do not have to be large in magnitude to have an impact; both major and minor events are predictors of positive symptom exacerbation and relapse in schizophrenia (Malla et al., 1990). Furthermore, daily hassles have been associated with increased subjective distress in schizophrenia (Norman and Malla, 1991).

Initial indications from analyses of a subsequent trial without maintenance antipsychotic medication suggest that independent life events may have less influence as triggers of psychotic exacerbations during this period. This raises the interesting possibility that the primary predictors of psychotic exacerbation for patients on maintenance antipsychotic medication may be different from the predictors during a medication-free period. The stronger role of stressors in influencing psychotic exacerbation during presence of antipsychotic

medication may at first seem counter-intuitive, because this medication would be expected to protect against return of psychotic
symptoms. However, it is consistent with a model in which antipsychotic medication has the effect of raising the threshold for
appearance of psychotic symptoms (Leff, 1987; Liberman, 1986). With
the threshold raised, major stressors would increase liability sufficiently to reach threshold for symptom formation. During a medication-free period, the relationship between life events and relapse
would be less salient given the patient's greater vulnerability to
many psychobiological and environmental fluctuations that might
lead to exacerbation. Thus, without antipsychotic medication, the
threshold is reached more easily in the absence of major life events.

Our finding that high levels of familial expressed emotion
predict psychotic relapse over a one-year period is consistent with
that of a recent study that shares many of the design considerations
and sample composition as the UCLA research program (Linszen
et al., 1997). In our sample, family members may have been reacting
critically to behavioral deficits secondary to negative symptoms of
schizophrenia, but which the family members believed were under
the ill relative's control (Weisman et al., 1998). This is consistent with
other findings that the burden of coping with a lower functioning
family member may contribute to the development of critical, hostile,
and emotionally overinvolved attitudes towards that individual
(Barrowclough and Parle, 1997; Bean et al., 1996; Nuechterlein
et al., 1992; Scazufca and Kuipers, 1996). In previous research,
relatives who were substantially bothered by, and felt unable to cope
with, the patient's behavior were also more likely to be high in EE
(Barrowclough and Parle, 1997). The inability to engage in paid
employment is another source of family burden; both poor premorbid
and current occupational functioning have been found to be associated with more negative attitudes towards that family member (Bean
et al., 1996; Bentsen et al., 1998). In fact, lack of paid employment
was a robust predictor of criticism and hostility, whereas three key
dimensions of psychiatric symptoms (positive, negative, and disorganized symptoms) were not predictive of negative attitudes by
family members (Bean et al., 1996). Thus, high-EE family members
report feeling more burdened by management issues common to
schizophrenia patients, some of which are distinctive and others
similar to those in other disorders (Barrowclough and Parle, 1997;
Holroyd and Guthrie, 1979; Walker et al., 1992).

The expressed emotion literature has usually emphasized the role of highly critical and emotionally overinvolved attitudes in raising relapse risk. However, we found that none of the patients from low expressed emotion environments had a psychotic relapse during the one-year period on antipsychotic medication (0 of 19 cases). Clearly the protective nature of a low expressed emotion environment deserves more attention. Our work suggests that the treatment of individuals with schizophrenia should involve family members whenever feasible. By doing so, a home environment in which there is a realistic understanding of the patient's disorder and functional capacity can be encouraged. Furthermore, family members can gain an awareness of the potentially deleterious impact of stressful life events on the individual with schizophrenia. Family members and patients may then together learn optimal strategies for coping with stressors in ways that minimize relapse risks and maximize effective functioning.

Acknowledgments

We would like to acknowledge the UCLA Aftercare Research Program patients who by participating in the research are helping us to better understand the early course of schizophrenia. We thank the clinicians and staff who helped in the collection and recording of the symptom information: Craig Childress, M.A., Rhonda Daily, Sally Friedlob, M.S.W., Debbie Gioia, Ph.D., Karen Hemmerling, Portia Loughman, B.A., David Lukoff, Ph.D., Mark McGee, B.A., Sandra Rappe, M.S.W., Karen Snyder, Ph.D., Mitchell Stoddard, Ph.D., Margie Stratton, M.S.W., Joseph Tietz, Ph.D., Kenneth Zaucha, Ph.D. We also thank Michael Gitlin, M.D., David Fogelson, M.D., and George Bartzokis, M.D., for their psychiatric care of the Aftercare Program patients. We acknowledge the statistical assistance of Jim Mintz, Ph.D., and Sun Hwang, M.S., of the Methodology and Statistical Support Unit (directed by Dr. Mintz) of the UCLA Center for Research on Treatment and Rehabilitation of Psychosis (directed by Robert P. Liberman, M.D.). This research was supported in part by National Institute of Mental Health Grants MH37705 and MH30911.

References

Barrowclough, C. and Parle, M. (1997): Appraisal, psychological adjustment and expressed emotion in relatives of patients suffering from schizophrenia. British Journal of Psychiatry 171: 26–30

Bean, G., Beiser, M., Zhang-Wong, J., and Iacono, W. (1996): Negative labeling of individuals with first episode schizophrenia: the effect of premorbid functioning. Schizophrenia Research 22: 111–118

Bebbington, P., Wilkins, S., Jones, P.B., Foerster A. et al. (1993): Life events and psychosis: Initial results from the Camberwell Collaborative Psychosis Study. British Journal of Psychiatry 162: 2–79

Bentsen, H., Notland, T.H., Munkvold, O., Boye, B. et al. (1998): Guilt proneness and expressed emotion in relatives of patients with schizophrenia or related psychoses. British Journal of Medical Psychology 71: 125–138

Brown, G.W. and Birley, J.L.T. (1968): Crisis and life change and the onset of schizophrenia. Journal of Health Social Behavior 9: 203–214

Brown, G.W., Birley, J.L.T., and Wing, J.K. (1972): Influence of family life on the course of schizophrenic disorders: A replication. British Journal of Psychiatry 121: 241–258

Burnett, P.L., Galletly, C.A., Moyle, R.J., and Clark, C.R. (1993): Low-dose depot medication in schizophrenia. Schizophrenia Bulletin 19: 155–164

Butzlaff, R.L. and Hooley, J.M. (1998): Expressed emotion and psychiatric relapse. Archives of General Psychiatry 55: 547–552

Cannon, T.D., Kaprio, J., Lönnqvist, J., Huttunen, M., and Koshenvuo, M. (1998): The genetic epidemiology of schizophrenia in a Finnish twin cohort. Archives of General Psychiatry 55: 67–74

Dawson, M.E., Nuechterlein, K.H., and Schell, A.M. (1992): Electrodermal anomalies in recent-onset schizophrenia: Relationships to symptoms and prognosis. Schizophrenia Bulletin 18: 295–311

Day, R., Nielsen, J.A., Korten, A. et al. (1987): Stressful life events preceding the acute onset of schizophrenia: A cross-national study from the World Health Organization. Culture, Medicine and Psychiatry 11: 123–205

Goldstein, M.J., Talovic, S.A., Nuechterlein, K.H., Fogelson, D.L., Subotnik, K.L., and Asarnow, R.F. (1992): Family interaction versus individual psychopathology: Do they indicate the same processes in the families of schizophrenics? British Journal of Psychiatry 161(Suppl. 18): 97–102

Hahlweg, K., Goldstein, M.J., Nuechterlein, K.H., Magaa, A.B., Mintz, J., Doane, J.A., Miklowitz, D.J., and Snyder, K. (1989): Expressed emotion and patient-relative interaction in families of recent onset schizophrenics. Journal of Consulting and Clinical Psychology 57(1): 11–18

Hardesty, J., Falloon, I.R.H., and Shirin, K. (1985): The impact of life events, stress, coping on the morbidity of schizophrenia. In: Family management of schizophrenia (Fallon, I.R.H., ed.), pp. 137–152. Baltimore and London: The Johns Hopkins University Press

Hirsch, S., Bowen, J., Emami, J., Cramer, P., Jolley, A., Haw, C., and Dickinson, M. (1996): A one year prospective study of the effect of life events and medication in the aetiology of schizophrenic relapse. British Journal of Psychiatry 168: 49–56

Holroyd, J. and Gurthrie, D. (1979): Stress in families of children with neuromuscular disease. Journal of Clinical Psychology 35: 734–739

Hooley, J.M., Orley, J., and Teasdale, J.D. (1986): Levels of expressed emotion and relapse in depressed patients. British Journal of Psychiatry 148: 642–647

Huguelet, P., Favre, S., Binyet, S., Gonzalez, C. et al. (1995): The use of the Expressed Emotion Index as a predictor of outcome in first admitted schizophrenic patients in a French speaking area of Switzerland. Acta Psychiatrica Scandinavica 92(6): 447–452

Kavanagh, D.J. (1992): Recent developments in expressed emotion and schizophrenia. British Journal of Psychiatry 160: 601–620

Kendler, K.S. and Diehl, S.R. (1993): The genetics of schizophrenia: A current, genetic-epidemiologic perspective. Schizophrenia Bulletin 19: 261–285

Leff, J. (1987): A model of schizophrenic vulnerability to environmental factors. In: Search for the causes of schizophrenia (Haefner, H., Gattaz, W.F., Janzarik, W., eds.), pp. 317–330. Berlin: Springer

Lewis, S.W. and Murray, R.M. (1987): Obstetric complications, neurodevelopmental deviance, and risk of schizophrenia. Journal of Psychiatric Research 21: 413–421

Liberman, R.P. (1986): Coping and competence as protective factors in the vulnerability-stress model of schizophrenia. In: Treatment of schizophrenia: Family assessment and intervention (Goldstein, M.J., Hand, I., Hahlweg, K., eds.), pp. 201–215. Berlin: Springer

Linszen, D.H., Dingemans, P.M., Nugter, M.A, Ven der Does, A.J.W., Scholte, W.F., and Lenior, M.A. (1997): Patient attributes and expressed emotion as a risk factor for psychotic relapse. Schizophrenia Bulletin 23: 119–130

Malla, A.K., Cortese, L., Shaw, T.S., and Ginsberg, B. (1990): Life events and relapse in schizophrenia: A one year prospective study. Social Psychiatry and Psychiatric Epidemiology 25: 221–224

Marder, S.R., Van Putten, T., McKenzie, J., Lebell, M., Faltico, G., and May, P.R.A. (1984): Costs and benefits of two doses of fluphenazine. Archives of General Psychiatry 41: 1025–1029

McCreadie, R.G., Robertson, L.J., Hall, D.J., and Berry, I. (1993): The Nithsdale schizophrenia surveys: XI. relatives' expressed emotion: Stability over five years and its relation to relapse. British Journal of Psychiatry 162: 393–397

Mednick, S.A., Machon, R.A., Huttunen, M.O., and Bonett D. (1988): Adult schizophrenia following prenatal exposure to an influenza epidemic. Archives of General Psychiatry 45: 189–192

Miklowitz, D.J. (1994): Family risk indicators of schizophrenia. Schizophrenia Bulletin 20(1): 137–149

Miklowitz, D.J., Goldstein, M.J., Nuechterlein, K.H., Snyder, K.S., and Mintz, J. (1988): Family factors and the course of bipolar affective disorder. Archives of General Psychiatry 45: 225–231

Moos, R.H. (1986): Coping responses inventory. Palo Alto, CA: Stanford University and Veterans Administration Medical Centers

Murray, R.M., O'Callaghan, E., Castle, D.J., and Lewis, S.W. (1992): A neurodevelopmental approach to the classification of schizophrenia. Schizophrenia Bulletin 18: 319–332

Norman, R.M.G. and Malla, A.K. (1991): Subjective stress in schizophrenic patients. Social Psychiatry and Psychiatric Epidemiology 26: 212–216

Nuechterlein, K.H. and Dawson, M.E. (1984): A heuristic vulnerability/stress model of schizophrenic episodes. Schizophrenia Bulletin 10: 300–312

Nuechterlein, K.H., Dawson, M.E., Gitlin, M., Ventura, J., Goldstein, M.J., Snyder, K.S., Yee, C.M., and Mintz, J. (1992): Developmental processes in schizophrenic disorders: Longitudinal studies of vulnerability and stress. Schizophrenia Bulletin 18: 387–425

Nuechterlein, K.H., Snyder, K.S., and Mintz, J. (1992): Paths to relapse: Possible transactional processes connecting patient illness onset, expressed emotion, and psychotic relapse. British Journal of Psychiatry 161(Suppl. 18): 88–96

Parnas, J. and Mednick, S.A. (1991): Early predictors of onset and course of schizophrenia and schizophrenia spectrum. In: Search for the causes of schizophrenia (Haefner, H. and Gattaz, W.F., eds.), Vol. II, pp. 34–47. Berlin: Springer

Rosenfarb, I.S., Goldstein, M.J., Mintz, J., and Nuechterlein, K.H. (1995): Expressed emotion and subclinical psychopathology observable within the transactions between schizophrenic patients and their family members. Journal of Abnormal Psychology 104: 259–267

Rosenfarb, I.S., Nuechterlein, K.H., and Goldstein, M.J. (2000) Neurocognitive vulnerability, interpersonal criticism, and the emergence of unusual thinking by patients with schizophrenia during family transactions. Archives of General Psychiatry 57: 1174–1179

Scazufca, M. and Kuipers, E (1996): Links between expressed emotion and burden of care in relatives of patients with schizophrenia. British Journal of Psychiatry 168(5): 580–587

Schulze Moenking, H.S., Hornung, W.P., Stricker, K., and Buchkremer, G. (1997): Expressed emotion in an 8 year follow-up. European Psychiatry 12: 105–110

Subotnik, K.L., Goldstein, M.J., Nuechterlein, K.H., and Mintz, J. (2001): Are communication deviance and expressed emotion related to family history of psychiatric disorders in schizophrenia? Manuscript submitted for publication

Ventura J., Nuechterlein, K.H., Hardesty, J.P., and Gitlin, M. (1992): Life events and schizophrenic relapse after withdrawal of medication. British Journal of Psychiatry 161: 615–620

Ventura, J., Nuechterlein, K.H., Lukoff, D., and Hardesty, J.P. (1989): A prospective study of stressful life events and schizophrenic relapse. Journal of Abnormal Psychology 98: 407–411

Ventura, J., Nuechterlein, K.H., Subotnik, K.L., Gitlin, M., Bartzokis, G., and Sharou, J. (1998, May 30–June 4). Coping responses and neurocognitive functioning in schizophrenia. Paper presented at the 151st meeting of the American Psychiatric Association, Toronto

Ventura, J., Nuechterlein, K.H., Subotnik, K.L., Pederson Hardesty, J., and Mintz, J. (2000). Life events can trigger depressive exacerbation in the early course of schizophrenia. Journal of Abnormal Psychology 109: 139–144.

Walker, L.S., Van Slyke, D.A., and Newbrough, J.R. (1992): Family resources and stress: A comparison of families of children with cystic fibrosis, diabetes, and mental retardation. Journal of Pediatric Psychology 17: 327–343

Weisman, A.G., Nuechterlein, K.H., Goldstein, M.J., and Snyder, K. (1998): Expressed emotion, attributions, and schizophrenia symptom dimensions. Journal of Abnormal Psychology 107(2): 355–359

Woo, S.M., Goldstein, M.J., and Nuechterlein, K.H. (1997): Relatives' expressed emotion and non-verbal signs of subclinical psychopathology in schizophrenic patients. British Journal of Psychiatry 170: 58–61

Zubin, J. and Spring, B. (1977): Vulnerability – A new view of schizophrenia. Journal of Abnormal Psychology 86: 103–126

8
Borderline Personality Disorder and the Family

Jill M. Hooley and George M. Dominiak

Borderline personality disorder (BPD) is a major clinical problem. It is arguably the most severe form of personality pathology that mental health professionals treat. It is also the most common personality disorder found in clinical settings worldwide (Loranger et al., 1994). With a prevalence of approximately 15% among psychiatric outpatients (Widiger and Weissman, 1991) and an estimated prevalence of 1–2% in the general population (Swartz et al., 1990), borderline patients are not few in number. Moreover, because BPD is typically a chronic form of psychopathology characterized by a high level of suffering on the part of the patient and a suicide rate of around 10% (Paris, 1999), it is a disorder that demands clinical and empirical attention.

Despite the obvious need to understand the nature and origins of BPD, researchers know surprisingly little about it. Although the psychoanalytic literature is rich with regard to theoretical discussions of BPD, the disorder was largely ignored by empirical researchers until the 1980s. In recent years, BPD has become the most researched of the DSM Axis II disorders. Much, however, remains to be learned.

During his long and distinguished career, Michael Goldstein never failed to acknowledge the importance of family transactions with respect to psychopathology. It therefore seems fitting that, in a book of papers written in his honor, the focus of this chapter is on family aspects of borderline personality disorder. Theoretical discussions of BPD place heavy emphasis on the role of the family in the development of the disorder. Recent data also suggest that family variables may play a role in the course of the illness. In this chapter we review what is known about the family environments of borderline patients from a theoretical and empirical perspective. Although space constraints make it impossible for us to provide a comprehensive summary of all aspects of all approaches to this fascinating disorder, we hope to leave readers with an appreciation of the importance of family variables for the understanding and treatment of BPD.

Clinical Perspective

The term "borderline" was first introduced by Adolf Stern, a psychoanalyst, in 1938. Stern used the word borderline to describe patients who appeared to be on the border between psychosis and neurosis. Yet the diagnosis remained of interest only within the psychoanalytic literature and was not incorporated into either DSM-I or DSM-II. The disorder was also slow in being incorporated into the ICD. The delay was due, in large measure, to the considerable resistance to the diagnosis in Europe (e.g., Tyrer, 1988). Increasingly, however, the diagnosis of BPD based on DSM criteria is now attracting the attention of European as well as American researchers and clinicians (e.g., Ryle, 1997; Waller, 1994).

The pathological features of BPD include impulsivity and affective instability as well as cognitive disturbances (Paris, 1999). Nine specific symptoms are recognized within DSM-IV. These include a pattern of intense unstable interpersonal relationships, intense anger, reactivity of mood, recurrent suicidality, and chronic feelings of emptiness. The disorder is more commonly diagnosed in women (75% of cases; see Gunderson, 1984; Swartz et al., 1990), although it appears to take a similar clinical form in men (Paris, 1994). It is also the case that patients with BPD are extremely likely to have additional Axis I diagnoses. For example, there is a high degree of co-morbidity between BPD and mood disorders (Pope et al., 1983). Many patients with BPD also suffer from eating disorders, particularly those that involve bulimic symptoms (Hull et al., 1993; Waller, 1994).

The Etiology of Borderline PD

Biological Perspectives

The etiology of borderline personality disorder is almost certainly multidimensional. At the very least, some form of biological vulnerability is likely to be necessary, a point acknowledged by most theorists regardless of orientation (e.g., Kernberg, 1984; Linehan, 1993). There is some preliminary evidence that BPD may run in families (Nigg and Goldsmith, 1994). However, virtually all of the studies to date have relied on patients' reports of psychopathology in their relatives rather than relying on interviews with the relatives themselves. This is a major methodological problem because border-line patients often view their families extremely negatively. Given the present state of knowledge, it is too soon to conclude that the disorder has a genetic basis. However, there is some reason to believe that the form of BPD characterized by impulsivity and affective instability may reflect a partly genetically influenced subsyndrome (Torgersen, 1994). It is also highly likely that abnormalities in several neuro-transmitter systems play a contributing role in BPD (Siever and Davis, 1991). Research has implicated acetylcholine (ACH), norepinephrine (NE), and gamma-aminobutyric acid (GABA) in the neurochemistry of affective instability. Neurotransmitters such as serotonin (5-HT) and arginine vasopressin (AVP) are also thought to be involved in the neurochemistry of impulsive aggression (Gurvitz et al., 2000).

These developments notwithstanding, disturbances or dys-regulations at the biological or temperamental level are not consid-ered sufficient to result in the development of BPD. Within the literature on BPD there is also a considerable focus on developmen-tal issues. In all cases, major theoretical approaches to BPD place heavy emphasis on the importance of the family environment and describe some form of disrupted early environment in the etiology of the disorder. In all probability, these factors interact with underlying biological vulnerability in a subtle and complex way.

Psychoanalytic Perspectives

Psychoanalytic theories of BPD primarily focus on disruptions in the process of psychological development. In particular, emphasis is placed on the experience of the parent-child relationship as it sup-ports, shapes or potentially disrupts personality development. Object relations theorists such as Klein (1948), Fairbairn (1952), Winnicott (1965), and Kernberg (1984) suggest that, by nature, humans seek deep personal attachment to caretakers. Over time, the dynamics of child-parent interactions set patterns of relating, social expectations and behaviors that can be recognized by clinicians in the adult patient. Clinically, it is hypothesized that social interactions in the present are experienced and distorted by the expectations fixed by childhood interactions with others. Patterns of behavior, psychological defense mechanisms and associated emotions are elicited in the present as predetermined by past experience. Specifically, internalized images of past familial relationships and the emotions associated with them are stimulated by present day human contacts.

BPD symptoms are seen as arising from a failure in the caretaking environment to meet the emotional developmental requirement of consistency, availability, and empathic attunement to personal needs. Basic trust in the family environment is altered and powerful emotions cannot be mitigated by the parent-child relationship. Patterns of certain defenses such as splitting (separating internal experiences) and projection (attributing self experiences as being located in others), failed attempts to mitigate impulses (see Kernberg, 1984) and negative self valuations become ingrained in the personality and manifest as borderline personality characteristics.

Similarly, self-psychology psychoanalytic theory as initially presented by Kohut (1971) emphasizes the importance of maternal attunement to the child's needs. In particular, empathic responses that mirror the child's strengths and efforts at exploration and that validate the child's sense of mastery are key components. When repeatedly disrupted, the child's need for a sense of safety and predictability in a responsive family environment is left unmet. The child reacts with hurt angry emotions that disrupt the development of positive self-regard and the capacity for interpersonal empathy (Adler, 1985). BPD is viewed as a developed pattern of maladaptive relating resulting from extremely conflicted relations with loved ones in the past. Finally, trauma theory (Herman, 1992) relates BPD symptoms to a history of childhood sexual, physical or psychological trauma and the attempts at mitigating the emotional upheaval that results. BPD per se is seen as one of many possible clusters of behavioral and psychological adaptations to trauma experiences.

Because most of the psychoanalytic theories of BPD are based on retrospective hypothesizing from adult clinical experience or, in the case of trauma theory, on describing the strong association of patient trauma histories with specified BPD-like symptoms, they have little predictive data based validity. However, the theories are seen as useful to clinicians using these descriptive models as a means of helping patients understand their present experience. They have also significantly influenced the clinical investigation of BPD.

The Families of Borderline Patients

As we note above, much of the thinking about the etiology of borderline pathology is based on extensive clinical experience. Yet, in the absence of empirical data, theoretical notions about the early environments of borderline patients remain nothing more than speculation. What researchers need to know is what pre-borderline children actually experienced in their families when they were growing up. Unfortunately, almost all efforts to assess the early environments of borderline patients have been based on patients' retrospective reports. Clearly, there are many methodological problems associated with this. The first is the problem of recall. Can we really obtain a reliable report of the patient's emotional environment at critical points in development by asking for this information, often decades later? Second, what impact might the patients' levels of symptomatology have on their retrospective reporting of their early childhood experiences? As Paris (1999) correctly points out, distortions of reports of recent life events are quite common in borderline patients. Therapists are also often strikingly aware of the tendency of borderline patients to blame others for their current problems and difficulties. Of course, this is not to say that borderline patients might not be reliable reporters of events that occurred to them earlier in their lives. As researchers, however, we need to remain cognizant of the limitations of using the self-reports of borderline patients about their early family environments. With this in mind, we now discuss the empirical literature with an eye to examining the developmental context of BPD.

Physical and Sexual Abuse

Beginning in the mid-1980s, many clinicians began to take note of the high rates of trauma that seemed to characterize the early lives of many of their patients. These clinical impressions were subsequently supported by several empirically-oriented studies that linked borderline PD and early abusive experiences. Westen et al. (1990) for example, noted that sexual or physical abuse was documented in the charts of more than half of a sample of 27 patients diagnosed with BPD. In a more systematic study, Ogata and her colleagues (Ogata et al., 1990) noted that 71% of a sample of 24 borderline patients reported a history of sexual abuse compared to 22% of a control sample of 18 depressed patients. A similar increased rate of sexual abuse in borderlines relative to psychiatric controls was also reported by Zanarini et al. (1989).

Neither Ogata et al. (1990) nor Zanarini and her colleagues (1989) found elevated rates of physical abuse in their borderline samples relative to controls. However, this is not invariably the case. Weaver and Clum (1993) for example, found that borderline patients reported higher rates of both sexual abuse and physical abuse than did a sample of non-borderline depressed controls. Interestingly, however, sexual abuse was a powerful predictor of later BPD even when physical abuse was statistically controlled.

It is, of course, important to keep in mind that not everyone who experiences physical or sexual abuse in childhood will go on to develop BPD. Childhood sexual abuse is also not a specific risk factor for BPD. Rather, early sexual or physical trauma is associated with a broad range of later clinical problems. A recent meta-analysis has also indicated that the effect size of the association between early sexual abuse and later BPD, although significant, is nonetheless modest ($r = 0.28$; see Fossati et al., 1999). Nonetheless, many patients with BPD report abusive experiences early in their lives. Whether these experiences are directly involved in the etiology of BPD remains unclear. What may be most important is that the family climate is one in which such abusive experiences can occur. Gunderson and Englund (1981) noted that the characteristic that most distinguished families of borderline patients from families of patients with other psychiatric disorders was some kind of neglect of the child, broadly defined. This raises the question of whether it is sexual or physical abuse per se that is so damaging with respect to the later development of BPD, or whether it is lack of care and parental protection that plays the most important etiological role. Ogata, Silk, Goodrich et al. (1990) noted that in their sample of borderline patients, sexual abuse was perpetrated not only by parents but also by siblings, relatives, and non-relatives. These authors regard the high rates of non-parental abuse as indicative of general disorganization, lack of protection, and pathological boundaries in the families of borderlines. In other words, the link between early abusive experiences in childhood and later BPD may reflect an underlying and severe form of parental failure. As we highlight below, failures of parenting have long been regarded as being at the heart of the development of BPD.

Parental Absence and Neglect

In many respects, BPD can be conceptualized as a disorder of attachment. Indeed, a hallmark of this disorder is marked difficulties in interpersonal relationships. Perhaps not surprisingly, evidence of disrupted early attachments can be found in the empirical literature. For example, in an early study, Bradley (1979) reported that separations from the mother of 3–4 weeks or more were more common in a sample of borderline children than they were in two samples of comparison children. 64% of the children who subsequently developed BPD experienced such separations during their first five years of life. In the 2 control samples, however, the combined rate of maternal separation was only 12%.

Continuing the theme of parental absence, it has also been noted, relative to depressed or schizophrenic controls, that borderlines are less likely to come from intact families (Soloff and Millward, 1983). In particular, Soloff and Millward noted the higher rate of paternal loss in the borderlines – typically from death or divorce. However, it must also be noted that evidence of parental absence is not invariably found. Several studies reported no significant differences with respect to early separation in borderlines relative to controls (Ogata et al., 1990a; Paris et al., 1988; Weaver and Clum, 1993). However, Ogata et al. noted that the borderlines in their study did have more parental separations of 2 or more weeks at some point in their childhoods and Paris et al. mention that the borderlines had more separation and loss experiences. Obviously much depends on which variables are selected for analysis and how specific or global the analyses are. Moreover, to the extent that early loss and depression are linked, selecting depressed patients as controls may make it harder to demonstrate greater rates of early separation and loss in BPD patients.

Periods of parental absence are clearly stressful for most children. However, even when they are physically present in the home, some parents may be emotionally unavailable. In such cases, the needs of the child may go unnoticed or be ignored. This climate of emotional deprivation may interact with temperamental vulnerabilities to create a context in which BPD may develop.

Consistent with this notion is evidence that families of borderline patients are more emotionally distant and less involved than are families of control patients. In an early and small-scale study, Gunderson and colleagues (Gunderson et al., 1980) observed that some kind of neglect of the child was a major factor discriminating the families of borderline patients from the families of schizophrenia patients or the families of patients diagnosed with neurotic conditions. Typically, this neglect took the form of under-involvement of the parent or a general tendency to deny problems, including the pathology of their offspring. Relative to the control patients, the borderline patients in Soloff and Millward's (1983) study also recalled their fathers as being more under-involved, while the borderline patients studied by Frank and Paris (1981) remembered their parents (particularly their fathers) as being less supportive and more disinterested in them than did a control sample of neurotic or other (non-BPD) Axis II patients. Emotional withdrawal of caretakers has also been shown to be more prevalent in families of borderline patients relative to families of antisocial PD controls (Zanarini et al., 1997). In short, much of the available empirical evidence points to problems with emotional expression and demonstrations of caring in the early childhood environments of borderline patients (see also Waller, 1994).

Abnormal Parenting

The failures in parenting that characterize the early home environments of borderline patients span an extremely wide range of severity. Experiences of abuse as well as separations from caretakers might well be expected to have a profound influence on the psychological development of any child. However, there is also evidence that other, less obviously pathological family environments, might also be involved in the development of BPD. Again, however, the central theme appears to be one of emotional neglect of the child. In some cases this may be deliberate. In other cases it may be the result of psychopathology in the parents themselves.

For example, Gunderson et al. (1980) observed that the mothers and fathers of borderline patients were more disturbed and less functional than were the parents of comparison patients. More specifically, he noted a tightness of the marital bond that essentially excluded the child. A similar pattern was described by Feldman and

Guttman (1984) based on a small study of 16 families. Here, the central finding that characterized the families of the borderlines was a "literal-minded" parent who lacked the ability to empathize with the child. Consistent with the notion of bi-parental failure, the other parent was too committed to the spouse or too under-involved generally to be emotionally committed to the child. Higher levels of verbal abuse, greater family conflict, less family cohesiveness, and psychopathology in the parents are also frequently noted in the families of borderlines relative to the families of control patients (Ogata et al., 1990b; Paris et al., 1988; Soloff and Millward, 1983; Weaver and Clum, 1993; Zanarini et al., 1997).

The consistent theme here is that the family is either unable or unwilling to devote emotional resources to the child. Although the reasons for this might vary, the result is that the child is raised in an environment that fosters a sense of emotional deprivation. Although some children may be temperamentally able to cope with this lack of emotional support or may have the skills to get their emotional needs met elsewhere, this is not invariably the case. When coupled with a vulnerable temperament, this kind of family context may well engender the later development of BPD.

Role of the Family in the Course of the Illness

Although the family environments of borderline patients have long been a focus of theoretical interest and empirical attention, the role of the family in the course of the illness has been little explored. Yet there are many reasons to expect that this might be a productive avenue of inquiry. Family factors are clearly highly relevant to a full understanding of BPD. It is also the case that many of the family variables that have been theoretically and empirically linked to BPD have much in common with the characteristics of the family environment captured in the expressed emotion (EE) construct. The literature on EE provides ample evidence that such family characteristics as criticism, hostility, and emotional overinvolvement (EOI) predict poor clinical outcomes in disorders such as schizophrenia, unipolar depression and bipolar disorder (see Butzlaff and Hooley, 1998). Because EE is a valid construct that can be measured reliably, it provides one way in which some hypotheses about the family variables important with respect to BPD might be explored (Links and Blum, 1990).

In the early 1990s, we began the first study of the predictive validity of EE in BPD (Hooley and Hoffman, 1999). We recruited a sample of 41 borderline patients during an inpatient hospitalization and assessed EE in their relatives in the conventional manner using the Camberwell Family Interview (Vaughn and Leff, 1976). One year after hospital discharge we re-contacted patients and their families and collected information on how patients had fared in the intervening period. We were successful in following up the majority (85%) of patients from our original sample and in collecting reliable outcome data on the patients. Clinical outcome was rated on a 1 (high) –5 (low) scale of global functioning based on the presence and severity of symptoms and overall social and occupational adjustment. Rehospitalization during the follow-up period was also used as a second (dichotomous) measure of outcome.

In keeping with what is typically found for patients with BPD, the one-year clinical outcomes of the patients was generally poor (see Fig. 1). More than half of the patients (54%) were rehospitalized again within the one-year follow-up period and 1 (3%) was treated in an Emergency Room but not hospitalized. A further 11% still had significant symptoms but had not experienced an exacerbation of symptoms that warranted hospitalization or treatment on an emergency basis. Despite these generally negative clinical

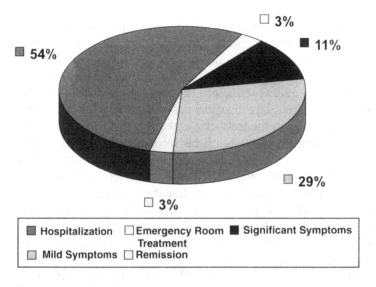

Fig. 1. 1-year clinical outcomes of borderline patients

outcomes, approximately one third of the sample was doing quite well in the year after hospital discharge; 29% of patients reported only mild symptoms and one patient (3%) experienced a full remission of symptoms.

It is interesting to note that, despite the considerable heterogeneity of clinical outcomes in our patients, the majority of clinical and demographic variables such as age, gender, socio-economic status, and chronicity of illness failed to predict how patients fared after leaving the hospital. Only the severity of the patients' symptoms during the index hospitalization was significantly and positively correlated with poorer clinical outcomes at 1-year follow-up. The more symptoms of BPD patients reported initially, the worse they tended to do in the months after leaving the hospital.

We then explored the predictive validity of the EE variables. Contrary to what is typically found for samples of patients with schizophrenia and mood disorders, high levels of family criticism and hostility were not associated with poor clinical outcome for the borderline patients. In fact, as can be seen in Fig. 2, the most critical family members of the borderline patients who did poorly made approximately the same number of critical comments as the most critical family members of the borderline patients who did well (means = 13.6 vs 12.5 criticisms respectively). What did predict patients' clinical outcomes, however, was the relatives' levels of emotional overinvolvement (EOI). EOI reflects an exaggerated or dramatic response to the patient's illness or a response that is characterized by extreme devotion and self-sacrifice. In schizophrenia, high levels of family EOI are associated with patients doing worse

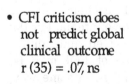

- CFI criticism does not predict global clinical outcome r (35) = .07, ns

- CFI criticism does not predict hospitalization r (35) = .05, ns

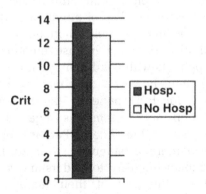

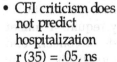

Fig. 2. Criticism and clinical outcome in BPD

- EOI predicts global
  clinical outcome
  r (35) = - .40, p < .02
- EOI predicts
  rehospitalization
  r (35) = - .44, p < .02
- Patients do better if
  their relatives are
  more emotionally
  overinvolved

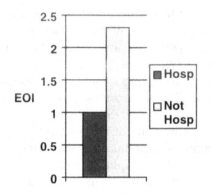

Fig. 3. EOI and clinical outcome in BPD

clinically during the period after hospital discharge. For borderline patients, however, the opposite appears to be the case. As can be seen in Fig. 3, patients whose relatives were rated as higher on EOI did better rather than worse during the follow-up period. Importantly, this was the case even when other factors such as severity or chronicity of illness were statistically controlled.

It should also be noted that EOI ratings of the relatives were made independently and were not based on patients' reports – a major limitation in many family studies of BPD. Yet precisely why borderline patients should do so much better in the context of an emotionally overinvolved family environment is not clear. However, these findings are particularly interesting when considered in light of research linking emotional under-concern and emotional neglect to borderline pathology. By definition, relatives high on EOI are not emotionally uninvolved with patients. Rather, they are paying a great deal of attention to their borderline family member and showing, in their emotional reactions, high levels of concern and distress. Such intense emotional reactions may be stressful for patients with conditions such as schizophrenia. For the borderline patient, however, they may be perceived quite differently. Indeed, for BPD patients, the presence of EOI may be viewed as a sign that the family is engaged and is, in some way, sharing the pain of the illness. Perhaps because the emotional range of the borderline patient is so broad, they require a similar level of emotional intensity to understand signals of concern and involvement on the part of their family. Alternatively, if the borderline patient tends to view his or her family as emotionally neglectful, extreme emotional reactions on the part of the family might be necessary to modify this perception. Quite clearly, gaining a more complete understanding of the meaning of EOI for the borderline patient should be a focus of empirical attention in the future.

Family-based Approaches to Treatment

Until quite recently, the standard treatment for borderline PD involved individual psychotherapy of some form, often combined with medication. Given the emphasis on family dynamics in BPD, however, it is hardly surprising that treatment approaches are now being developed that address family issues more directly. These approaches are still very much in their infancy, and none has yet been studied in a formal clinical trial. However, there is every reason to expect that family-based approaches to the treatment of BPD will provide clinical benefit to patients. Given the high prevalence of psychopathology in the families of borderlines (Zanarini et al., 1990) and, as noted in our review, the high level of problems in these families, there is also every reason to expect some direct benefit for the relatives themselves.

The most well-developed family-based approaches to the treatment of BPD are those of Hoffman and colleagues (Hoffman et al., 1999) and Gunderson and colleagues (Gunderson et al., 1997). Both of these groups view families as allies in the treatment of the patient and use the multi-family group (MFG) treatment format that has been so successful with families of patients with schizophrenia (e.g., McFarlane et al., 1995).

Gunderson et al.'s approach begins with psycho-educational workshops. Families then attend biweekly group meetings that involve 5–6 families and last 90 minutes each. Interestingly, the patient is not present. During these meetings each family talks about their current situation and then a specific problem is selected for general discussion. Although the selected problem is one presented by one particular family, the best situation is when the targeted problem occurs in several other families also. Families then work together in the group format to generate possible solutions about how to manage the problem. The meetings are designed to be relatively informal, and the duration of the MFG treatment is approximately 12–18 months.

The approach used by Hoffman et al. is broadly similar, although there are some important differences. Perhaps the most important of these is that the treatment is based on the principles of Dialectical Behavior Therapy, or DBT (Linehan, 1993). Dialectical Behavior Therapy-Family Skills Training (DBT-FST) involves weekly meetings over 6 months, with each meeting lasting 90 minutes. The first 45 minutes of each meeting are devoted to a didactic component that emphasizes traditional and family-specific DBT skills such as interpersonal effectiveness, emotion regulation, and validation skills. The second part of each group meeting involves consultation, discussion, and an opportunity to put some of the learned DBT skills into practice. One family presents a problem or issue and then the group leaders and other group participants try to help the target family work on their selected issue (see Hoffman and Hooley, 1998). This part of the treatment has much in common with Gunderson's treatment model. However, one important difference is that although patients attend the DBT-FST groups of Hoffman et al., this is not the case in the Gunderson treatment approach.

Although no formal tests of either of these treatment approaches have yet been conducted, preliminary evidence is positive. Gunderson et al. (1997) note that families report increased communication 6 months after the start of treatment. Informal reports for families in DBT-FST also suggest that this treatment is well received and that the drop out rate from the groups is low (Hoffman et al., 1999). Although such observations in no way substitute for empirically-based demonstrations of treatment efficacy, family-based approaches to the treatment of BPD appear to have considerable promise.

Concluding Remarks

Borderline PD is characterized by marked difficulties in interpersonal relationships. Nowhere is this perhaps more striking than in the family context. The retrospective reports of borderline patients point to high levels of family pathology and noxious or abusive early family relationships compared to control families.

We must keep in mind, however, that some of these family problems might well be engendered by emerging psychopathology in a child. It is also important to remember that most of the empirical studies in this area have placed heavy reliance on the self-reports of borderline patients with respect to the early family experiences. To the extent that family factors are involved in the development of borderline PD, they most likely interact with temperamental or otherwise inborn vulnerabilities in a complex way.

Rather than joining with patients and blaming families, clinicians and researchers would do well to focus more specifically on the role of the family in the course and treatment of BPD. Recent evidence suggests that certain characteristics of families might be linked to patients having a better clinical outcome. Much work now needs to be done to understand why this is. In a related vein, involving relatives in family-based treatments for BPD is an idea whose time has clearly come. Regardless of whether they are directly or indirectly involved in the development of the disorder, family members of borderline patients need to be helped to become part of the clinical solution. Although we still have much to learn about how best to do this, this is clearly an important direction for the future.

References

Adler, G. (1985): Borderline psychopathology and its treatment. New York: Jason Aronson

Bradley, S.J. (1979): The relationship of early maternal separation to borderline personality in children and adolescents: A pilot study. American Journal of Psychiatry 136(4): 424–426

Butzlaff, R.L. and Hooley, J.M. (1998): Expressed emotion and psychiatric relapse. Archives of General Psychiatry 55: 547–552

Fairbairn, W.R.D. (1952): Psychoanalytic studies of personality. London: Routledge

Feldman, R.B. and Guttman, H.A. (1984): Families of borderline patients: Literal-minded parents, borderline parents, and parental protectiveness. American Journal of Psychiatry 141: 1392–1396

Fossati, A., Madeddu, F., and Maffei, C. (1999): Borderline personality disorder and childhood sexual abuse: A meta-analytic study. Journal of Personality Disorders 13: 268–280

Frank, H. and Paris, J. (1981): Recollections of family experience in borderline patients. Archives of General Psychiatry 38: 1031–1034

Gunderson, J.G. (1984): Borderline personality disorder. Washington, D.C.: American Psychiatric Press

Gunderson, J.G., Berkowitz, C., and Ruiz-Sancho, A. (1997): Families of borderline patients: A psychoeducational approach. Bulletin of the Menninger Clinic 61: 446–457

Gunderson, J. and Englund, D. (1981): Characterizing the families of borderlines. Psychiatric Clinics of North America 4: 159–168

Gunderson, J.G., Kerr, J., and Englund, D.W. (1980): The families of border-lines: A comparative study. Archives of General Psychiatry 37: 27–33

Gurvitz, I.G., Koenigsberg, H.W., and Siever, L.J. (2000): Neurotransmitter dysfunction in patients with borderline personality disorder. Psychiatric Clinics of North America 23: 27–40

Herman, J.L. (1992): Trauma and recovery. New York: Basic Books

Hoffman, P.D., Fruzzetti, A.E., and Swenson, C.R. (1999): Dialectical behavior therapy-family skills training. Family Process 28(4): 399–414

Hoffman, P.D. and Hooley, J.M. (1998): Expressed emotion and the treatment of borderline personality disorder. In Session 4: 39–54

Hooley, J.M. and Hoffman, P.D. (1999): Expressed emotion and clinical outcome in borderline personality disorder. American Journal of Psychiatry 156(10): 1557–1562

Hull, J.W., Clarkin, J.F., and Kakuma, T. (1993): Treatment response of borderline inpatients: A growth curve analysis. Journal of Nervous and Mental Disease 181: 503–508

Kernberg, O.F. (1984): Severe personality disorders: Psychotherapeutic strategies. New Haven, CT: Yale University Press

Klein, M. (1948): Contributions to psycho-analysis, 1921–1945. London: The Hogarth Press

Kohut, H. (1971): The analysis of the self. New York: International University Press

Linehan, M.M. (1993): Cognitive behavioral treatment of borderline personality disorder. New York: Guilford Press

Links, P.S. and Blum, H.M. (1990): Family environment and borderline personality disorder: Development of etiologic models. In: Family environment and borderline personality disorder (Links, P.S., ed.), pp. 3–24. Washington, D.C.: American Psychiatric Press

Loranger, A.W., Sartori, N., Andreoli, A., Berger, P., Bucheim, P., and Channabasavanna, S.M. (1994): The international personality disorder examination. Archives of General Psychiatry 51: 215–224

McFarlane, W.R., Lukens, E., Link, B., Dushay, R., Deakins, S.A., Newmark, M., Dunne, E.J., Horen, B., and Toran, J. (1995): Multiple-family groups and psychoeducation in the treatment of schizophrenia. Archives of General Psychiatry 52: 679–687

Nigg, J.T. and Goldsmith, H.H. (1994): Genetics of personality disorders: Perspectives from personality and psychopathology research. Psychological Bulletin 115: 346–380

Ogata, S.N., Silk, K.R., and Goodrich, S. (1990a): The childhood experience of the borderline patient. In: Family environment and borderline personality disorder (Links, P.S., ed.). Washington, D.C.: American Psychiatric Press

Ogata, S.N., Silk, K.R., Goodrich, S., Lohr, N.E., Westen, D., and Hill, E.M. (1990b): Childhood sexual and physical abuse in adult patients with borderline personality disorder. American Journal of Psychiatry 147(8): 1008–1013

Paris, J. (1994): Borderline personality disorder: A multi-dimensional approach. Washington, D.C.: American Psychiatric Press

Paris, J. (1999): Borderline personality disorder. In: Oxford textbook of psychiatry (Millon, T., Blaney, P.H., and Davis, R.D., eds.). New York: Oxford University Press

Paris, J., Nowlis, D., and Brown, R. (1988): Developmental factors in the outcome of borderline personality disorder. Comprehensive Psychiatry 29: 147–150

Pope, H.G., Jonas, J.M., Hudson, J.I., Cohen, B.M., and Gunderson, J.G. (1983): The validity of DSM-III borderline personality disorder. Archives of General Psychiatry 40: 23–30

Ryle, A. (1997): The structure and development of borderline personality disorder: A proposed model. British Journal of Psychiatry 170: 82–87

Siever, L.J., and Davis, K.L. (1991): A psychobiological perspective on the personality disorders. American Journal of Psychiatry 148: 1647–1658

Soloff, P.H., and Millward, J.W. (1983): Developmental histories of borderline patients. Comprehensive Psychiatry 23: 574–588

Stern, A. (1938): Psychoanalytic investigation of and therapy in the borderline group of neuroses. Psychoanalytical Quarterly 7: 467–489

Swartz, M., Blazer, D., George, L., and Winfield, I. (1990): Estimating the prevalence of borderline personality disorder in the community. Journal of Personality Disorders 4: 257–272

Torgersen, S. (1994): Genetics in borderline conditions. Acta Psychiatrica Scandinavica 89(Suppl. 379): 19–25

Tyrer, P. (1988): Personality disorders: Diagnosis, management, and course. Boston: Wright

Vaughn, C.E., and Leff, J.P. (1976): The measurement of expressed emotion in the families of psychiatric patients. British Journal of Social and Clinical Psychology 15: 157–165

Waller, G. (1994): Borderline personality disorder and perceived family dysfunction in the eating disorders. Journal of Nervous and Mental Disease 182: 541–546

Weaver T.L., and Clum, G.A. (1993): Early family environments and traumatic experiences associated with borderline personality disorder. Journal of Consulting and Clinical Psychology 61: 1068–1075

Westen, D., Ludolph, P., Misle, B., Ruffins, S., and Block, J. (1990): Physical and sexual abuse in adolescent girls with borderline personality disorder. American Journal of Orthopsychiatry 60: 55–66

Widiger T.A., and Weissman, M.M. (1991): Epidemiology of borderline personality disorder. Hospital and Community Psychiatry 10: 1015–1021

Winnicott, D.W. (1965): The maturational process and the facilitating environment: Studies in the theory of emotional development. New York: International University Press

Zanarini, M.C., Gunderson, J.G., Marino, M.F., Schwartz, E.O., and Frankenburg, F.R. (1989): Childhood experiences of borderline patients. Comprehensive Psychiatry 30: 18–25

Zanarini, M.C., Gunderson, J.G., Marino, M.F., Schwartz, E.O., and Frankenburg, F.R. (1990): Psychiatric disorders in the families of borderline outpatients. In: Family environment and borderline personality disorder (Links, P.S., ed.). Washington, D.C.: American Psychiatric Press

Zanarini, M.C., Williams, A.A., Lewis, R.E., Reich, R.B., Vera, S.C., Marino, M.F., Levin, A., Yong, L., and Frankenberg, F.R. (1997): Reported pathological childhood experiences associated with the development of borderline personality disorder. Archives of General Psychiatry 154: 1101–1106

Part III

Intervention Strategies in Schizophrenia, Depression and Bipolar Disorder

9
Principles and Results of Family Therapy in Schizophrenia*

Kurt Hahlweg and Georg Wiedemann

Psychosocial Factors in Relapse

Long-term neuroleptic treatment has been shown to be effective in preventing relapse, but even with continuous medication, about 40% of patients relapse during the first year of discharge from the hospital compared with about 70% of patients taking placebo (Hogarty, 1984). The high rate of relapse has stimulated research on contributing factors: apart from medication non-compliance (Kissling, 1992), social stressors, in particular life events and/or a family environment high on "Expressed Emotion" (EE, Leff and Vaughn, 1985) seem to be important. High EE (HEE) relatives emit more than six critical comments during the semistructured Camberwell Family Interview (CFI) and/or receive a rating of three or more in the "Emotional Overinvolvement" (EOI) scale. Otherwise, relatives are categorized as low on EE (LEE). The predictive validity of the EE rating has been investigated in about 27 studies worldwide resulting in a relapse rate nine months after discharge of 52% for patients living with a HEE relative in contrast to 22% for patients living in a LEE family (Butzlaff and Hooley, 1998).

Of the 27 studies published, 24 showed a positive association between EE and relapse, with higher levels of EE in families being associated with greater rates of relapse in patients. The mean effect size was 0.31. This effect size is quite impressive when compared

---

*This paper has also been published in European Archives of Psychiatry and Clinical Neuroscience 1999, 249 (Suppl. 4), 108–115.

with data from medical studies: In the Physicians Health Study the effect of aspirin on the prevention of heart attacks was clearly established. However, the effect size for aspirin in that study was 0.034!

In a recent well-controlled study, Nuechterlein and his colleagues (1998) investigated the predictors of the early course of schizophrenic and schizo-affective patients. Patients were treated with fluphenazine, individual case management, skills-focused group therapy and family education. During a period of ongoing antipsychotic medication and psychosocial intervention, discrete stressful life events and highly critical or emotionally overinvolved attitudes towards patients and a higher symptom level were highly significant predictors of the chances of getting a psychotic relapse. The predictive role of these psychosocial stress variables is not accounted for by factors that would be expected to index genetic factors (family history, neurocognitive vulnerability factors), suggesting that these environmental stress variables operate through separate processes.

The EE concept essentially measures the key relative's attitudes towards the patient, but since the CFI interview is only conducted with that relative, it is not clear whether or not HEE relatives actually emit negative behavior in real life interaction with the patient. In several studies, the research group of the late Michael J. Goldstein at UCLA (see Strachan et al., 1986) were able to show that a critical attitude of the relative toward the patient correlates with critical interactional behavior when the family was asked to discuss family problems in the video laboratory. These findings were replicated using a different coding system in the US by Hahlweg et al. (1989) and with a German sample by Müller et al. (1992b). These studies also demonstrated that HEE families build up negative escalation patterns for extended parts of the discussion while LEE families were able to escape such vicious circles. Furthermore, detailed analysis demonstrated that the patient contributed to the development and sustainment of these negative escalation patterns just as much as the relatives (Hahlweg et al., 1989).

At least two consequences emerge from these results:

(a) The findings clearly indicate the active role of the patient in establishing a positive or negative family atmosphere and argue against a tendency to blame the relatives for being responsible for a relapse (see Hatfield et al., 1987; Mintz et al., 1987).

(b) In order to be able to modify the behavior of all family members simultaneously, the patient should be included in family management.

Psychoeducational Approaches in Preventing Relapse

The cited results emphasize the impact of family interaction on the course of the schizophrenic disorder, and fit well in recent heuristic vulnerability-stress models (Nuechterlein and Dawson, 1984; Zubin and Spring, 1977). Several consequences for prevention of relapse with schizophrenic patients ensue from this model and from the results of EE research: neuroleptic medication seems to be necessary to control positive symptoms of the disorder, probably by lowering autonomic hyperarousal, while psychosocial intervention to modify unfavorable familial factors seems to be indispensible for effective prevention of relapse.

Several anglo-american intervention programs based on the vulnerability-stress model have been developed which combine family intervention and neuroleptic medication as a means of preventing relapse in schizophrenia (Falloon et al., 1984; Goldstein et al., 1978; Hogarty et al., 1986, 1991; Leff et al., 1982, 1985; Tarrier et al., 1988, 1989). Although the individual concepts differ in their procedures, there are several common components:
(a) The patients are on neuroleptic medication; (b) Intervention is relatively brief (15–25 sessions in the first year) and starts with informational sessions on psychosis and neuroleptic medication; (c) The main focus is on lowering EE variables like criticism and over-involvement; (d) The aim is to resolve current areas of conflict in the family, with the goal of minimizing social stress; (e) Therapy is not only directed at problems of the patient, but aims to alleviate the whole family's burden.

The results from these different studies are very consistent in showing a marked reduction in relapse for patients in family treatment when compared with patients in standard psychiatric care. Relapse rates in the first year varied from 44% to 53% (mean: 49%) in the control groups in contrast to 6% and 23% (mean: 13%) in patients with family intervention. After two years the mean relapse rates were 72% in the control groups and 31% in the experimental groups. Furthermore, these interventions, in particular the Behavioral Family Management (BFM) approach by Falloon et al. (1984), seem to increase the level of social competence of the patient, decrease the subjective burden of relatives, change the communication patterns in the family, and are cost-effective in comparison to routine psychiatric treatment.

Psychoeducational approaches seem to be effective also in other cultural backgrounds. In a study conducted in China, Xiong et al. (1994) found that family intervention was significantly more effective than standard care in terms of rates and duration of hospitalization.

McFarlane et al. (1995) investigated in an uncontrolled study the effectiveness of psychoeducational Multiple Family Groups (MFG) on the outcome in schizophrenia. After four years, the relapse rate was 50%, averaging 12.5% per year. When compared to the above mentioned relapse rates in the control groups, the result points toward a long-term therapeutic effect for multiple family groups.

Recently, Falloon and his colleagues (1998) conducted a meta-analysis of 20 controlled and uncontrolled family management studies. Results showed that the clinical outcome (hospitalization and major episodes combined) is clearly associated with the strength of treatment, that is the intensity, and length of treatment. Clinical outcome is also associated with the type of family strategy used for treatment, favoring the cognitive behavioral approaches.

Alternative Neuroleptic Dosage-strategies

The efficacy of standard-dose antipsychotic neuroleptic medication in the long-term maintenance treatment of schizophrenia has been established. However, concerns about the adverse effects of neuro-leptic medication, in particular the development of tardive dyskine-sia, have led to a search for alternative long-term medication regimens, in particular **low dose** (Goldstein et al., 1978; Hogarty et al., 1988; Johnson et al., 1987; Kane et al., 1983, 1985; Marder et al., 1984, 1987) and **targeted** (or **intermittent**) treatment (Carpen-ter et al., 1990; Herz et al., 1991; Jolley et al., 1989, 1990; Müller et al., 1992a). In low dose therapy, patients receive about 10%–20% of the usual standard dose, while in targeted treatment medication is in most cases discontinued gradually. If clinical deterioration is noted, e.g. the occurrence of prodromal signs (Herz and Melville, 1980), medication is promptly reinstituted.

The cited studies have confirmed the feasibility of these strategies in that outcome with low dose or targeted treatment is in many respects comparable to continuous treatment at least for the **first** year of treatment. While more symptom exacerbations are noted, this worsening is usually brief when treated with an increase of dosage. However, during the second year relapse rates and families' burden are significantly higher in patients treated with intermittent treatment.

The Munich Study

In the following, the results of a study conducted in Munich, Germany are summarized, in which the effectiveness of different alternative treatment strategies in combination with Behavioral Family Management was investigated. This open clinical trial was conducted with the following main aims (see Hahlweg, Dürr and Müller, 1995):

(a) Replication of the BFM results (Falloon et al., 1984) in Germany.

(b) Investigating the feasibility of the targeted approach in combination with Behavioral Family Management (BFM) as suggested by Jolley et al. (1990).

It was hypothesized that the inclusion of the family would lower the relapse rates considerably since more persons are involved in detecting prodromal signs. Therefore the reinstitution of medication and an increase of concurrent psychosocial measures would occur early enough to prevent psychotic exacerbation. Over the study period, patients with targeted medication should receive less medication and experience fewer side-effects than patients with standard dose.

An open 18 month clinical trial was used in order to investigate the **clinical** feasibility of these treatment approaches using the existing lines of treatment. In Germany the treatment of schizophrenic patients is primarily done by psychiatrists in private practise. So the treatment approach was adopted for the private practitioner model.

In contrast to the previous psychoeducational studies both HEE- and LEE families were included. Since the effectiveness of BFM in everyday clinical practise was the focus of the study, inclusion of LEE families seems appropriate. On the one hand, in clinical routine it does not seem possible to use the lengthy CFI to identify the EE status of families because of the costs involved. On the other hand, LEE families may not constitute a homogenous group of families with a benign environment to the patient. It may well be that a subgroup of relatives is not rated as critical or overinvolved simply because they do not care about the patient any longer. Results by Buchkremer et al. (1986) showing that relative's **indifference** toward the patient is correlated with relapse support this notion.

Originally the study was planned as a controlled 2 × 2 design, assigning patients randomly to one of the following 4 groups: a) BFM plus standard dose, b) BFM plus targeted medication as the control conditions, c) standard dose alone, d) targeted medication alone. However, when the first six patients/families were assigned to the control groups, all of the patients refused to take part in the study after reading the informed consent letter. These patients had to be excluded from the study despite the fact that they were quite willing to be treated by BFM. Since patient/family recruitment had been generally difficult, the study design was changed omitting both control groups.

Study Entry Criteria

Consecutive admissions to the Max-Planck Institute of Psychiatry (MPIP) were recruited for the study between September 1988 and July 1991. Patients in the age range of 17 to 50 years had to meet Research Diagnostic Criteria (RDC, Spitzer, Endicott and Robins, 1978) for either schizophrenia or schizoaffective (mainly schizophrenic) disorder. For at least three months before admission, the patient had to live with or had to be in close contact (defined as at least 10 hours per week) with a relative and was likely to return to that household after discharge. Exclusion criteria were: a) evidence of an organic central nervous system disorder; b) recent history of alcohol or substance abuse; c) mental retardation (IQ less than 70); d) a history of more than two relapses per year after the withdrawal of maintenance neuroleptic medication.

Procedure

After the patient had satisfied the RDC criteria, the closest relative (-s) was administered the Camberwell Family Interview (CFI, Leff and Vaughn, 1985) in order to establish the EE status of the family. After informed consent was obtained from patient and family members, patients were randomly assigned to receive Behavioral Family Management (BFM) either in combination with continuous standard dose (SD) or with targeted medication (TM). The random allocation was done in a stratified manner with EE status and sex as factors. In most cases randomization took place within 6 weeks after hospital admission and in all cases before discharge.

Behavioral Family Management started at discharge and lasted in a structured form for one year. Thereafter families were seen on their request. All patients received individualized standard-dose medication for at least three months after hospital discharge. Whenever stabilization was achieved it was attempted to withdraw medication gradually for TM-patients. Once prodromal signs occurred medication at the psychiatrist's discretion was reinstituted.

Patients

The recruitment procedure and the drop-out rates are reported by Wiedemann et al. (1994). There was a total of 51 patients with an average age of 29.4 years (SD = 9.0); 60.8% were male. With regard to marital status, 57% were single, 39% married or cohabitating, and 4% divorced or separated; 58% lived in a parental household. Educational levels were Hauptschule (primary school) 16%, Mittlere Reife (secondary school) 27%, Abitur (high school) 37%, and Fachhochschule/Universität (university) 20% (an average of 11.6 years of school education). Occupational status: fulltime employment = 25%, parttime = 12%, unemployed = 12%, sick-leave = 14%, housewife = 10%, in education = 27%. 16% belonged to the lower, 66% to the middle, and 18% to the upper social class.

The clinical characteristics of the patients were: diagnosis: schizophrenia: 46 (90%), schizoaffective, mainly schizophrenia: 5 (10%). First admission: 43%, 2nd admission: 31%, 3 or more admissions: 26%; mean number of admissions: 2.1 (SD = 1.7); mean age of onset: 26.1 (SD = 7.6); median days in hospital (index admission): 56; mean GAS score at admission: 39.9 (SD = 15.6), at discharge: 72.8 (SD = 12.7).

Of the patients, 27 were randomly allocated to the BFMSD and 24 to the BFMTM group. There were no significant differences between the two groups with regard to sociodemographic and symptom variables.

Relatives

In total, 73 relatives (49% males) were included with a mean age of 49 years; 22 (43%) households contained two relatives. The relationship of relative to patient was: mother: 27 (37%), father: 22 (31%), husband: 13 (18%), wife: 10 (14%). The relatives belonged mainly to the middleclass. The family EE status as assessed by the CFI was: Low EE = 21 (42%), High EE-critical: 21 (42%), and High EE-EOI: 8 (16%).

Assessment

Major assessments were made at admission (diagnosis and psychopathology), discharge, and 6, 12 and 18 months after discharge. The major outcome measures were: the **Brief Psychiatric Rating Scale** (BPRS; Overall and Gorham, 1962; Lukoff, Nuechterlein and Ventura, 1986) and the **Global Assessment Scale** (GAS, Endicott, Spitzer, Fleiss and Cohen, 1976).

Behavioral Family Management (BFM)

The goal of BFM (BFM; Falloon et al., 1984; Hahlweg, Dürr and Müller, 1995) is to provide comprehensive long-term community care for persons suffering from schizophrenia by utilizing the problem solving potential of their natural support systems. While the patient is hospitalized an extensive **assessment** of the patient and the family is done including the CFI and the videotaping of the family's interaction discussing a family problem. One important task is to establish the patient specific prodromal signs.

Education

After discharge, the first two sessions are directed towards the education of the patient and his/her family about the nature, course, etiology, and treatment of schizophrenia. Individuals who develop symptoms of schizophrenia are probably born with a vulnerability to this and are neither responsible nor to blame for it, nor is their family. It is an illness similar, in a sense, to diabetes or hypertension, in that although there is no cure, there are very effective treatments that can reduce and often eliminate symptoms for long periods of time, allowing in many cases a gradual return to premorbid levels of functioning.

Although families do not *cause* schizophrenia, they can influence its *course*. Since it is a stress related illness, the amount of tension and stress in the home environment is a critical factor. There are many ways in which families can help maximize the patient's level of functioning, as well as minimize the chances of relapse; therein lies the rationale for a family management approach.

The second session is devoted to discussing issues related to medication. A cost-benefit analysis is presented with the principal advantages being (1) reduction or elimination of psychotic symptoms, (2) reduction of morbidity due to stressful life events, and (3) prophylaxis against relapse. Disadvantages discussed include bothersome side effects and possible long-term complications such as tardive dyskinesia. Strategies for coping with side effects are discussed.

Communication Skills Training

Following the two educational sessions, the treatment goals for each family shift to enhancing the problem solving potential of that family unit. Because a minimally sufficient repertoire of interpersonal communication skills is a prerequisite to effective problem solving, several sessions usually focus on improving family communication. Behavioral rehearsal strategies are employed to shape effective expression of positive and negative feelings, reflective listening, making requests for behavioral change in a positive manner, and reciprocity of conversation.

This communication skills training is accomplished primarily via behavioral rehearsal and concomitant instruction, modeling, coaching, social reinforcement, and performance feedback. Families are encouraged to practice newly-learned communication techniques and are given specific homework assignments to facilitate the daily use of these skills.

Problem Solving Training

When families show competency of basic communication skills, the problem solving model is introduced as a means to enhance coping with stressful life events and reduce family tension. Family members are taught a six step problem-solving method that involves (1) discussing and coming to an agreement on the exact nature of the problem, (2) generating a list of five or more alternative solutions without judging their relative merits as of yet, (3) discussing, in turn, the pros and cons of each proposed alternative, (4) choosing the best solution or combination of solutions, (5) formulating a specific plan of how to implement the solution, and (6) subsequent review of successfulness and praise for people's efforts implementing the solution.

The major focus is on the enhancement of problem resolution beyond sessions, unassisted by the therapist. Once the family has demonstrated competent problem solving the therapist reduces the frequency of sessions and eventually withdraws completely, although he/she will remain available for consulting and further coaching upon request.

Time Schedule BFM

Overall 10 therapists were involved and one therapist was treating a family. Weekly sessions were held during the first three months followed by biweekly sessions for another three months period. Thereafter monthly sessions were conducted for at least one year according to the families' needs. The mean number of sessions was $M = 26$ (SD = 5.7), HEE families received on average 27.2, LEE families 24.6 sessions (n.s.). In contrast to Falloon et al. BFM sessions were conducted in the outpatient clinic. Home visits were too costly, averaging up to three hours for one session due to travel time. Whenever possible, at least one home visit was conducted during the first phase of BFM.

Neuroleptic Treatment

Neuroleptic treatment was preliminary conducted by psychiatrists in private practice using standard oral or depot neuroleptics (Haldol, Fluphenazine, Clozapine). The project psychiatrist kept close contact to the treating psychiatrist in particular with TM patients in order to enhance drug withdrawal.

Results

Relapse

Relapses were defined as a reoccurrence of psychotic symptoms with or without subsequent hospitalization and operationalized following the recommendations of Nuechterlein et al. (1986): A rating of 5 or higher in any of the BPRS scales "Unusual Thought Content", "Conceptual Disorganization", "Suspiciousness" or "Hallucinations" given the patient was previously in remission (a rating of less than 3 on the scales). According to this criterion all patients were remitted at hospital discharge. Assessment of relapse was based on an unanimous team decision. Three treatment takers dropped out of treatment, two patients were assigned to Behavioral Family Management with Standard Dose (BFMSD), and one patient was assigned to BFM with Targeted Medication (BFMTM). Percentages of relapse were calculated based on the remaining sample ($N = 48$). Nine patients (6 male, 3 female; n.s.) relapsed, 8 in BFMTM and 1 patient in BFMSD; eight patients had to be hospitalized. These patients had a mean number of days at the hospital during index-admission of 80 days, and of 70 days for rehospitalization. The cumulative relapse rates are as follows: 6 month: BFM SD: 0%, BFMTM: 13.4% (3); 12 month: BFMSD: 4% (1), BFMTM: 17.4% (4); 18 month: BFMSD: 3.9% (1), BFMTM: 34.8% (8). The latter difference was significant.

Medication (Dose Levels)

Because a variety of neuroleptics were administered to the patients the actual prescribed drug dose for each day was transformed into "chlopromazine equivalents" (CPE) according to the conversions used in the Pietzcker et al. (1986) study. From the second month on, dose levels for BFMTM patients were significantly lower than for BFMSD patients. The mean daily dosage during the first year after discharge amounted to: BFMSD = 266 mg CPE (SD = 140) and BFMTM = 148 (SD = 127). This difference was highly significant.

Only two BFMSD patients were without prescribed medication for 1 or 2 months during the first year. In the BFMTM group the number of neuroleptic-free months varied considerably: 7 patients

(30.4%) received medication continuously, and only 7 patients were drug free for more than 5 months.

Psychopathology and Social Adjustment

The pattern of results were similar for the various measures and assessment points: Patients in both groups improved significantly from hospital discharge to the 6, 12, and 18 month follow-ups with regard to psychopathology (BPRS) and social adjustment (GAS). There were no significant differences in any of the global variables.

This general pattern of results was also obtained for the **relatives**: significant improvements in SCL-90 GSI and family burden from hospital discharge to the follow-ups and no significant differences between the two groups with regard to self-rated psychopathology.

Discussion

This study examined the efficacy of standard dose or targeted medication in combination with Behavioral Family Management for relapse prevention in schizophrenic patients living in high or low EE families. A major aim was to replicate the results of the Falloon et al. study (1984) with a German sample. Our 4% relapse rate after 18 months for BFM in combination with standard dose neuroleptic treatment clearly points to the crosscultural efficacy of this psychosocial approach and is in line with the results reported by Falloon et al. (1984; 9 month: 6%, 24 month: 17%), and by Hogarty et al. (1986, 1991), Leff et al. (1982, 1985), and Tarrier et al. (1988, 1989). Besides the low relapse rate within-analysis showed that patients and relatives improved on a number of other variables, e.g. psychopathology, social adjustment and family burden, again replicating the results reported by Falloon et al. (1984).

The major focus of BFM is to improve the family's ability to solve problems in order to lower familial stress. It is therefore important to show that the treatment is able to change family communication in the long run. To investigate these questions further, families were asked to discuss family conflicts in the video laboratory after discharge (pre), and at 6, 12, and 18 months. At six months, significant reductions in negative verbal and nonverbal behavior, notably in criticism, concomitant with significant increases in positive communication, notably in problemsolving and acceptance, were observed (Rieg et al., 1991). These findings parallel those reported by Doane et al. (1986) using the Falloon et al. sample.

Obviously control groups are missing in order to attribute these changes definitely to the treatment. In order to estimate relapse rates in patients hospitalized in comparable university or research clinics and later on treated in private practice as outpatients, the results of two naturalistic studies may be helpful. Laessle et al. (1987) retrospectively investigated the clinical course of 40 schizophrenic patients living with relatives who were hospitalized in the Max-Planck-Institute of Psychiatry six years ago. The relapse rate 18 months after discharge was 45%. A prospective study with 65 schizophrenic patients is currently underway at the "Zentralinstitut für seelische Gesundheit", a research facility in Mannheim. Preliminary results yielded a relapse rate of 48% 18 months after discharge (Olbrich, personal communication, 1992).

These relapse rates are very much in line with the outcomes of the control groups of patients living with high-EE families used in the psychoeducational studies yielding a mean relapse rate 12 months after discharge of 49%, and 72% 24 months later. Taking these findings together, it seems warranted to attribute our low relapse rate to the combined approach of standard dose treatment and Behavioral Family Management. Whether a better drug compliance, a more benign family atmosphere due to the enhanced capability of the family to solve their problems and to communicate more positively, or the combination of both factors is responsible for the very encouraging results remains unclear.

The second aim of the study was to investigate the feasibility of the targeted approach in combination with Behavioral Family Management (BFM). It was hypothesized that, beside the positive effects of the psychosocial approach, the inclusion of the family would enhance the capability to monitor prodromal signs and would consequently lower the otherwise reported higher relapse rates. This hypothesis has to be rejected since our results showed a significantly higher relapse rate of 34% 18 months after discharge in contrast to the 4% for patients with standard dose and BFM. These results are in line with the published reports by Carpenter et al. (1990), Herz et al. (1991), Jolley et al. (1989, 1990), and Müller et al. (1992a). While these studies differ with regard to patient selection, methodology, and criteria for relapse, all reported a significantly higher relapse rate two years after discharge for TM-patients in contrast to SD-patients ranging from 36% (Herz et al., 1991) to 62% (Carpenter et al., 1990). The German study by Müller et al. (1992a) reported relapse rates of 39% (12 months) and 49% (24 months), respectively. Our results clearly indicate that targeted medication even in combination with BFM is not a viable alternative as a routine outpatient treatment for schizophrenic patients. This conclusion is supported by the results of the recent NIMH study, in which the effects of dose reduction and family treatment were investigated (Schooler et al., 1997). The two year relapse rate was 19% for patients treated with BFM and standard dose, 26% for patients treated with low dose and BFM, and 43% for patients treated with targeted medication and BFM. However, targeted medication may be an alternative treatment for patients unwilling to be on standard medication for an extended period of time.

Apart from the significant differences with regard to relapse between the two groups any of the other variables used did not show significant differences – a finding also reported by Carpenter et al. (1990), Herz et al. (1991), Jolley et al. (1990), and Müller et al. (1992a). Despite the higher relapse rates TM-patients improved as well as SD-patients in psychopathology, side-effects, social competence, and were less burdened by the family. The same pattern of results was true for the relatives.

Over the 18 months TM-Patients received significantly less medication than SD-patients and about 50% did not receive any medication for at least 4 months. This parallels the findings by Carpenter et al. (1990), who reported that TM patients were drug free for 48% of the study time. Contrary to expectations the two groups did not differ significantly with regard to side-effects. This may be due to the generally low dosage in the SD-group. Anyway, side-effects were very mild generally and tardive dyskenisia was not reported at all in our sample of comparatively young schizophrenic patients.

A crucial limitation of new approaches to health services lies in the cost, which often exceeds that of previous approaches and, despite the advantages of improved effectiveness, restricts general implementation. In the Falloon et al. study all direct and indirect costs of community management to patients, families, health, welfare, and community agencies were recorded. The results after

1 year showed that the overall costs of the family approach were 19% less than those of the control condition (Cardin et al., 1985). In the Tarrier et al. study (1991) the family intervention resulted in a 27% decrease in mean cost per patient mainly due to fewer hospitalizations.

In Germany BFM could be provided by clinical psychologists or psychiatrists in private practise. Insurance companies would have to pay approximately 2,500 DM per case treated by BFM (25 session of 100 DM; not taking costs for seeing the psychiatrist and for medication into account). Readmitted patients stayed on average 70 days in the hospital. A day at hospital costs at least 350 DM = 24,500 DM. Taking a 40% relapse rate for standard medication only over an 18 month period into account (relapse for 10 out of 26 patients = 245,000 DM) in our study the BMFTSD treated patients would saved approximately 145,000 DM (1 relapse = 24,500 plus 65,000 DM for BFM) calculating only hospital costs!

These reductions in cost do not even take the benefits for the patient and the family into account of not being disrupted by hospital admissions. Less frequent admissions would probably lead to less stigmatization and better self-esteem in the long run.

In conclusion: There is a lot of positive evidence to support the broad scale application of psychoeducational family treatment in schizophrenia. Unfortunately, after 15 years of research, virtually no one is using the treatments in everyday practise; this is true for Germany and England as well as for the US.

What are the barriers to implement family management? Several issues may be relevant (Johnson, 1998):

(i)   Mental health providers are not convinced by the scientific evidence, or may not be influenced by the scientific evidence. They basically rely on personal experience.
(ii) Other, not empirically investigated theories like psychoanalytic theories, systemic and strategic family therapy, humanistic theories are too powerful.
(iii) Not interested in families. Families continue to be ignored by mental health professionals in many treatment facilities in most parts of the world.
(iv) Too many people have to be persuaded to implement these new approaches.
(v)   Implementation requires highly trained staff. The trainings costs may be high; programs require more time; clinical

routine has to be changed; psychiatrists in free practise may be afraid of loosing patients.

Obviously systematic training and supervision in these new multidisciplinary psychosocial approaches are necessary in order to offer these treatment strategies to many more families in need. Health care managers should seriously consider financing these training courses so that chronically ill patients and their families will be able to obtain better service in the near future.

Acknowledgement

Supported by a grant from the Bundesministerium für Forschung und Technologie (BMFT; PSF 20 0701620 5).

References

Buchkremer, G., Schulze-Mönking, H., Lewandowski, L., and Wittgen, C. (1986): Emotional atmosphere in families of schizophrenic outpatients: relevance of a practice-oriented assessment instrument. In: Treatment of schizophrenia. Family assessment and intervention (Goldstein, M.J., Hand, I., Hahlweg, K., eds.), pp. 79–84. Heidelberg: Springer

Butzlaff, R.L. and Hooley, J.M. (1998): Expressed emotion and psychiatric relapse: A meta-analysis. Archives of General Psychiatry 55: 547–552

Cardin, V.A., McGill, C.W., and Falloon, I.R.H. (1985): An economic analysis: Costs, benefits, and effectiveness. In: Family management of schizophrenia (Falloon, I.R.H. et al., eds.), pp. 115–123. Baltimore: John Hopkins University Press

Carpenter, W.T., Jr., Hanlon, T.E., Heinrichs, D.W., Kirkpatrick, B., Levine, J., and Buchanan, R.W. (1990): Continuous vs. targeted medication in schizophrenic outpatients: Outcome results. American Journal of Psychiatry 147: 1138–1148

Doane, J.A., Goldstein, M.J., Miklowitz, D.J., and Falloon, I.R. (1986): The impact of individual and family treatment on the affective climate of families of schizophrenics. British Journal of Psychiatry 148: 279–289

Endicott, J., Spitzer, R.L., Fleiss, J.L., and Cohen, J. (1976): The Global Assessment Scale. A procedure for measuring overall severity of psychiatric disturbance. Archives of General Psychiatry 33: 766–771

Falloon, I.R.H., Boyd, J.L., and McGill, C.W. (1984): Family care of schizophrenia. New York: Guilford

Falloon, I.R.H., Coverdale, J.N., Roncone, R., Held, T., Laidlaw, T.M., and Barbaro, A. (1998): Meta-analysis of psychoeducational family treatments for schizophrenia. Unpublished manuscript, paper at the 6th World Congress for Psychosocial Rehabilitation, Hamburg

Goldstein, M.J., Rodnick, E.H., Evans, J.R., May, P.R.A., and Steinberg, M.R. (1978): Drug and family therapy in the aftercare of acute schizophrenics. Archives of General Psychiatry 35: 1169–1177

Hahlweg, K., Dürr, H., and Müller, U. (1995): Familienbetreuung schizophrener Patienten. Ein verhaltenstherapeutischer Ansatz zur Rückfallprophylaxe. Weinheim: Beltz Psychologie Verlags Union

Hahlweg, K., Goldstein, M.J., Nuechterlein, K.H., Magana, A.B., Mintz, J., Doane, J.A., Miklowitz, D.J., and Snyder, K.S. (1989): Expressed emotion and patient-relative interaction in families of recent onset schizophrenics. Journal of Consulting and Clinical Psychology 57: 11–18

Hatfield, A.B., Spaniol, L., and Zipple, A.M. (1987): Expressed emotion: A family perspective. Schizophrenia Bulletin 13: 221–226

Herz, M.I., Glazer, W.M., Moster, M.A., Sheard, M.H., Szymanski, H.V., Hafez, M., Mirza, M., and Vaha, J. (1991): Intermittent vs. maintenance medication in schizophrenia. Two year results. Archives of General Psychiatry 48: 333–339

Herz, M.I. and Melville, C. (1980): Relapse in schizophrnia. American Journal of Psychiatry 137: 801–805

Hogarty, G.E. (1984): Depot neuroleptics: The relevance of psycho-social factors. Journal of Clinical Psychiatry 45: 36–42

Hogarty, G.E., Anderson, C.M., Reiss, D.J., Kornblith, S.J., Greenwald, D.P., Javna, C.D., Madonia, M.J., and the EPICS Schizophrenia Research Group (1986): Family psychoeducation, social skills training and maintenance chemotherapy in the aftercare treatment of schizophrenia: I. One year effects of a controlled study on relapse and expressed emotion. Archives of General Psychiatry 43: 633–642

Hogarty, G.E., Anderson, C.M., Reiss, D.J., Kornblith, S.J., Greenwald, D.P., Ulrich, R.F., Carter, M., and the environmental-personal indicators in the course of schizophrenia (EPICS) (1991): Family psychoeducation, social skills training, and maintenance chemotherapy in the aftercare treatment of schizophrenia. II. Two-year effects of a controlled study on relapse and adjustment. Archives of General Psychiatry 48: 340–347

Hogarty, G.E., Goldberg, S.C., Schooler, N.R., and Ulrich, R.F. (1974): The collaborative study group: Drug and sociotherapy in the aftercare of schizophrenic patients: II. Two year relapse rates. Archives of General Psychiatry 31: 603–608

Hogarty, G.E., McEvoy, J.P., Munetz, M., DiBarry, A.L., Bartone, P., Cather, R., Cooley, S.J., Ulrich, R.J., Carter, M. Madonia, M.J., and Environmental/ Personal Indicators in the Course of Schizophrenia Research Group (1988): Dose of fluphenazine, familial expressed emotion, and outcome in schizophrenia. Results of a two-year controlled study. Archives of General Psychiatry 45: 797–805

Jolley, A.G., Hirsch, S.R., McRink, A., and Manchanda, R. (1989): Trial of brief intermittent prophylaxis for selected schizophrenic outpatients: Clinical outcome at one year. British Medical Journal 298: 985–990

Jolley, A.G., Hirsch, S.R., Morrison, E. et al. (1990): Trial of brief intermittend neuroleptic prophylaxis for selected schizophrenic outpatients: clinical and social outcome at two years. British Medical Journal 301: 837–842

Johnson, D. (1998): The major barriers to implement the findings. Paper at the 6th World Congress for Psychosocial Rehabilitation, Hamburg

Johnson, D.A.W., Ludlow, J.M., Street, K., and Taylor, R.D.W. (1987): Double-blind comparison of half-dose and standard-dose Flupenthixol Decanoate in the maintenance treatment of stabilised out-patients with schizophrenia. British Journal of Psychiatry 151: 634–638

Kane, J.M., Rifkin, A., Woerner, M., Reardon, G., Sarantakos, S., Schiebel, D., and Ramos-Lorenzi, J. (1983): Low-dose neuroleptic treatment of outpatient schizophrenics. Archives of General Psychiatry 40: 893–896

Kane, J.M., Riftkin, A., Woerner, M., Kreisman, D., Blumenthal, R., and Borenstein, M. (1985): High - dose versus low-dose strategies in the treatment of schizophrenia. Pharmacological Bulletin 21: 533–537

Kavanagh, D.J. (1992): Recent developments in expressed emotion and schizophrenia. British Journal of Psychiatry 160: 601–620

Kissling, W. (1992): Ideal and reality of neuroleptic relapse prevention. British Journal of Psychiatry 161 (Suppl. 18): 133–139

Laessle, R., Pfister, H., and Wittchen, H.-U. (1987): Risk of rehospitalization of psychotic patients. A 6-year follow-up investigation using the survival approach. Psychopathology 20: 48–60

Leff, J., Kuipers, L., Berkowitz, R., Eberlein-Fries, R., and Sturgeon, D. (1982): A controlled trial of intervention in the families of schizophrenic patients. British Journal of Psychiatry 141: 121–134

Leff, J.P., Kuipers, L., Berkowitz, R., and Sturgeon, D. (1985): A controlled trial of social intervention in the families of schizophrenic patients: two year follow-up. British Journal of Psychiatry 146: 594–600

Leff, J.P. and Vaughn, C.E. (1985): Expressed emotion in families. New York: Guilford

Lukoff, D., Nuechterlein, K.H., and Ventura, J. (1986): Manual for the Expanded Brief Psychiatric Rating Scale (BPRS): Schizophrenia Bulletin 12: 594–602

Marder, S.R., Van Putten, T., Mintz, J., Lebell, M., McKenzie, J., and May, P.R.A. (1987): Low and conventional dose maintenance therapy with fluphenazine decanoate: Two year outcome. Archives of General Psychiatry 44: 510–517

McFarlane, W.R., Link, B., Dushay, R., Marchal, J., and Crilly, J. (1995): Psychoeducational multiple family groups: Four-year relapse outcome in schizophrenia. Family Process 34: 127–144

Mintz, L.I., Liberman, R.P., Miklowitz, D.J., and Mintz, J. (1987): Expressed Emotion: A call for partnership among relatives, patients, and professionals. Schizophrenia Bulletin 13: 227–235

Müller, P., Bandelow, B., Gaebel, W., Köpke, W., Linden, M., Müller-Spahn, F., Pietzcker, A., Schaefer, E., and Tegeler, J. (1992a): Intermittend medication, coping and psychotherapy. Interactions in relapse prevention and course modification. British Journal of Psychiatry 116 (Suppl. 18): 140–144

Müller, U., Hahlweg, K., Feinstein, E., Hank, G., Wiedemann, G., and Dose, M. (1992b): Familienklima (Expressed Emotion) und Interaktionsprozesse in Familien mit einem schizophrenen Mitglied. Zeitschrift für Klinische Psychologie 21: 332–351

Nuechterlein, K.H. and Dawson, M.E. (1984): A heuristic vulnerability/stress model of schizophrenic episodes. Schizophrenia Bulletin 10: 300–312

Nuechterlein, K.H., Ventura, J., Snyder, K.S., Gitlin, M., Subotnik, K.L., Dawson, M.E., and Mintz, J. (1998): The role of stressors in schizophrenic relapse: Longitudinal evidence and implications for psychosocial interventions. Unpublished manuscript, University of California, LA

Overall, J.E. and Gorham, D.R. (1962): The Brief Psychiatric Rating Scale. Psychological Reports 10: 799–812

Pietzcker, A., Gaebel, W., Kopcke, W., Linden, M., Muller, P., Müller-Spohn, F., Schussler, G., and Tegeler, J. (1986): A German multi-center study on the neuroleptic long-term therapy of schizophrenic patients' preliminary report. Pharmacopsychiatry 19: 161–166

Rieg, C., Müller, U., Hahlweg, K., Wiedemann, G., Hank, G., and Feinstein, E. (1991): Psychoedukative Rückfallprophylaxe bei schizophrenen Patienten: Ändern sich die familiären Kommunikationsmuster? Verhaltenstherapie 1: 283–292

Schooler, N.R., Keith, S.J., Severe, J.B., Matthews, S.M., Bellack, A.S. et al. (1997): Relapse and rehospitalization during maintenance treatment of schizophrenia. The effects of dose reduction and family treatment. Archives of General Psychiatry 54: 453–463

Spitzer, R.L., Endicott, J., and Robins, E. (1978): Research Diagnostic Criteria: Rationale and reliability. Archives of General Psychiatry 35: 773–782

Strachan, A.M., Goldstein, M.J., and Miklowitz, D.J. (1986): Do relatives express expressed emotion? In: Treatment of schizophrenia. Family assessment and intervention (Goldstein, M.J., Hand, I., Hahlweg, K., eds.), pp. 51–58: Heidelberg: Springer

Tarrier, N., Barrowclough, C., Vaughn, C., Bamrah, J.S., Porceddu, K., Watts, S., and Freeman, H. (1988): The community management of schizophrenia. A controlled trial of a behavioural intervention with families to reduce relapse. British Journal of Psychiatry 153: 532–542

Tarrier, N., Barrowclough, C., Vaughn, C., Bamrah, J.S., Porceddu, K., Watts, S., and Freeman, H. (1989): Community management of schizophrenia. A two-year follow-up of a behavioral intervention with families. British Journal of Psychiatry 154: 625–628

Tarrier, N., Lowson, K., and Barrowclough, C. (1991): Some aspects of family interventions in schizophrenia. II: Financial considerations. British Journal of Psychiatry 159: 481–484

Wiedemann, G., Hahlweg, K., Hank, G., Feinstein, E., Müller, U., and Dose, M. (1994): Deliverability of psychoeducational family management for schizophrenia. Schizophrenia Bulletin 20: 547–556

Xiong, W., Phillips, M.R., Hu, X. et al. (1994): Family based intervention for schizophrenia patients in China: A randomised controlled trial. British Journal of Psychiatry 165: 239–247

Zubin, J. and Spring, B. (1977): Vulnerability – a new view of schizophrenia. Journal of Abnormal Psychology 86: 103–126

10

A Controlled Trial of Couple Therapy versus Antidepressant Medication for Depressed Patients with a Critical Partner

Julian Leff

Introduction

Michael J. Goldstein initiated the first study which showed that family work for schizophrenia could be effective. The publication document-ing this research appeared in 1978 (Goldstein et al., 1978) two years after our own replication of the association between relatives' Expressed Emotion (EE) and the outcome of schizophrenia (Vaughn and Leff, 1976a). Following this successful replication we began to plan a controlled trial of intervention with the families of schizophrenic patients, unaware of Goldstein's ongoing study of the same kind. His publication encouraged us because up till then there had been no convincing evidence of the efficacy of this kind of approach. Since then at least eight randomised controlled trials have been published all demonstrating that family work in conjunction with maintenance antipsychotic medication is better at preventing relapse of schizo-phrenia than medication alone. The accumulating evidence has been endorsed by the Cochrane Collaboration as substantiating the value of family work for schizophrenia (Anderson and Adams, 1996).

We originally embarked on our first intervention study (Leff et al., 1982) with two aims in mind: the first was to investigate the direction of cause and effect in the association between EE and relapse of schizophrenia. We argued that if we could change the emotional environment in the home in the desired direction and that if this was then accompanied by a reduction in relapse rate, it was reasonable to infer that EE played a causal role in relapse. Testing the efficacy of our intervention was only a secondary aim, although if the intervention was unable to effect change in the family, the first aim could not be pursued. We were quite surprised to find that our target of reducing EE from high to low and/or lowering face-to-face contact was achieved in three quarters of the experimental families in both of our trials. Furthermore, in families which changed, the relapse rate of the patients was significantly lower than in families which did not (Leff, 1989). The meta-analysis conducted by the Cochrane Collaboration led to the conclusion that lowering of EE was not essential for a therapeutic effect (Mari and Streiner, 1996). However, this analysis did not include changes in face-to-face contact, partly because they were not reported in every study included. In view of the importance of this factor in modifying the effect of EE and the fact that it is a target of most interventions, its omission from an analysis of this area of research weakens any conclusions drawn about the mechanisms by which therapy achieves its beneficial effects on the relapse rate.

Christine Vaughn and I felt we ought to attempt to replicate Brown, Birley and Wing's (1972) demonstration of an association between EE and the outcome of schizophrenia because it was potentially of great importance to an understanding of this myste- rious condition and because no other research group had taken it up in the succeeding ten years. However, we deemed it essential to include a comparison group suffering from a psychiatric illness which was as different as possible from schizophrenia in order to determine how specific the EE effect was. In the event we chose to study depressive neurosis, excluding patients with psychotic symp- toms of any sort. We found that one component of EE, critical comments, predicted relapse of depression, although at a different threshold from schizophrenia (Vaughn and Leff, 1976b). Whereas a level of six critical comments separated patients with high and low relapse rates of schizophrenia, the distinguishing level for depres- sion was as low as two critical comments. This suggested to us that patients with depression were *more* sensitive to criticism than patients with schizophrenia, but we were unable to pursue this line of research any further because the effort required to develop and test the family intervention for schizophrenia was very demanding.

The unfinished work on depression was always at the back of my mind and loomed even larger as replications of the association between critical comments and the course of depression appeared in print. The first was a study from Oxford by Hooley, Orley and

Teasdale (1986) which replicated our findings perfectly. The next to be published was, surprisingly, a replication in Egypt by Okasha and colleagues (1994). They found a different threshold to be linked to relapse, but a level of three rather than two critical comments was found to produce a significant difference in relapse rates, a relatively trivial variation. However, the next study to appear was a failure to replicate our findings (Hayhurst et al., 1997). This research was conducted in Cambridge and was focused largely on middle class depressed women, a somewhat different sample from the previous studies. Whether this accounts for the disparate result must remain speculative until further attempts are made to replicate the work with samples varying in social class and gender. However, I considered that sufficient support had accumulated for our original findings to justify an intervention study.

Planning the Intervention

The context for planning an intervention to lower EE in depression differed in many ways from that for schizophrenia. The prophylactic efficacy of antipsychotic medication for schizophrenia had been firmly established and there was no suggestion that any social treatment could substitute for medication. Consequently all the trials based on EE research tested family work in combination with maintenance medication. By contrast, there is a substantial body of literature indicating that various kinds of social intervention are as effective as medication in treating acute episodes of depression, including cognitive therapy (Hollon et al., 1991), interpersonal therapy (Klerman and Weissman, 1992), and marital therapy (Emanuels-Zuurveen and Emmelkamp, 1996). All these trials, though, were relatively brief and none had continued for long enough to investigate the prophylactic efficacy of the social therapies. This body of research supported a design in which a social intervention was tested against antidepressant medication, and which included a prophylactic as well as a treatment phase.

Another major difference from schizophrenia concerned the type of household. Whereas about half the patients with schizophrenia in our original study lived with parents, only one of the depressed patients did so. This is largely due to the fact that schizophrenia commonly begins in adolescence or early adulthood, disrupting the achievement of independence from parents. Hence we knew that the social intervention for depression should be focused on couples.

Possible Mechanisms Maintaining Depression

The psychological processes mediating the effect of relatives EE on schizophrenic symptoms were unknown and remain obscure, apart from some evidence that they operate through non-specific physiological arousal (Tarrier et al., 1979; Sturgeon et al., 1984). For depression, however, a substantial body of theory and research had developed which identified low self esteem as the psychological substrate of depressive symptoms (Beck et al., 1961, Brown et al., 1990). As with schizophrenia, my prime interest in mounting an intervention study was to investigate the possible causal link between critical comments and depressive symptoms and the mechanisms by which this might operate. I drew up a simple diagram incorporating depressive symptoms, self esteem and partner's critical attitude and the possible relationships between them (see Fig. 1).

Low self esteem could give rise to depressive symptoms which in turn could provoke criticism in a partner. The partner's critical attitude could affect the patient both by further lowering self esteem and by worsening depression. It appeared to me that a productive way of investigating these relationships was to employ three different interventions, each of which was primarily directed at one of the components of the system. Antidepressant medication is claimed to relieve the symptoms of depression, cognitive therapy is mainly directed at improving the patient's self esteem, while couple

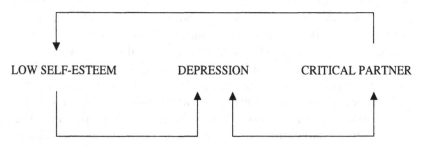

Fig. 1. Possible mechanisms for the maintenance of depressive symptoms

therapy attempts to improve the relationship between the patient and partner. The use of these three therapies as alternative interventions appeared to offer the best chance of teasing out the mechanisms of maintenance of depression. Of course a trial comparing these three interventions would also be a test of their relative efficacy.

Design of the Trial

The design of the trial was initially a three way comparison between antidepressant medication, cognitive therapy and couple therapy for a year of active treatment, followed by a second year in which no treatment would be given in order to study the prophylactic efficacy of the interventions. Subjects had to be over the age of 18, suffering from depression of moderate severity (a Hamilton Depression Rating Scale score of 14 or above), and living in stable union (more than one year) with a heterosexual partner. The partner was interviewed with the Camberwell Family Interview (CFI) and had to make two or more critical comments in the course of the interview. In fact only a tiny proportion of subjects was excluded as failing to meet this criterion: less than 5 percent.

Nature of the Treatments

We were concerned to provide the best treatment possible in each modality as this was a trial of efficacy, not of effectiveness. The antidepressant regime was chosen after consultation with an international authority on the drug treatment of depression. The initial choice of medication was a tricyclic antidepressant, desipramine. The dose was gradually increased over a few weeks, titrating it against side effects and symptom reduction. Compliance was monitored by checking serum levels of the drug at 4 weeks, 8 weeks, 6 months and one year. For the first two sessions of drug treatment the partner was seen with the patient and an educational programme about depression and antidepressants was given to maximise compliance. If the first line drug failed to relieve symptoms within 6 weeks, or intolerable side effects developed, a second line antidepressant, fluvoxamine, was substituted. Once an effective dose was achieved and symptoms had remitted, the medication was continued on this dose for four months, after which it was gradually reduced to a maintenance dose. Patients were maintained on this lower dose for the rest of the first year. During this period patients were seen between 12 and 20 times, for 20 to 30 minutes per session. At the end of one year the antidepressant was tailed off over two weeks, although two patients opted to remain on medication and two others relapsed as soon as it was discontinued, requiring a reintroduction.

In order to ensure that the cognitive therapy was of the highest quality, we selected only therapists who were trained in Aaron Beck's unit. The first two therapists we engaged in the study worked with six patients during a pilot phase. They were unhappy with the type of patients they saw, whom they perceived as suffering primarily from personality disorders, with depression as a secondary issue. Consequently they withdrew from the study before the experimental phase began. Faced with the difficulty of finding a replacement therapist, we sent one of our research psychologists to Beck's unit for four months to be trained as a cognitive therapist. Once the definitive study began, we soon became aware of a high drop-out rate from cognitive therapy. Of the first 11 patients who were randomly assigned to cognitive therapy, eight dropped out before the treatment was completed. At this point the rate of recruitment to the trial was worryingly slow, so that we felt impelled to delete the cognitive therapy arm, even though this meant losing a vital component of the aetiological investigation.

The couple therapy was developed for this trial by two experienced couple and family therapists. Their approach was based on a systemic formulation that close relationships both influence and are influenced by the patient and his/her symptoms. Systemic couple therapy aims to help the patient and partner to gain new perspectives on the presenting problems, to attach different meanings to the depressive behaviors and to experiment with new ways of relating to each other. A manual for the couple therapy was constructed which specifies the techniques to be used and their approximate sequence (Jones and Asen, 1999). These include observation and enactment of couple issues, attempts to interrupt problematic cycles of behavior in order to shift negative attributions, and the setting of tasks to promote more rewarding interactions. Attempts were made in a pilot phase to reduce the partner's critical comments, but as these seemed to make no impact on depressive symptoms they were not incorporated in the manual. The therapy is divided into three distinct phases in which specific interventions are used, but enough flexibility is built in to avoid the therapy becoming too rigid. The protocol allowed for 12 to 20 sessions, each lasting around 50 minutes.

Assessments

A full psychiatric history was taken from the patients who were also interviewed with the Present State Examination. These data were processed with the CATEGO program (Wing et al., 1974) to generate the Index of Definition. Levels of 5 and above are used to identify psychiatric cases in community surveys, and this was included as a criterion for entry into the trial. The patients also had to receive a primary classification of depression from the CATEGO program and score 14 or more on the Hamilton Depression Rating Scale (HRSD) (Hamilton, 1960). The partners had to make at least two critical comments in the course of the CFI (Vaughn and Leff, 1976b), but in fact less than 5 percent of the referrals were excluded on this account. The Self Esteem and Social Support Schedule (SESS) (Brown et al., 1990) was used to monitor changes in self esteem, while the Beck Depression Inventory (BDI) (Beck et al., 1961) was selected as the outcome measure for depression. It was chosen in preference to the HRSD because it is a more extended scale and is more focused on depressive symptoms, whereas the HRSD has a broader coverage including anxiety and somatic symptoms.

A full assessment was conducted at entry into the study, and then the outcome measures were repeated at the end of treatment at about one year, and again at the end of the second year without treatment.

Subjects

Suitable subjects were sought from psychiatric out-patient clinics and from general practitioners working in groups in north and south London. When it became evident that the referral rate was too slow, advertisements were placed in local newspapers. Just under one quarter of the subjects were responders to the advertisements. These patients did not differ from the professional referrals on age of onset of first depression, PSE score, BDI score, and a significant history of depression (current symptoms for more than six months or a previous treated episode in the past three years). However, they scored significantly lower on the HSRD.

Of the 88 subjects who entered the trial, 11 were randomly assigned to cognitive therapy and will not be considered further here. The other 77 were split between 37 assigned to medication and 40 to couple therapy. The two groups did not differ on any of the demographic, relationship or clinical variables measured, confirming the effectiveness of the randomisation procedure.

Dropouts

After randomisation but before any treatment was received, 12 patients dropped out of the trial: nine of these were assigned to drug treatment. This suggests that even though they had consented to randomisation in principle they were probably hoping to be randomised to couple therapy and were not really prepared to accept medication. Another 12 patients dropped out of drug treatment before an adequate course had been completed. Three of these were withdrawn by the pharmacotherapist on account of side effects. After treatment began three patients dropped out of couple therapy, making a total of six drop-outs or 15 percent. This is in dramatic contrast to the drug arm, from which the drop-out rate was 57 percent, a highly significant excess ($X^2 = 14.72$, $df = 1$, $p < 0.001$). The proportion of drop-outs from drug treatment appears remarkably high, but reference to other standard trials of antidepressants shows that drop-out rates of around 40% are common (Hollyman, 1988; Elkin et al., 1985). Furthermore our study was unusual in continuing treatment for as long as one year, whereas few previous trials have exceeded six months. In addition it is well documented that the general public is antipathetic to medication for depression, which many misperceive as addictive (Scott and Freeman, 1992; Whitton et al., 1996). Although we included education sessions to counter this prejudice and to provide other information about drugs, patients who dropped out on randomisation would have missed this.

Drop-outs were found to be significantly younger than completers (34.3 vs. 41.6, $t = 3.30$, df 75, $p < 0.002$) and to have higher BDI scores initially (29.4 vs. 25.2, $t = 2.99$, df 75, $p < 0.004$). In order to accommodate for this potential bias, treatment group and age were included as covariates in the analysis of outcome.

Data Analysis

The outcome variable chosen for the analysis was the BDI as this is more focused on depressive symptoms than the HRSD and is a more extended scale. Data were available at three time points; baseline, one year and two year follow-ups. Because of the loss of data through drop-outs, it was decided to use the likelihood approach described by Schluchter (1988). This method allows for drop-outs and produces valid parameter estimates and standard errors as long as the drop-outs are representative of the original sample (Everitt, 1998). Even when the drop-outs differ from the completers, as in this instance, the likelihood method will produce a less biased analysis than commonly used alternatives such as analysing completers only or replacing missing values with the last available measurement (Diggle, 1998).

Results

Efficacy of treatment

The likelihood approach was used to fit a variety of models for the mean profiles of the BDI outcome variable. Main effects of treatment group and time and the interaction of treatment group and time were considered. In addition the initial value of the BDI was introduced as a covariate, along with age and a small number of additional covariates such as sex and history of depression. Only treatment group was found to be significant (95% C.I. 1.62–11.54). This implies that from initial assessment to the one year follow-up the mean BDI score in the couple therapy group fell to between 1.62 and 11.54 points lower than the corresponding mean in the medication group. This difference was maintained from the one year to the two year follow-up. Hence we can infer that couple therapy was not only more acceptable to the subjects recruited to the trial, but was also more efficacious in the treatment and prophylaxis of depression.

Mechanism of action of the treatments

Changes in partner's critical comments and in patient's self esteem over time were analysed for both treatment groups. At baseline, the mean number of partner's critical comments was 8.30 (S.D.1.02) for the couple therapy group and 8.76 (S.D. 1.61) for the medication group, comparable with the mean of 7.20 from the study of Vaughn and Leff (1976b). During the first year of treatment the mean number of critical comments fell to 4.69 (0.90) for those in couple therapy and 3.92 (0.96) for the medication group, both reductions being significant, but no difference emerging between them. The same pattern was found for improvements in negative self esteem over time. Hence neither modification of partner's critical attitude nor improvement in self esteem can account for the better outcome of the patients receiving couple therapy. Inspection of the data suggested that there might be differences between the treatment groups in the effect on hostility. Therefore an analysis was conducted of changes in partner's hostility during the treatment. Couples in which the partner was initially hostile but who separated during the two year follow-up period were included since the patients would no longer have been exposed to the hostility. In all there were nine separations in the couple therapy group and four in the medication group, a nonsignificant difference. Of the eight partners who were initially hostile and received couple therapy, all either lost their hostility or separated from the patient. However, two partners developed hostility in the course of the study. Including these two, there is still a significant reduction in hostility for the couple therapy group over the two years. No such change occurred in the medication group.

Thus it appears that some of the effect of the couple therapy in relieving depression can be attributed to a reduction in the exposure of the patient to hostility. This cannot be the total explanation since only a minority of partners (20%) were rated as showing hostility initially. We must conclude that we failed to identify the main mechanism by which systemic couple therapy achieved its clinical benefit. The fact that in the medication group the partner's critical comments reduced and the patient's low self esteem increased alongside the improvement in symptoms does not support the hypothesis that they are instrumental in maintaining depression. At best we could postulate an interactional process between these factors in patient and partner and the depressive symptoms.

In conclusion, in contrast to the family interventions developed for schizophrenia, which reinforced EE and face-to-face contact as influential factors in relapse, this intervention for depression leaves the question of the mechanisms maintaining symptoms wide open. In some ways this is disappointing, but on the other hand, as with schizophrenia, the research on EE and depression has lead to the development of a new form of therapy which has proven efficacious.

References

Anderson, J. and Adams, C. (1996): Family interventions in schizophrenia. British Medical Journal 313: 505–506

Beck, A.T., Ward, C.H., Mendelson, M., Mock, J.E., and Erbaugh, J.K. (1961): An inventory for measuring depression. Archives of General Psychiatry 4: 561–571

Brown, G.W., Bifulco, A., Veiel, H.O.F., and Andrews, B. (1990): Self-esteem and depression. II. Social correlates of self-esteem. Social Psychiatry and Psychiatric Epidemiology 25: 225–234

Brown, G.W., Birley, J.L.T., and Wing, J.K. (1972): Influence of family life on the course of schizophrenic disorders: A replication. British Journal of Psychiatry 121: 241–258

Diggle, P.J. (1998): Dealing with missing values in longitudinal studies. In: Statistical analysis of medical data (Everitt, B.S., and Dunn, G., eds.). London: Arnold

Elkin, I., Morris, B., Parloff, S., Hadley, W., Joseph, H., and Autry, M.D. (1985): NIMH-treatment of depression collaborative research program: Background and research plan. Archives of General Psychiatry 42: 305–316

Emanuels-Zuurveen, L. and Emmelkamp, P.M. (1996): Individual behavioural cognitive therapy versus marital therapy for depression in maritally distressed couples. British Journal of Psychiatry 169(2): 181–188

Everitt, B.S. (1998): Analysis of longitudinal data: Beyond MANOVA. British Journal of Psychiatry 172: 7–10

Goldstein, M.J., Rodnick, E.H., Evans, J.R., May, P.R.A., and Steinberg, M.R. (1978): Drug and family therapy in the aftercare treatment of acute schizophrenia. Archives of General Psychiatry 35: 169–177

Hamilton, M. (1960): A rating scale for depression. Journal of Neurology, Neurosurgery and Psychiatry 23: 59–61

Hayhurst, H., Cooper, Z., Paykel, E.S., Vearnals, S., and Ramana, R. (1997): Expressed emotion and depression: A longitudinal study. British Journal of Psychiatry 171: 439–443

Hollon, S.D., Shelton, R.C., and Loosen, P.T. (1991): Cognitive therapy and pharmacotherapy for depression. Journal of Consulting and Clinical Psychology 59: 88–99

Hollyman, J.A., Freeling, P., Paykel, E.S., Bhat, A., and Sedgewick, P. (1988): Double-blind, placebo-controlled trial of amitriptyline among depressed patients in general practice. Journal of the Royal College of General Practitioners 38: 393–397

Hooley, J.M., Orley, J., and Teasdale, J.D. (1986): Levels of expressed emotion and relapse in depressed patients. British Journal of Psychiatry 148: 642–647

Jones, E. and Asen, E. (1999): Systemic couple therapy and depression. London: Karnac Books

Klerman, G.L. and Weissman, M. (1992): Interpersonal psychotherapy. In: Handbook of affective disorders (Paykel, E.S., ed.), 2nd ed., pp. 501–510. London: Churchill Livingstone

Leff, J. (1989): Controversial issues and growing points in research on relatives' expressed emotion. International Journal of Social Psychiatry 35: 133–145

Leff, J.P., Kuipers, L., Berkowitz, R., Eberlein-Fries, R., and Sturgeon, D. (1982): A controlled trial of social intervention in the families of schizophrenic patients. British Journal of Psychiatry 141: 121–134

Mari, J.J. and Streiner, D. (1996): Family intervention for those with schizophrenia. In: Schizophrenia module of the Cochrane database of systematic reviews (Adams, C., Anderson, J., and De Jesus Mari, J., eds.)

Okasha, A., El Akabawi, A.S., Snyder, A.S., Wilson, A.K., Youssef, I., and El Dawla, A.S. (1994): Expressed emotion, perceived criticism, and relapse in depression: A replication in an Egyptian community. American Journal of Psychiatry 151: 1001–1005

Schluchter, M.D. (1988): Analysis of incomplete multivariate data using linear models with structured covariance matrices. Statistics in Medicine 7: 317–324

Scott, A.I.F. and Freeman, C.P.L. (1992): Edinburgh primary care depression study: treatment outcome, patients satisfaction, and cost after 16 weeks. British Medical Journal 304: 883–887

Sturgeon D., Turpin, D., Kuipers, L., Berkowitz, R., and Leff, J. (1984): Psychophysiological responses of schizophrenic patients to high and low expressed emotion relatives: a follow-up study. British Journal of Psychiatry 145: 62–69

Tarrier, N., Vaughn, C., Lader, M.N., and Leff, J.P. (1979): Bodily reactions to people and events in schizophrenics. Archives of General Psychiatry 36: 311–315

Vaughn, C. and Leff, J.P. (1976a): The measurement of expressed emotion in families of psychiatric patients. British Journal of Social and Clinical Psychology 15: 157–165

Vaughn, C. and Leff, J.P. (1976b): The influence of family and social factors on the course of psychiatric illness: a comparison of schizophrenic and depressed neurotic patients. British Journal of Psychiatry 129: 125–137

Whitton, A., Warner, R., and Appleby, L. (1996): The pathway to care in post-natal depression: women's attitudes to post-natal depression and its treatment. British Journal of General Practice 46: 427–428

Wing, J.K., Cooper, J.E., and Sartorius, N. (1974): The measurement and classification of psychiatric symptoms. Cambridge: Cambridge University Press

11

Bipolar Disorder and Family Psychoeducational Treatment:

A Comparison of One-Year Effects Using Repeated Measures Analysis of Variance and Random Regression Models

Jeffrey A. Richards and David J. Miklowitz

Introduction

Bipolar disorder manifests over time in a recurrent or episodic manner. Symptoms progress and recede in fluctuating patterns of frequency, severity and duration, as well as shifts in mood valence (Goldberg et al., 1995). Investigators interested in describing bipolar disorder longitudinally, particularly those assessing outcome in treatment efficacy research, must determine how best to capture these fluctuations (Coryell and Winokur, 1992). One may conceptualize the course of the disorder in various ways, each of which carries strengths and weaknesses. One common approach is to address symptom severity, which is assessed at select time points, and measure change from baseline to a specific time (e.g., percentage decrease at 12 months) or across select time points. Others have focused on understanding the bipolar symptom course in terms of events. For example, Frank et al. (1991) proposed operational criteria for the course event descriptors *remission, recovery, relapse,* and *recurrence* based on symptomatic variation in severity and duration. Thus, treatment efficacy may be shown by establishing a longer time to relapse or shorter time to remission, by comparing duration of time spent in a symptomatic state, or simply by counting the number of episodes occurring during a follow-up period. These methods are informative, yet each shares the common problem of reducing potentially rich streams of data into less informative units.

Analyses that make use of all or most of the available longitudinal data improve upon this situation.

Fluctuations in symptoms over time among groups are typically compared using some form of analysis of variance (ANOVA). One basic strategy is to assess symptoms at a baseline (e.g., pre-treatment) and then again at a specified time (e.g., post-treatment) and test for mean differences among treatment and control groups via analysis of covariance (ANCOVA). This method may indicate improvement or decline at follow-up, but symptoms occurring outside the assessment period are not considered. This limitation may be mitigated by increasing the number of assessments.

Event-based outcome assessment suggests another statistical strategy. Survival analyses (Cox, 1972) make use of continuously recorded data to examine time elapsed to specific events (e.g., relapse, recovery, or hospitalization). One may compare groups with respect to the time to an outcome event and the probability of occurrence of the event. Given the recurrent nature of bipolar disorder, psychosocial treatments generally aim to affect the course of the illness by either delaying relapse, quickening recovery, or both. Thus, a statistical technique that measures treatment impact on such events is well-suited. Survival analysis has the advantage of taking the entire period of follow-up into consideration, but it is limited to examining discrete, usually dichotomous events. It is not suited to a direct examination of changes in symptomatic outcome over time.

Repeated measures analyses of variance (and covariance) allow one to test for time effects and their interactions with treatment effects at discrete time points over a longitudinal follow-up period. Also, statistical contrasts may be tested; for example, time by treatment interactions may be decomposed into polynomial (i.e., linear, quadratic, etc.) components with increased statistical power (and perhaps with a better fit to the hypotheses being tested). Although the fixed-effect repeated measures ANOVA technique is an improvement over standard univariate ANOVA procedures, the technique is limited in that it requires uniform assessment periods across participants. Perhaps more importantly, participants with missing data are excluded from analyses (Gibbons et al., 1993).

Research that takes advantage of a longitudinal design, such as the treatment efficacy study on which the current report is based, can be subject to complexities that render more difficult the traditional statistical methods. First, as discussed above, discrete outcome events such as relapse or remission do not capture the variability in course patterns over time. Second, participants may not be assessed at similar times, despite the best efforts of the investigators. Third, participant attrition is common. Excluding incomplete or irregular data from analyses can contribute to misleading or biased interpretations of treatment efficacy. For example, although a protocol may dictate regular follow-up assessments at selected time points, participants may have difficulty adhering to the schedule and so introduce variability into the data. Similarly, participants who drop out of treatment may do so because their treatment has been ineffective. Thus, analyzing data derived only from those who complete the treatment protocol may lead to inflated estimates of efficacy.

These concerns may be addressed by the use of mixed-effect random regression models (RRMs, Gibbons et al., 1988; Gibbons and Hedeker, 2000). In addition to measuring average change over time at the population level, random regression models also account for heterogeneous individual responses. For example, whereas the fixed-effect repeated measures ANOVA ignores individual variability among participants within groups, the RRM estimates individual differences that go beyond group differences. Individual effects are estimated by taking weighted averages of the participant's own data and the average group data. So, individual effects for participants with more data are weighted more heavily than the group data, but effects for participants with missing data may still be modeled by weighing the group data more heavily (Gibbons et al., 1993). Thus, an investigator may examine the degree of individual variation in the sample relative to group variation. Given the difficulties that can occur in treatment efficacy studies, such an approach seems well-suited to evaluating outcomes.

The current treatment efficacy study compared a family-focused psychoeducational treatment for bipolar disorder (Miklowitz and Goldstein, 1997) with a standard care crisis management condition. Psychosocial interventions for bipolar disorder are increasingly important as evidence accumulates that pharmacotherapy alone is insufficient. Although medication-based interventions are improving, even the most aggressive may fail to prevent relapse or poor functional outcomes (e.g., Gitlin et al., 1995). Miklowitz and Frank (1999) detail a variety of supporting arguments for adjunctive psychosocial interventions for bipolar patients, among which is addressing medication nonadherence and enhancing the protective effects of the family and social environment. Given the variable course of bipolar disorder, one must consider not only whether treatments produce improvement initially but also whether such improvements exceed what may be expected in the natural course of the illness over time.

The purpose of the present study is to analyze symptom outcome data from the first year of a 2-year treatment efficacy study of bipolar disorder using random regression modeling and to compare the results to those from fixed-effect repeated measures analyses of variance. Consistent with earlier findings from this study (Miklowitz et al., 2000), it is predicted that among participants who complete the protocol, those who received the family-focused psychosocial intervention will show better symptomatic outcome over time than those in the crisis management condition, and that this difference will be present at the conclusion of treatment (i.e., at the 12-month assessment). It is further predicted that this effect will not be significantly altered by unmeasured effects (i.e., individual variation). Finally, it is predicted that a re-analysis of the data including participants who did not complete the protocol will yield similar treatment effects.

Patients (Material) and Methods

Participants

Participants (N = 101) were psychiatric inpatients (N = 82) and outpatient referrals (N = 19) from the Boulder/Denver, CO area who were recruited to participate in a two year longitudinal treatment protocol for bipolar disorder (cf. Miklowitz et al., 2000). Research interview assessments covering symptom severity, medication compliance, and social and occupational functioning, were conducted every 3 months over the first year of the study. Of the 101 participants recruited into the study, 79 continued their involvement to the 12 month assessment (the 1-year completer sample). Of the 22 participants who dropped out of the study in the first year, 19 completed at least one research assessment, and 3 were not assessed subsequent to admission. Thus, research outcome data were available for 98 participants (the intent-to-treat sample). Table 1 shows demographic and illness history characteristics of the intent-to-treat sample.

Table 1. Demographic and illness history characteristics of 98 patients with bipolar disorder

	All (N = 98) Mean (SD)	CM (N = 67) Mean (SD)	FFT (N = 31) Mean (SD)
Age (years)	35.4 (10.2)	35.3 (10.7)	35.7 (9.2)
SES	2.4 (1.1)	2.4 (1.1)	2.5 (1.1)
Education (years)	13.7 (2.4)	13.8 (2.3)	13.5 (2.7)
% Female	63%	66%	58%
Onset age	24.1 (9.2)	24.4 (9.9)	23.4 (7.6)
Prior episodes	4.8 (4.9)	4.4 (4.5)	5.5 (5.5)
Prior hospitalizations	2.5 (3.0)	2.4 (2.8)	2.7 (3.4)

Socioeconomic status computed according to Hollingshead and Redlich, 1958.

To be accepted into the study, participants were required to meet diagnostic criteria for bipolar I disorder according to the Diagnostic and Statistical Manual of Mental Disorders, Revised Third Ed. (DSM-III-R, American Psychiatric Association, 1987). The 101 participants met DSM-III-R criteria within the preceding 3 months for a bipolar manic (N = 51), mixed (N = 35) or depressed (N = 15) episode based on the Structured Clinical Interview for DSM-III-R, Patient Version (SCID-P, Spitzer et al., 1992). Participants also met the following inclusion criteria: age between 18 and 60; absence of neurological disorders or developmental disabilities; absence of DSM-III-R psychoactive substance abuse or dependence diagnoses in the preceding 6 months; regular contact with a close relative willing to participate; willingness to follow a pharmacological treatment plan; and willingness of patients and relatives to provide informed consent.

Study Design

On completion of the evaluation protocols (including a baseline symptom assessment) and acceptance into the study, participants and their family members engaged in an interactional assessment (for details see Simoneau et al., 1999), approximately 4–5 weeks after the baseline diagnostic assessment. After this family assessment, participants were randomly assigned to one of two 9-month psychosocial treatment protocols (in a 1:2 ratio): family-focused treatment (FFT) with pharmacotherapy (N = 31) or a crisis management comparison condition (CM) with pharmacotherapy (N = 70). (All three participants who withdrew from the study before completing any research assessments were in the CM condition.) The protocol assignment ratio was in accordance with the ratio of available clinicians to participants (see also Miklowitz et al., 2000).

The 31 participants assigned to FFT participated in upto 21 one-hour sessions ($M = 18.1 \pm 6.2$) of family therapy over the next 9 months (12 weekly sessions, followed by 6 biweekly sessions, concluding with 3 monthly sessions). Sessions were conducted in the families' homes by a cotherapy team, following an FFT manual (Miklowitz and Goldstein, 1990; 1997). Therapists ($N = 19$) were trained first by observing therapy sessions and attending weekly supervision sessions, then by serving as a cotherapist to a trained FFT clinician for at least 2 cases. Levels of previous clinical experience among the therapists varied ($M = 3.5 \pm 3.8$ years), as did educational background (3 with PhDs in psychology, 14 with MA degrees, 2 with BA degrees). The training protocol was sufficient to establish adherence to the treatment (Nelson, 1999).

The FFT treatment protocol consisted of three modules of 7–10 sessions each. The emphasis on each module was left flexible to adapt to the needs of individual families. The first module was centered around education about bipolar disorder (e.g., causes and symptoms), focusing on the family's unique experiences. The second FFT module concentrated on enhancing communication skills (e.g., active listening, giving positive and negative feedback) to reduce intrafamilial stress. Training in problem-solving skills was provided in the third FFT module to help families cope with common conflicts in the post-episode period.

Participants assigned to the CM condition were provided two sessions of family education about bipolar disorder (using a format similar to that of the FFT condition) and emergency counseling sessions as needed. Monthly telephone contact was also maintained, but participants were otherwise followed in a naturalistic manner. This condition was modeled after standard community care.

Pharmacotherapy

Participants were required to maintain pharmacological treatment throughout the study and were referred to such treatment at study entry if not already receiving it. At baseline, 91% ($N = 92$) were prescribed either a primary ($N = 70$) mood stabilizer or a combination ($N = 22$) of mood stabilizers (lithium carbonate, carbamazepine, valproate or in rare cases, verapamil). In addition to the mood stabilizer(s), participants also received adjunctive antipsychotics ($N = 36$), antidepressants ($N = 17$), and anxiolytics ($N = 21$). Three of the remaining nine participants were treated without a primary mood stabilizer, one refused medication, and five withdrew from the study before the medication regime could be assessed.

Symptom Severity Assessment Measure

Symptom severity status was assessed in clinical interviews using the Schedule for Affective Disorders and Schizophrenia, Change Version (SADS-C, Spitzer and Endicott, 1978). The SADS-C contains 36 Likert-scaled items, although for this study only the 18 items that assess depression and mania symptoms were included. Scores range from 1 to 6 or 7. Depression items include depressed mood, loss of interests, suicidal tendencies, self-reproach, negative self-evaluations, discouragement, insomnia, lack of energy, poor appetite, psychomotor retardation, and weight loss. Mania items include overt irritability, elevated mood, increased activity, grandiosity, agitation, less need for sleep, and increased energy. Separate scores for depression and mania symptom severity were computed as average ratings from the appropriate items. An overall affective symptom severity score was generated from the average rating for all mood disorder items.

Assessments were conducted at 6 time points during the first year: during the baseline diagnostic period, during the pretreatment family assessment (approximately 1 month after study entry), and at 3, 6, 9, and 12 months post-intake. The 9-month FFT treatment started shortly following the family assessment and lasted until 10 months after the baseline assessment. Interviews always covered the period since the preceding interview. The most severe ratings given during the assessment period were chosen to characterize the entire period. Potential relapses occasioned additional assessments. Inter-rater reliability for SADS-C scores was evaluated for the outcome assessors on the basis of at least 10 independent ratings. Intraclass r's for the overall affective symptom severity score ranged from 0.81 to 0.92 ($p < 0.0001$) across 11 outcome assessor/criterion rater pairs.

Statistical Analyses

Parallel analyses were performed on the three SADS-C severity rating scores (depression symptoms, mania symptoms, and overall affective symptoms). A repeated measures ANOVA was performed on the first-year data (which corresponded to the period of active psychosocial treatment) to test whether symptoms varied differentially between the conditions over time. Because the repeated measures ANOVA does not allow missing data, the 22 participants who withdrew prior to the 12 month follow-up were not included, resulting in a first-year completer sample of 79 participants. It was expected that changes in symptom severity would follow a linear course of improvement. Thus, linear trends were examined primarily, with the higher-order effects of time examined secondarily.

Random regression models (RRMs) were constructed using the MIXREG random regression program (Hedeker, 1993). The models, following the same structure as the repeated measures ANOVA, examined whether symptom severity differed between the FFT and CM conditions over time. These analyses were first performed using only the first-year completer sample ($N = 79$) to assess the impact of including individual effects on the group comparisons. Two individual effects were included: baseline symptom severity and symptom change over time. The data for the first-year period were then reanalyzed using the total ($N = 98$) intent-to-treat sample to test whether the comparison between conditions was significantly affected by the inclusion of participants who withdrew from the study. For example, if participant dropouts were differentially distributed across treatment conditions, their inclusion in data analyses might cancel out the effects observed with treatment completers alone. Finally, effect sizes were compared with those from the repeated measures ANOVA, and the potential advantages of random regression models (modeling individual variation and including participants with missing data) were considered.

Results

Repeated Measures Analyses

Three sets of repeated measure ANOVAs were conducted, using overall affective severity scores, depression severity scores and mania severity scores as the dependent variables. Mean overall symptom severity scores are given in Table 2. (See Miklowitz et al., 2000). Time effects represent changes in scores per month.

Table 2. Overall affective symptom scores: means and (standard deviations)

Assessment	1-Year completer ($N = 79$)		Intent-to-treat ($N = 98$)	
	CM ($N = 51$)	FFT ($N = 28$)	CM ($N = 67$)	FFT ($N = 31$)
Baseline	2.82 (0.68)	3.10 (0.81)	2.81 (0.67)	3.07 (0.80)
1 Month	2.19 (0.59)	2.23 (0.61)	2.21 (0.63)	2.22 (0.61)
3 Months	2.31 (0.74)	2.41 (0.79)	2.31 (0.75)	2.39 (0.79)
6 Months	2.17 (0.78)	2.24 (0.94)	2.19 (0.79)	2.24 (0.94)
9 Months	2.17 (0.77)	1.92 (0.64)	2.17 (0.77)	1.92 (0.64)
12 Months	2.21 (0.81)	2.04 (0.74)	2.21 (0.81)	2.04 (0.74)

The analysis of overall severity scores yielded no main effect of FFT versus CM treatment ($F_{1,77} = 0.01$, n.s.), a highly significant main effect of time across conditions ($F_{5,385} = 25.86$, $p < 0.001$), and a treatment by time interaction between conditions ($F_{5,385} = 2.19$, $p = 0.05$). Examination of linear time trends revealed a highly significant linear main effect of time ($F_{1,77} = 40.00$, $p < 0.001$) as well as a significant linear treatment by time interaction between conditions ($F_{1,77} = 5.30$, $p = 0.024$) that indicated greater improvement in the FFT condition.

The repeated measures ANOVA on the depression severity scores showed a significant main effect of time ($F_{5,385} = 7.10$, $p < 0.001$), no significant main effect of treatment condition ($F_{1,77} = 0.01$, n.s.), and a significant treatment by time interaction between conditions ($F_{5,385} = 2.36$, $p = 0.040$), again indicating greater improvement in the FFT condition. A significant linear main effect of time was found ($F_{1,77} = 15.84$, $p < 0.001$), though the linear treatment by time interaction ($F_{1,77} = 3.70$, $p = 0.058$) was of borderline significance.

The repeated measures ANOVA on mania severity scores also showed a significant main effect of time ($F_{5,385} = 27.66$, $p < 0.0001$), but no significant main effect of treatment condition ($F_{1,77} = 0.00$, n.s.), or treatment by time interaction between conditions ($F_{5,385} = 0.74$, n.s.), indicating no differential improvement in the FFT condition. A significant linear main effect of time was found ($F_{1,77} = 24.37$, $p < 0.001$), although the linear treatment by time interaction ($F_{1,77} = 1.20$, $p = 0.277$) was not significant.

The repeated measures ANOVAs confirmed the hypothesis that participants who received FFT would show a greater reduction in symptoms over time. This effect was true for overall symptom severity and for depression severity, but not for mania severity. No higher order time by treatment interaction effects (i.e., beyond linear) were found in any of the above analyses, regardless of symptom type. Thus, the repeated measures analysis of the completer sample supported the assumption that symptom change follows a simple linear trajectory. Consequently, random regression models tested only linear time effects.

Random Regression Analyses

Several comments regarding the random regression models are appropriate. First, assessment time points are not required to be fixed (e.g., at 3 months exactly) but may vary as the actual time an individual's assessment occurred (e.g., 3.25 months). For these data, results from models using variable time points did not appreciably differ from those using fixed time points. Thus, the simpler fixed-time models are presented here. Second, the random regression technique allows the application of autocorrelation of errors of measurement within participants, and all models were calculated with and without autocorrelation components. Fixed group effects did not substantially differ based on this component, though in some cases the random time component was marginally affected. For greater simplicity, the analyses presented do not include an autocorrelation component. Finally, parameter estimates should be interpreted according to the following: treatment condition was contrast coded for these analyses (CM = –1, FFT = +1), and time effects represent linear change in scores per month.

Table 3 presents the population and individual parameter estimates for the random regression analyses of symptomatic outcome at 12 months. Parameter estimates predicting overall severity scores for the first-year completer sample ($N = 79$) are quite close in value to those for the full intent-to-treat sample ($N = 98$). This similarity suggests that the participants who withdrew from the study were not following a substantially different course trajectory from those who remained in the study. Analyses of completer and intent-to-treat samples showed significant population effects of initial severity and time, no main effect of treatment condition, and significant treatment by time interactions (see Table 3). The results indicated that participants entered the study at an average overall symptom severity level of 2.6 (indicating mild severity based on the 18 SADS-C items used), which is not surprising given that participants were recruited

Table 3. 12-Month random regression parameter estimates for population and individual effects

	Population effects				Individual effects			
	Baseline severity	Time	Treatment	Time × treatment	Baseline severity	Time	Time × severity	Residual variance
Completer (N=79)								
Overall symptoms	2.607*	−0.053*	0.087	−0.017*	0.201*	−0.001#	0.001	0.348*
Depression symptoms	2.678*	−0.044*	0.132	−0.021#	0.603*	−0.024*	0.004*	0.479*
Mania symptoms	2.509*	−0.071*	0.029	−0.011	0.032	0.000	0.000	0.969*
Intent-to-treat (N=98)								
Overall symptoms	2.613*	−0.054*	0.078	−0.016*	0.185*	0.001#	−0.000	0.355*
Depression symptoms	2.623*	−0.041*	0.160	−0.022*	0.596*	−0.024*	0.004*	0.482*
Mania symptoms	2.586*	−0.079*	−0.027	−0.006	0.037	0.000	0.000	1.014*

* $p < 0.05$.
# p between 0.05 and 0.10.

in the midst of or immediately following a bipolar episode. The time effect suggested that all participants' symptom scores tended to improve over time (by about 0.05 per month). The time by treatment interaction suggested that the FFT group improved differentially over the CM group (by about 0.03 per month).

With respect to individual effects, significant individual variation in initial severity was found, and individual variation in improvement over time was marginally significant ($p < 0.10$). No significant covariation between these individual effects was observed. Thus, a better estimate of a participant's overall symptom scores (beyond that estimated by the population effects) was obtained by considering individual baseline severity levels and rates of improvement. The lack of covariation between the individual effects suggested that participants' initial severity scores did not determine the degree of improvement over time.

Results from the random regression analysis of the depression severity scores from the first-year completer sample ($N = 79$) and intent-to-treat sample ($N = 98$) are also quite similar. Both indicate significant population effects of initial severity and time, no main effects of treatment, and significant (borderline significant in the completer cases) treatment by time interactions. Significant individual effects on initial severity and improvement over time were found. A significant (but relatively small) positive covariation between these individual effects was observed, suggesting that depression scores decrease to a lesser degree for participants with higher baseline depression.

Random regression analyses of the first-year completer sample ($N = 79$) and intent-to-treat sample ($N = 98$) with respect to mania severity scores were quite similar as well. The only significant effects found were population effects of initial severity and time. The addition of individual effects did not result in better estimates of mania severity scores.

Repeated Measures ANOVA versus Random Regression

Table 4 lists effect sizes (R^2) for the linear time by treatment effect of interest in the 12-month completer sample from the repeated measures ANOVAs and the random regression models. These models differ in that the former have no individual random effects, but the

Table 4. Effect sizes (R^2) for linear time by treatment effects: repeated measures ANOVA versus random regression

	Repeated measures completer sample	Random regression completer sample	Random regression intent-to-treat sample
Overall symptoms	0.064*	0.057*	0.043*
Depression symptoms	0.046#	0.048#	0.045*
Mania symptoms	0.015	0.014	0.003

* $p < 0.05$.
# p between 0.05 to 0.10.

latter do. In the present study the effect sizes are roughly comparable in magnitude and significance level between the two approaches. These results suggest that although significant individual variation in symptom severity is present, it is relatively independent of the simple linear change effects of treatment over time.

Table 4 also lists random regression effect sizes (R^2) for the linear time by treatment effect of interest, in the intent-to-treat sample. These effect sizes are comparable to those from the random regression analyses of the completer samples at those time points, although they are numerically smaller. The fact that they are smaller does raise the possibility that effects are overestimated in the completer analyses, although the largest difference in effect sizes was only 0.014. Nevertheless, further investigation of the sources of such differences may be helpful in understanding participant attrition. For example, participants who withdraw from treatment may not experience as high a level of symptom reduction over time as those who choose to stay in treatment.

Discussion

This study examined the first-year symptomatic outcome of bipolar patients who participated in a randomized study of a psychosocial treatment and mood-stabilizing medications. The study compared a family-focused psychoeducational approach with pharmacotherapy

(FFT) to a standard care crisis management, education, and pharmacotherapy condition (CM) for patients who had recently experienced a bipolar episode. Symptom assessments were conducted at
six time points over the course of the first year. The efficacy of FFT
was evaluated for 12 months after intake into the study (shortly
following treatment completion).

Bipolar patients recovering from a recent episode fared
better following FFT than did those who received standard crisis
management care. Participation in FFT resulted in less severe overall
affective symptoms during the course of the first year following the
episode. Decomposition of the overall symptom scores into constit-
uent depression and mania components revealed that the advantage
was greater for depression scores than for mania scores (for which
treatment effects were nonsignificant).

Other studies (e.g., Clarkin et al., 1998; Goldstein and
Miklowitz, 1995) have reported benefits in delivering psychosocial
treatments in conjunction with pharmacotherapy (cf. Miklowitz, 1996,
and Miklowitz and Frank, 1999 for more thorough discussions of
psychosocial interventions for bipolar disorder). FFT treatment did
not produce differential improvement in manic symptoms beyond that
attributed to medication (and the natural course of bipolar episodes).
In contrast, pharmacological interventions for bipolar disorder (i.e.,
lithium, divalproex, carbamazepine) tend to be more effective in
reducing or preventing the occurrence of mania symptoms than the
occurrence of depression symptoms (Keck and McElroy, 1996).

Beyond confirming the efficacy of FFT in reducing bipolar
symptom severity, this study compared two statistical methodologies
to analyze the effects of treatment: repeated measures analysis of
variance and random regression modeling. Certain unique features of
random regression proved to be unnecessary. First, the introduction
of an autocorrelation component (i.e., within-subject correlations
among time sequential data) to the prediction estimates did not
produce a better fit to the outcome data than models which did not
include an autocorrelation effect. Even when the autocorrelation
models made significantly better outcome predictions, the differences
with the other, simpler models were very small. Second, calculations
made using very specific assessment time points (i.e., the week rather
than the month post-intake of the follow-up assessment) yielded
virtually identical estimations of the population and individual
effects. One explanation for this negative result is that in the present
study the actual week of follow-up assessment occurred reason-

ably closely to the scheduled week (on average, a difference of 2.5 weeks).

A major incentive for using random regression modeling is to increase the accuracy of outcome predictions by considering not only group and sample-wide (or population) fixed effects, but also individual-specific random effects. Individual variation in baseline symptom severity was found to increase estimates of symptomatic outcome significantly beyond the population effects for the depression and mania composite total scores and the depression scores alone. Mania scores did not show such an effect. Individual effects for time were also found to be significant or of borderline significance, beyond the population effects for the composite total scores and the depression scores. The same was not true for the mania scores.

These effects suggest that there is value in attending to individual variation in symptom severity. Although the effects are small relative to the population effects, they suggest that the assumption of equivalent variation across participants within a group may be inaccurate. That is, predictions of individual symptomatic outcome based on a sample average of initial severity are less accurate than those calculated on the basis of the sample and the individual. These results, for depression symptomatology in particular, are consistent with Elkin et al.'s (1995) re-analysis of data from the National Institute of Mental Health Treatment of Depression Collaborative Research Program (TDCRP) using random regression models.

Elkin et al. (1995) found that the baseline severity of depression symptoms predicted differential responses to psychosocial and pharmacological treatments, but only in a high initial severity subgroup. Earlier survival analyses of data from the same sample (Elkin et al., 1989; Shea et al., 1992) had not found this effect. Elkin et al. (1995) also found significant treatment comparisons using random regression models that had not reached significance in earlier analyses. They attributed their different results to the increased power of the random regression methodology, especially the use of all available outcome data.

Participant attrition is a typically unavoidable occurrence in longitudinal research, so a methodology that can utilize all existing data, however incomplete, is welcome. Another incentive for using random regression techniques is the ability to include participants with incomplete data in a repeated measures format. A repeated measures ANOVA limits the investigation of fixed time effects to participants who contribute a full complement of scores, but random regression modeling has no such restrictions. This flexibility allows the very useful comparison of intent-to-treat samples with completer samples. With respect to the course of symptom severity, it does not appear that in this study the participants who withdrew substantially differed from those who did not. Parameter estimates (population and individual) were quite similar when compared in random effect models across the completer and intent-to-treat samples. These findings give greater assurance that the treatment effects observed among this study's protocol completers are not markedly biased by participant attrition.

The present findings, and those described in Miklowitz et al. (2000), suggest that FFT with pharmacotherapy is associated with greater improvements in symptom severity than CM with pharmacotherapy, over a one year period of treatment and evaluation. However, the effects of FFT are limited to depression symptoms. In parallel, Frank (1999) compared interpersonal psychotherapy with medication to clinical management with medication in a sample of bipolar patients and also found greater effects on depressive than manic symptoms. Whether adjunctive psychosocial interventions can produce reductions in mania symptoms beyond those afforded by pharmacological interventions deserves further investigation.

With respect to the time effects used in the random regression models, it is possible that considering only linear time trends is too simplistic. For example, symptomatic recovery from a bipolar episode can follow a complex course of gradual recovery with occasional worsening (Coryell and Winokur, 1992). Although it is possible that some patients do follow a nonlinear symptomatic course, significant polynomial time by treatment effects were not observed in this sample.

As Elkin et al. (1995) noted, the increased statistical power of random regression models can more clearly delineate differences among treatments in longitudinal designs. In particular, treatment studies could take advantage of the flexibility of the random regression methodology by paying greater attention to individual differences, beyond average group effects, in symptomatic profile and treatment response. For example, the apparent efficacy of a treatment could be impacted by relatively large differences in individual treatment response based on initial symptom severity. Parsing out these unique effects could more clearly highlight treatment effects and lead to refinements in tailoring the intensity or timing of the treatment to the individual.

References

American Psychiatric Association (1987): Diagnostic and statistical manual of mental disorders. 3rd revised ed. Washington, DC

Clarkin, J.F., Carpenter, D., Hull, J., Wilner, P., and Glick, I. (1998): Effects of psychoeducational intervention for married patients with bipolar disorder and their spouses. Psychiatric Services, 49: 531–533

Coryell, W. and Winokur, G. (1992): Course and outcome. In: Handbook of affective disorders (Paykel, E., ed.), pp. 89–108. New York: Guilford Press

Cox, D.R. (1972): Regression models and life tables. Journal of the Royal Statistical Society, Ser B 34: 187–220

Elkin, I., Shea, M.T., Watkins, J.T., Imber, S.D., Sotsky, S.M., Collins, J.F., Glass, D.R., Pilkonis, P.A., Leber, W.R., Docherty, J.P., Fiester, S.J., and Parloff, M.B. (1989): National Institute of Mental Health Treatment of Depression Collaborative Research Program: General effectiveness of treatments. Archives of General Psychiatry 46: 971–982

Elkin, I., Shea, M.T., Watkins, J.T., Gibbons, R.D., Sotsky, S.M., Pilkonis, P.A., and Hedeker, D. (1995): Initial severity and differential treatment outcome in the National Institute of Mental Health Treatment of Depression Collaborative Research Program. Journal of Consulting and Clinical Psychology 63: 841–847

Frank, E. (1999): Interpersonal and social rhythm therapy prevents depressive symptomatology in bipolar I patients (abstract). Bipolar Disorders 1(Suppl. 1): p. 13

Frank, E., Prien, R.F., Jarrett, R.B., Keller, M.B., Kupfer, D.J., Lavori, P.W., Rush, A.J., and Weissman, M.M. (1991): Conceptualization and rationale for consensus definitions of terms in major depressive disorder. Archives of General Psychiatry 48: 851–855

Gibbons, R.D. and Hedeker, D. (2000): Applications of mixed-effects models in biostatistics. Sankhya Ser B, 62: 70–103

Gibbons, R.D., Hedeker, D., Elkin, I., Waternaux, C., Kraemer, H.C., Greenhouse, J.B., Shea, M.T., Imber, S.D., Sotsky, S.M., and Watkins, J.T. (1993): Some conceptual and statistical issues in analysis of longitudinal psychiatric data. Archives of General Psychiatry 50: 739–750

Gibbons, R.D., Hedeker, D., Waternaux, C., and Davis, J.M. (1988): Random regression models: a comprehensive approach to the analysis of longitudinal psychiatric data. Psychopharmacology Bulletin 24: 438–443

Gitlin, M.J., Swendson, J., Heller, T.L., and Hammen, C. (1995): Relapse and impairment in bipolar disorder. American Journal of Psychiatry 152: 1635–1640

Goldberg, J.F., Harrow, M, and Grossman, L.S. (1995): Course and outcome in bipolar affective disorder: A longitudinal follow-up study. American Journal of Psychiatry 152: 379–384

Goldstein, M.J. and Miklowitz, D.J. (1995): The effectiveness of psychoeducational family therapy in the treatment of schizophrenic disorders. Journal of Marital Family Therapy 21: 361–376

Hedeker, D. (1993): MIXREG: A FORTRAN program for mixed-effects linear regression models [Computer program]. Chicago: Prevention Research Center, University of Illinois

Hollingshead, A. and Redlich, F. (1958): Social class and mental illness. New York: Wiley

Keck, P.E. and McElroy, S.L. (1996): Outcome in the pharmacologic treatment of bipolar disorder. Journal of Clinical Psychopharmacology 16(Suppl 1): 15S–23S

Miklowitz, D.J. (1996): Psychotherapy in combination with drug treatment for bipolar disorder. Journal of Clinical Psychopharmacology 16(Suppl 1): 56S–66S

Miklowitz, D.J. and Frank, E. (1999): New psychotherapies for bipolar disorder. In: Bipolar disorders: Clinical course and outcome (Goldberg, J.H. and Harrow, M., eds.), pp. 57–84. Washington, DC: American Psychiatric Press

Miklowitz, D.J. and Goldstein, M.J. (1990): Behavioral family treatment for patients with bipolar affective disorder. Behavior Modification 14: 457–489

Miklowitz, D.J. and Goldstein, M.J. (1997): Bipolar disorder: A family-focused treatment approach. New York: Guilford Press

Miklowitz, D.J. Goldstein, M.J., Nuechterlein, K.H., Snyder, K.S., and Mintz, J. (1988): Family factors and the course of bipolar affective disorder. Archives of General Psychiatry 45: 225–231

Miklowitz, D.J., Simoneau, T.L., George, E.A., Richards, J.A., Kalbag, A., Sachs-Ericsson, N., and Suddath, R. (2000). Family-focused treatment of bipolar disorder: One-year effects of a psychoeducational program in conjunction with pharmacotherapy. Biological Psychiatry 48: 581–592

Nelson, J. (1999): Evaluating therapist adherence and competence to a family-focused psychoeducational treatment for bipolar patients. Unpublished manuscript, University of Colorado at Boulder

Shea, M.T., Elkin, I., Imber, S.D., Sotsky, S.M., Watkins, J.T., Collins, J.F., Pilkonis, P.A., Beckham, E., Glass, D.R., Dolan, R.G., and Parloff, M.B. (1992): Course of depressive symptoms over follow-up: Findings from the National Institute of Mental Health Treatment of Depression Collaborative Research Program. Archives of General Psychiatry 49: 782–787

Simoneau, T.L., Miklowitz, D.J., Richards, J.A., Saleem, R., and George, E.L. (1999): Bipolar disorder and family communication: Effects of a psycho-educational treatment program. Journal of Abnormal Psychology 108: 588–597

Spitzer, R.L. and Endicott, J. (1978): Schedule for affective disorders and schizophrenia, change version (SADS-C). New York: New York State Psychiatric Institute

Spitzer, R.L., Williams, J.B.W., Gibbon, M., and First, M.B. (1992): The structured clinical interview for DSM-III-R (SCID), I. History, rationale, and description. Archives of General Psychiatry 49: 624–629

12
Family Intervention for Severe Mental Illness and Substance Use Disorder

Kim T. Mueser, Lindy Fox and Carolyn Mercer

Introduction

Alcohol and drug use disorders (including both abuse and dependence) are a major problem that plagues the lives of many persons with severe mental illness (SMI) such as schizophrenia or bipolar disorder. Epidemiological research has repeatedly shown that individuals with SMI are at increased risk to develop substance use disorders (Cuffel, 1996; Regier et al., 1990). Surveys of the prevalence of substance abuse among the SMI population indicate that on average between 40 and 60 percent of clients have a disorder over their lifetime, and 25 to 40 percent have a current substance use disorder (Mueser et al., 1995a).

The problem of substance abuse is important because alcohol and drug use can have a deleterious effect on the course of psychiatric illnesses. Substance use disorders in psychiatric clients are associated with many negative consequences, including more relapses (Drake et al., 1996; Haywood et al., 1995), arrests and incarceration (Barry et al., 1996), medication non-compliance (Miner et al., 1997), aggressive or violent behavior (Swartz et al., 1998), engagement in HIV risky behaviors (Cournos et al., 1991), homelessness (Susser et al., 1989), and utilization of costly psychiatric services (Dickey and Azeni, 1996). Thus, addressing substance abuse in the SMI is critical in order to improve the long term outcome of these disorders.

Prior to the mid-1980s, most programs for dually diagnosed clients provided mental health and substance abuse treatments in either a parallel fashion (i.e., simultaneous treatments provided by different programs) or sequentially (i.e., one disorder treated first followed by another) (Minkoff, 1991; Ridgely, Goldman and Willenbring, 1990). The lack of treatment integration posed numerous obstacles to families and professionals alike. Concerned family members often experienced difficulty obtaining assistance from professionals involved in the management of a dually diagnosed relative. Professionals themselves were often at odds with one another about treatment philosophy, the boundaries of responsibility, and perceptions of the role of families. Recognition of the inadequacy of the parallel and sequential treatment approaches for dually diagnosed clients led to the development of integrated treatment approaches in which interventions are provided by the same clinicians that simultaneously address both substance use and psychiatric disorders (Carey, 1989; Drake et al., 1993; Mueser et al., 1998).

As integrated treatment programs for dually diagnosed clients have developed, there have been some forays into family work with this population. Among 13 local Community Support Program (CSP) demonstration projects of dual diagnosis treatment for young adults with SMI, ten established the goal of reaching out and working with families (Mercer-McFadden et al., 1997). Several studies reported disappointing results of their efforts to involve families. However, Edwards et al. (1991) reported that engaging families early correlated with progress in clients' substance abuse, and Johnsen et al. (1992) reported that culturally specific family work was successful in engaging families and improving client outcomes. A notable problem is that few projects described specific interventions for families.

In this chapter we begin with a discussion of the importance of involving family members in the treatment of dually diagnosed clients. Next, we introduce the concept of stages of treatment, and explain how an understanding of the process of recovery from substance abuse in persons with SMI can be used to determine appropriate treatment goals and interventions in family work. We then describe a family intervention model developed for dual disorders. We conclude with a case example of a family who participated in this program, and preliminary data from a pilot study of its effectiveness.

The Importance of Families

Working with the families of dually diagnosed clients may be beneficial for several reasons. First, many dually diagnosed clients have regular contact with their relatives (Clark, 1996). Between 25% and 60% of persons with SMI live at home (Goldman, 1984; Talbott, 1990), and many others maintain contact with relatives. Clients with SMI tend to have constricted social networks (Cresswell et al., 1992; Sokolove and Trimble, 1986) so that relatives are often the most important social relationships in their lives. This special relationship enables family members to encourage clients to take steps towards recovery and greater self-sufficiency.

Second, there are many challenges in maintaining a relationship with a dually diagnosed individual. Caring for a person with SMI is associated with high levels of distress (Hatfield and Lefley, 1987; Lefley and Johnson, 1990). Furthermore, dually diagnosed clients create even more tension and interpersonal conflict in their families (Dixon et al., 1995; Salyers and Mueser, in press), which is further exacerbated by violence directed at family members (Steadman et al., 1998). The net effects of chronic caregiver stress can be a weakening of family support, leading to housing instability and homelessness (Caton et al., 1994; Caton et al., 1995). Family intervention that reduces stress on relatives, including the negative impact of substance abuse, can avoid overwhelming the coping efforts of families, averting the loss of their support. In addition, reducing family tension due to substance abuse may decrease clients' vulnerability to relapse (Butzlaff and Hooley, 1998).

Third, family intervention is important because relatives often know little about the interactions between substance use and severe mental illness. Substance use disorders are more common in families of dually diagnosed clients (Noordsy et al., 1994), and relatives may unintentionally enable clients' use of substances. Families need practical information about dual disorders, and help in both recognizing the signs of substance abuse and developing strategies for its management (Clark and Drake, 1992; Mueser and Gingerich, 1994).

Finally, there is abundant evidence that family intervention for clients with SMI has a positive effect on the course and outcome of the disorders, especially in preventing relapses and rehospitalizations (Dixon et al., 2000). In addition, research shows that family therapy is more effective than individual counseling or therapy, peer group therapy, or family psychoeducation in improving substance abuse outcomes (Stanton and Shadish, 1997). The evidence supporting the effects of family intervention for the SMI and primary substance abuse populations suggests that working with families may also improve the course of dual disorders.

Stage-wise Treatment for Families

In recent years, integrated programs for dual disorders have adopted a stage-wise approach to treatment. Stage-wise approaches are based on the assumption that recovery from a substance use disorder takes place over a series of stages, and that the goals and treatment strategies vary from one stage to the next (Osher and Kofoed, 1989).

One widely used formulation of the stages of treatment identifies four stages: engagement, persuasion, active treatment, and relapse prevention (e.g., Mueser et al., 1998). During the *engagement stage*, the client does not have a therapeutic relationship with a clinician, nor does he or she recognize substance abuse as a problem. Therefore, the goal of this stage is to establish a working relationship with the client. Notably, at this stage the relationship is not strong and the clinician does *not* try to convince the client that substance abuse is a problem. At the *persuasion stage*, the client and clinician have established a strong relationship, but the client does not recognize substance abuse as a problem. Therefore, the primary goal of this stage is for the client to identify substance abuse as a problem that he or she wants to address.

In the *active treatment* stage, the client is motivated to work on substance abuse and the focus of treatment is on reducing (or eliminating) alcohol and drug use. When clients achieve a sustained level of harmless substance use or abstinence they enter the *relapse prevention stage*. The aim of treatment in this stage is to help clients maintain an awareness of their vulnerability to relapses of substance abuse, while expanding recovery to other areas of functioning, such as social relationships, work, and health.

The concept of stages of treatment can also be useful for working with families. At the beginning of treatment during the *engagement stage* clinician reach out to families, provide them with practical assistance, and begin the educational process in order to establish a collaborative working relationship. Clinicians may inadvertently drive family members away from treatment "jumping the gun" too quickly by trying to address substance abuse before the family is ready. Similarly, the clinician may alienate the client from treatment if he or she colludes with relatives' belief that *all* the client's problems stem from substance abuse rather than the mental illness.

As the relationship solidifies and the family enters the *persuasion stage*, the clinician begins to educate families about the effects of substances on the course of psychiatric illness in order to develop motivation to address the substance abuse. In addition to educating family members, clinicians can employ motivational strategies (Miller and Rollnick, 1991) to inform family members about the impact of substance abuse. For example, helping families articulate specific client-related goals and exploring the possible obstacles (including substance abuse) to achieving these goals is often effective at fostering motivation to change.

When family members recognize the impact of substance abuse and enter the *active treatment stage*, the focus shifts to developing strategies for decreasing substance abuse in the dually diagnosed member. A wide range of different methods can be employed to achieve this goal, depending on the client's motivation to change, the circumstances of the client's substance abuse, and the family's communication and problem solving skills. Following successful reduction of substance abuse, family work in the *relapse prevention stage* aims at minimizing vulnerability to relapses of substance abuse and expanding recovery to other areas of functioning.

One important feature of taking a stage-wise approach to working with families is that clients and relatives may differ in their stage of treatment at any particular point in time. Such differences may have important implications for the clinical strategies used with individuals and their families. For example, the client may be at the persuasion stage, not yet convinced that he or she has a substance abuse problem, while other family members are in the active treatment stage, attempting to decrease the client's substance use. In such a case, individual and group work with a client needs to focus on developing awareness about how substance abuse can interfere with obtaining personal goals, while family work can address strategies for reducing the client's propensity to use substances or the effects of substance use on the family. It is also possible for the *same* family member to be at a different stage of treatment with respect to different family members' substance abuse. For example, a wife with a drinking problem may recognize that her dually diagnosed husband has a substance use disorder, but may not view her own drinking as problematic.

Family Intervention for Dual Disorders Program

We describe next the family intervention program for dual disorders (FIDD) program. This program, which is based on the concept of stage-wise family intervention, includes both single and multiple-family group formats. Although families can participate in either format alone, their combination offers unique advantages over either one alone.

Single family intervention involves outreach and engagement of the family, and is focused on psychoeducation and training in problem-solving for addressing the substance abuse and its impact on the family. An immediate goal of the intervention is to maintain family involvement and to buffer relatives against the impact of substance abuse on them. A longer term goal is to decrease the client's substance abuse, and to help everyone make progress towards personal and shared goals. The multiple-family group is provided on a time-unlimited basis, and serves the goal of providing continued psychoeducation about dual disorders and their management, and developing social support from other families with similar experiences, including both relatives and clients. Although multiple-family groups may be helpful in assisting individual families in dealing with specific problems, their primary functions are to provide validation and support for the experiences of family members, and to maintain a connection with the treatment team.

Single Family Treatment

Single family intervention is based on the behavioral family therapy model developed for schizophrenia by Falloon, Boyd, and McGill (1984) and adapted for other psychiatric disorders by Mueser and Glynn (1999). For the FIDD program, the single family treatment is divided into five phases, including connecting with the family, assessment, psychoeducation, problem solving training, and termination. Table 1 provides a summary of the different phases of the single family intervention, and the approximate number of sessions devoted to each phase. We address the logistical aspects of the

Table 1. Phases of single family treatment for dual disorders

	Component	# Meetings	Time-frame
1.	Engagement	3–4	2 weeks
2.	Assessment	1/member	2–3 weeks
3.	Psychoeducation	6	6 weeks
4.	Problem solving	10–15	9 months
5.	Termination	1	1 week

single family intervention model, followed by a description of each of the phases of treatment.

Logistics

Sessions can be conducted in either the home of a family member or the clinic. Although home-based sessions may be less convenient for the clinician, they facilitate engagement of family members in treatment who might not otherwise receive services. In addition, home based sessions provide valuable information to the clinician about the family environment, and provide clues regarding ongoing substance abuse. For many families, conducting some sessions at home, and then shifting the locus of sessions to the clinic is a viable compromise.

Family sessions usually last for one hour and occur on a declining contact basis, usually starting with weekly sessions for about three months, followed by sessions every other week for several months, and then monthly sessions. Although single family treatment is usually time-limited, lasting for a duration of usually at least six months to up to two years, ongoing maintenance sessions can be scheduled.

The participants in family sessions include the client and any relatives who are involved in the client's life, or who want to become more involved. Typical relatives include parents, siblings, spouses, and children. If the client has a long-standing boyfriend or girlfriend, or other important people in his or her social network (e.g., member of the clergy, landlord) those persons can be included in sessions.

Connecting

Connecting with family members and engaging them in treatment often involves outreach. In motivating clients to involve their families in treatment it is helpful to emphasize that working with the family is intended to help all members understand the nature of the client's difficulties, to decrease stress in the family, and to help them solve problems or achieve goals. Establishing a working alliance with families is facilitated by explaining the goals of the FIDD program, and assuring them that sessions are focused on education and solving problems, and not on dredging up the past. Both clients and relatives are responsive to clinicians who invite them to become "members of the treatment team." Such an offer conveys the clinician's respect for the family, his or her willingness and desire to work with everyone, and the understanding that families can make an important contribution to the client's treatment.

The first contact with the family may come during a crisis, such as a symptom relapse, an alcohol or drug binge, an episode of violence, or the loss of housing for the client. In these situations, successful connecting with the family must involve resolving the crisis, which can then be used to continue the relationship through mutual work in family sessions. When engaging the family, clinicians need to be mindful that relatives are often not concerned about the client's use of substances, and may see many other problems as more important (Mueser, Bellack, Wade, Sayers and Rosenthal, 1992). Therefore, it is important when connecting with the family not to emphasize substance abuse as a focus of family work, unless the client or relatives express a concern and desire to work on it. Goals of family work that most members endorse include education, avoiding relapses and rehospitalizations, and promoting more independence for the client.

Assessment

After family members have agreed to participate in family sessions, but before sessions begin, the clinician meets individually with each person. The purpose of these meetings is to build rapport with each member, and to obtain information about his or her perspectives on the strengths and weaknesses of the family. During the individual assessments the clinician explores the family member's understanding of the psychiatric illness and substance use problems, and perceptions of what helps and hinders the disorders. Family work is most successful when it focuses on improving the functioning and well-being of all members, not just the client. In addition to developing an understanding of each person's perceptions of the family, the clinician prompts members to identify goals for family sessions that are personally meaningful and not exclusively focused on the client.

A final goal of assessment is to develop an understanding of the factors which appear to maintain the client's substance abuse, and which prevent him or her from changing to a healthier, more substance-free lifestyle. This "functional analysis" is based on the assumption that substance use is reinforced by the positive consequences, and that decreasing substance use or achieving abstinence is associated with negative consequences (or perceived "costs") in related areas. For example, a client's substance use may occur in social settings and facilitate relationships with others. A cost of giving up substances may be the difficulties in negotiating relationships with others who are substance users, or the need to establish new relationships with non-users. Other examples of functions that substance use may play in persons with a SMI include coping with symptoms (e.g., hallucinations) or negative mood states (depression, apathy), recreation and leisure (e.g., "getting high"), or creating meaning in life (i.e., needing to get money in order to "score" and "get high"). Successful treatment of the substance abuse requires helping clients develop new ways of getting their needs met other than by using substances.

Psychoeducation

A series of eight educational topics are covered in the sessions devoted to psychoeducation, including: 1) Psychiatric diagnosis; 2) Medication; 3) The stress-vulnerability model; 4) The role of the family; 5) Basic facts about alcohol and drugs; 6) Alcohol and drugs: Motives and consequences; 7) Treatment of dual disorders; 8) Good communication.

The primary goal of psychoeducation is to help the family understand the nature of the psychiatric illness and its interactions with substance abuse in order to motivate them to work together on both disorders. Psychoeducation is conducted in a lively, interactive manner. A series of educational handouts are provided to family members that summarize the pertinent information (see Mueser and Glynn, 1999). The clinician connotes the client as the "expert" to help explain facts about the illness, and acknowledges the expertise of the relatives who contribute their own observations. Disagreements between members are acknowledged, but concerted efforts are not made towards their resolution. Rather, the clinician strives to develop a safe atmosphere in the family with a minimum of tension in which free discussion is encouraged, differences in opinion are accepted, and there is a mutual respect for each person's opinion.

By the end of psychoeducation, many families are persuaded to work on substance abuse, and they are in the active stage of treatment. Some families continue to be uncertain about working on substance abuse, and remain in the persuasion stage. Regardless of their stage of treatment, when the educational sessions have been completed the clinician begins training in problem-solving skills.

Problem-solving Training

The focus of problem-solving training is to teach families how to solve problems on their own. Families elect a chairperson to lead them through problem-solving, and a secretary to keep track of the problem solving efforts. Although the clinician may choose to get involved in solving problems with families, the emphasis is on the family acquiring the skills for solving problems on their own. Family members are taught the following sequence for solving problems: (1) Define the problem to everyone's satisfaction; (2) Generate possible solutions; (3) Evaluate advantages and disadvantages of solutions; (4) Select the best solution; (5) Plan on how to implement the selected solution; (6) Meet at a later time to follow-up on the plan.

When families are still in the persuasion stage, problem-solving is aimed at developing motivation to address substance abuse, or reducing it effects on the family. Taking a motivational interviewing approach (Miller and Rollnick, 1991), the clinician identifies goals or problems that family members want to work on. Then, using problem-solving, the clinician explores with the family how to achieve the desired goal or resolve the specific problem. During this process the clinician looks for opportunities to prompt family members to consider whether the client's substance abuse interferes with achieving the goal. Developing a discrepancy between substance abuse and a desired goal can instill motivation to address the problem of substance abuse. For example, a client who wants to work, but does not view his alcohol use as a problem, may experience performance difficulties on a job on days after a bout of heavy drinking. Family problem-solving about improving the client's job performance, or obtaining a more rewarding job, may lead to a decision to reduce drinking on certain days, or to stop drinking altogether.

When families are in the active treatment stage, the focus of problem-solving is often directly on reducing substance use (e.g., self-monitoring urges to use), anticipating high risk situations for continued abuse or that pose a threat to relapse (e.g., going to a family celebration), or developing skills or strategies for getting needs met that were formally met by using substances (e.g., places to meet people who are not substance users, ways of dealing with anxiety). In relapse prevention, the focus of problem-solving shifts to other areas, such as work, independent living, health, and close relationships.

Termination

The decision to terminate is based on a combination of factors, including improvements in the client's substance abuse, skill with the problem-solving method, decreased family stress, and improved ability of the family to manage the dual disorder. The family is involved in determining with the clinician when sessions will end. Termination does not signify an end of the family's role as members' of the treatment team; long-term partnerships between families and treatment providers are necessary to optimize client outcomes.

The clinician reviews with the family the accomplishments they have made, and prompts them to consider future needs. Plans for responding to an impending relapse of either disorder are reviewed. For some families, a regular informal follow-up can be arranged, such as monthly or bimonthly phone calls. If the family is participating in a multiple-family group, as described in the next section, this can provide ongoing social support and regular contact with clinicians. Regardless of the exact arrangements made for social support and involvement with the client's treatment team, the most crucial feature of termination is that relatives feel comfortable with the end of single family sessions, and know that their collaboration with professionals will continue.

Multiple-family Groups

Multiple-family group intervention is based on the model developed for the Treatment Strategies for Schizophrenia study (Schooler et al., 1997), which we have adapted for a wider range of psychiatric disorders. Group meetings are focused on providing ongoing education to families about dual disorders and their management, while facilitating a free exchange that validates each others' experiences, motivates families to directly address the client's dual disorders, and encourages the sharing of coping strategies.

Logistics

Multiple-family groups are conducted on a monthly, time-unlimited basis. Both relatives and clients are invited to participate. If one member declines to participate, the others are still free to attend. Meetings usually last 75–90 minutes. At least three families are needed to begin a multiple-family group. The maximum number of participants in a group should not exceed twenty to thirty. Groups are conducted in a physical space that is well-lit, publicly accessible, and reasonably quiet. The space should permit chairs to be arranged in a circle or semi-circle to facilitate direct interaction among the participants.

Groups are co-led by two leaders. The leaders are professionals from the agency providing treatment to the client. Leaders should be either members of clients' treatment teams or in regular contact with the team to ensure open communication with the family in the event of a relapse. Each month reminder letters are sent out to all participants about two weeks before the next group. Leaders contact family members who miss group meetings in order to express their concern, to evaluate whether any current problems need attention, and to troubleshoot obstacles that may interfere with future participation.

The Structure of Group Meetings

The structure of meetings is summarized in Table 2. Following greetings and introductions the leaders facilitate brief informal discussions among families about how things have been going for them over the past month. This conversation warms the group members up, identifies any critical issues that the leaders may need to address later, and sets the stage for ongoing interaction among families during the remainder of the group.

Table 2. Structure of multiple-family group meetings

Time	Activity
First 5–10 minutes	Greetings, introductions, caring and sharing
Next 20–35 minutes	Presentation on educational topic
Next 20–35 minutes	Group discussion
Final 5–10 minutes	Wrap-up, discuss future topics for groups

When the introductions have been completed, the leaders focus on the educational topic for that meeting. For the first several group sessions, one of the leaders gives the presentation. These presentations by the leaders help to build group cohesion necessary for an effective multiple-family group. After several sessions, the leaders can begin to invite outside speakers to present educational topics, while interspersing such presentations with others done by themselves. When invited speakers present on a topic, the leaders act as group facilitators to stimulate discussion and sharing among family members.

The presentation on the educational topic is prepared in advance and supplemented in the session with posters, overhead transparencies, or flipcharts. Information is provided in a semi-didactic fashion, with the presenter frequently pausing to solicit questions from participants and helping them in understanding its relevance for their own families. For example, beginning a presentation about coping with depression, the presenter might ask group members to list different symptoms of depression, and write down the answers on a flipchart. The presentation transitions into a group discussion, with families sharing their experiences and perspectives.

Sometimes conflict among the members of a family becomes evident, such as relatives commenting on the destructive effects of the client's substance use, but the client denying or minimizing such effects. The leaders explore with other families their experiences with similar situations, and elicit suggestions or examples of how they have dealt with those problems. When facilitating a discussion of specific problems or conflicts experienced by a group member or family, the leaders strive to maintain a mutually respectful, upbeat atmosphere in the group, while acknowledging the frustrations of the members who are involved.

Educational Topics for Multiple-family Groups

Each multiple-family group includes a presentation and discussion of a topic relevant to coping with dual disorders. The presentation need not be lengthy, but should both provide some basic information which serves to stimulate discussion among group members.

A wide variety of sources of information can be tapped to help leaders develop the curriculum for educating family members about a particular topic. Useful sources of information included books for families about coping with mental illness, self-help books, books and periodicals for professionals, and educational videos. Examples for topics for multiple-family groups include: dealing with cravings; improving communication; managing stress; coping with holiday stress; dealing with high risk situations; coping with depression; self-help groups (e.g., AA); dealing with anxiety; finding and improving relationships; resolving conflicts; recreational and leisure activities; work: finding and keeping jobs; planning for the future; new advances in medication treatment; money management. Examples of outside speakers include a doctor from the mental health center to talk about new medications, someone from the social security agency to discuss rules about benefits, an addiction specialist to discuss biological aspects of addiction, or a mental health consumer to discuss the concept of recovery from mental illness.

Pilot Study of the FIDD Program

We conducted a pilot study of the FIDD program at a community mental health center. Clients were enrolled in the program who had: (a) DSM-IV diagnosis of schizophrenia, schizoaffective disorder, bipolar disorder, or major depression, (b) DSM-IV diagnosis of substance use disorder within the past six months; and (c) weekly contact with a relative or long-term conjugal partner. Diagnoses were based on the Structured Clinical Interview for DSM-IV (First et al., 1996).

Ten families have been enrolled in the FIDD program. One family dropped out of treatment, one client died, and six families have completed at least one year of treatment. We describe preliminary findings for these six clients. Three clients were male, three had diagnoses of schizophrenia, one had schizoaffective disorder, one had bipolar disorder, and one had major depression. Five clients had an alcohol use disorder at baseline and five had a drug use disorder. Clients were an average of 30.0 years old (range 20 to 40), had an onset of their SMI at the age of 19.4 (range 15 to 23), and had an onset of their substance use disorder at the age of 16.6 (range 14 to 19). Five families included one or both parents and one included a long-term girlfriend.

Families participated in an average of 29 single family treatment sessions (range 16–50). The majority of sessions were conducted at home for four families and at the clinic for two families. Four families attended the multiple-family groups regularly.

Changes in substance use problems were evaluated with two rating scales: the Alcohol Use Scale (AUS) and the Drug Use Scale (DUS). Progress in stages of treatment were evaluated with the Substance Abuse of Treatment Scale (SATS) (Mueser et al., 1995b). Consensus ratings for each scale were completed at baseline and every six months based on all available data, including clinician reports, records, significant others, and client self-reports.

Changes in the SATS over the course of treatment for each client, and for the overall group, are summarized in Fig. 1. This figure indicates that all clients made significant progress in their stage of treatment, with 3 clients achieving relapse prevention, and 2 clients reaching the active treatment stage. Figure 2 depicts changes over treatment in the AUS and DUS for each client and the overall

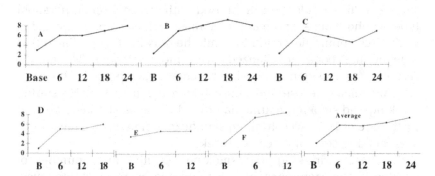

Fig. 1. Changes in individual clients' stage of treatment, and the overall group, on the Substance Abuse of Treatment Scale (SATS). Scores on the SATS correspond to the four stages of treatment, with higher numbers reflecting more progress in dual disorder treatment: 1–2 = early and late *engagement*, 3–4 = *persuasion*, 5–6 = *active treatment*, and 7–8 = *relapse prevention*

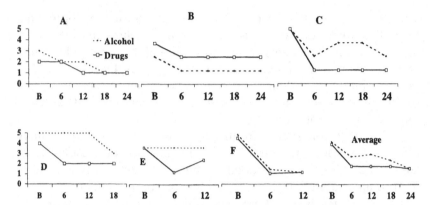

Fig. 2. Changes in substance abuse for individual clients, and the overall group, on the Alcohol Use Scale (AUS) and Drug Use Scale (DUS). For the AUS and DUS, 1 = abstinence for the past 6 months, 2 = use without impairment, and 3 = abuse, 4 = dependence, and 5 = dependence with institutionalization group. All of the clients improved in their substance abuse. These findings suggest that the FIDD program may be helpful in treating dual disorders.

Case Vignette

Jack is a 26 year old man diagnosed with schizophrenia, paranoid type, alcohol abuse, and marijuana abuse. He was first hospitalized for his schizophrenia at age 22 while he was in college. Since that time he has been hospitalized twice more, at ages 24 and 25. Although Jack began to develop psychiatric symptoms in his early 20s, his substance use and abuse began much earlier. He started drinking and smoking marijuana around the ages of 15 and 16, and by the age of 19 he was drinking significant amounts on a daily basis and smoking several times per week.

Jack's drinking and smoking resulted in a number of problems. His symptoms of schizophrenia were only tenuously controlled, and he experienced persistent delusions of reference, poor attention, and disorganization which were exacerbated by his substance abuse. Jack had not worked in several years. His substance use led to frequent conflicts with his mother and stepfather, and limited his ability to form friendships with new people, despite a desire to do so. When Jack was enrolled in the family program he was drinking alcohol every few days, in quantities ranging between three and eight drinks at a time. Jack indicated that he had been abstinent from marijuana for two months, but prior to that he had been smoking every other day for four months. Jack was also a heavy cigarette smoker, averaging about two packs per day.

Jack is the youngest in the family with seven other siblings. Jack was living with his mother and stepfather when he was engaged in the FIDD program. Jack was in contact with his biological father, who lives in a different state. Jack's mother stated that his father is an alcoholic, which is why she divorced him. One of Jack's brothers also has an alcohol problem and has been in and out of treatment for it over the past ten years.

During Jack's individual assessment, and in subsequent meetings, it was noted that he had difficulty organizing his thinking and staying on track. Because of this, his social functioning was low as he had trouble relating to other people. Jack stated one goal during the assessment of making some friends, and expressed an interest in having a girlfriend. He recognized that his drinking was a problem, and wanted to cut down. In the assessment of Jack's mother, she expressed extreme anxiety over his psychiatric illness and the effects of alcohol on it. She felt that Jack was unable to take care of himself or to manage his illness, and that he required daily monitoring, even if it meant sacrificing some of her own needs. Jack resented what he perceived to be his mother's overinvolvement in his life, which led to conflict between them. Nevertheless, there was a close bond between mother and son, and they both indicated enjoying the other's company. Jack's mother expressed a desire to spend less time managing Jack's illness and more on herself (e.g., taking an exercise class) and with her husband. Jack's stepfather was supportive of his mother's concern for Jack, but had a more strained relationship with Jack. He tended to be highly critical of Jack, which often led to arguments, and he had only a limited understanding of Jack's schizophrenia. Jack's mother was often stuck between Jack and his stepfather, "protecting" Jack from criticism while trying to communicate her and her husband's concerns to Jack. Jack's stepfather expressed an interest in learning more about Jack's illness, and a desire for Jack to live more independently so that he and his wife could travel more.

The family treatment began with the six educational sessions. During the session on "What is Schizophrenia?," Jack talked openly about his symptoms, and his stepfather began to see what the experience was like for Jack. During the educational sessions on substance use, Jack gained a better understanding of how he used substances to escape from feelings of failure. The whole family was interested in the concept of integrated dual diagnosis treatment and looked forward to becoming active members of Jack's treatment team.

After being introduced to problem-solving, the first problem the family worked on was getting Jack enrolled in a course at a local community college. Jack's mother was worried that the stress might be too great because he first became ill while in college, but she was able to suspend her concerns and encourage him to pursue his education. Over the first year of treatment, Jack successfully completed two courses. Another problem the family worked on was to increase Jack's independence. Following several problem-solving discussions, Jack moved into supervised housing, and then several months later into his own apartment. As part of the problem-solving, the family members also agreed on how often Jack's mother would check on him.

Over the course of treatment, Jack had several months of sobriety and then began drinking again. Jack stopped taking his medication and began to show signs of decompensation, including hallucinations and disorganization. Jack's mother called the family clinician and a special appointment was made to see the family. A problem-solving session was conducted to address Jack's drinking. Jack agreed to decrease his alcohol use and take his medications. The clinician also arranged for Jack to meet with the doctor and for the case manager to do daily monitoring of Jack's medication adherence. These steps were successful in stemming Jack's drinking, improving his compliance with medication, and averting a full-blown relapse of his schizophrenia.

Several problem-solving sessions were also spent helping Jack find a job. Soon after beginning the family program Jack obtained a job as a janitor. Although he changed jobs twice over the following two years, he was continuously employed. Later in family sessions he expressed interest in a finding a more rewarding job, which became a focus of problem solving.

After one year of sessions, training in problem-solving ended. Two-and-a-half years after beginning family sessions the family continues to meet with the family clinician once every one to

two months. Jack and his parents have also been regular participants at the monthly multiple-family group meetings. Jack's parents
appreciate the support from other relatives and have learned more
about his illness from other group participants who have schizophrenia. Jack also seems to benefit from this setting where he has
talked very eloquently about what it means to develop a mental
illness and how he has had to deal with the loss of some hopes and
dreams.

Jack has succeeded in decreasing his drinking and his
alcoholism has been in remission for one-and-a-half years; he
currently drinks one or two beers on occasion, and he actively
contemplates abstinence. He has been abstinent from marijuana use
since the beginning family sessions. Jack's mental illness has been
stable for almost two years and he has not been hospitalized since
the beginning of family work. In the past year Jack has become
interested in improving his health. He has been running regularly for
the past eight months and he has competed in two races. Jack has
also cut down his cigarette smoking from two packs per day to less
than one pack. His current goals are to find a better job, resume
taking college courses, and to find a girlfriend. Jack's parents have
achieved their goal of having more time for themselves, and have
taken several vacations on their own.

Conclusions

Substance use disorders are common in persons with severe mental
illness and often have a deleterious impact on family relationships.
The effect of these dual disorders on relatives is an increase in the
burden of caregiving and greater vulnerability to violent victimiza-
tion, which often leads to overwhelming their coping capacity, and
the subsequent withdrawal of emotional and material support. The
long-term consequences of this loss of support are a worse course of
both disorders, housing instability, and homelessness.

In this chapter we described the family intervention for dual
disorders (FIDD) program. The FIDD program includes both single
family and multiple-family group treatment formats. The single
family format, which is based on the behavioral family therapy
model, is divided into five separate phases, including: connecting
with the family, assessment, psychoeducation, problem-solving
training, and termination. The specific phases of the program are

tailored to the family's level of motivation to work on the substance use problem (or their stages of treatment). Single family treatment is designed to be given on a time-limited basis. The multiple-family group format is oriented to providing ongoing psychoeducation to families, social support and validation, and to promote the sharing of coping strategies among different families. Multiple-family groups are provided on a time-unlimited basis.

We described a pilot study of the FIDD program that suggests it is effective in treating substance use disorders in persons with severe mental illness, and we provided a case example of a client's progress in this program. Preliminary experience with the program suggests that it benefits families. Controlled research is needed to evaluate the effects of the program for families with a dually diagnosed client.

References

Barry, K.L., Fleming, M.F., Greenley, J.R., Kropp, S., and Widlak, P. (1996): Characteristics of persons with severe mental illness and substance abuse in rural areas. Psychiatric Services 47: 88–90

Butzlaff, R.L. and Hooley, J.M. (1998): Expressed emotion and psychiatric relapse. Archives of General Psychiatry 55: 547–552

Carey, K.B. (1989): Treatment of the mentally ill chemical abuser: Description of the Hutchings day treatment program. Psychiatric Quarterly 60(4): 303–316

Caton, C.L., Shrout, P.E., Eagle, P.F., Opler, L.A., Felix, A.F., and Dominguez, B. (1994): Risk factors for homelessness among schizophrenic men: A case-control study. American Journal of Public Health 84(2): 265–270

Caton, C.L. M., Shrout, P.E., Dominguez, B., Eagle, P.F., Opler, L.A., and Cournos, F. (1995): Risk factors for homelessness among women with schizophrenia. American Journal of Public Health 85: 1153–1156

Clark, R.E. (1996): Family support for persons with dual disorders. In: Dual diagnosis of major mental illness and substance abuse disorder II: Recent research and clinical implications. New directions for mental health services (Drake, R.E., Mueser, K.T., eds.), Vol. 70, pp. 65–77. San Francisco: Josssey-Bass

Clark, R.E. and Drake, R.E. (1992): Substance abuse and mental illness: What families need to know. Innovations and Research 1(4): 3–8

Cournos, F., Empfield, M., Horwath, E., McKinnon, K., Meyer, I., Schrage, H., Currie, C., and Agosin, B. (1991): HIV prevalence among patients admitted to two psychiatric hospitals. American Journal of Psychiatry 148(9): 1225–1229

Cresswell, C.M., Kuipers, L., and Power, M.J. (1992): Social networks and support in long-term psychiatric patients. Psychological Medicine 22: 1019–1026

Cuffel, B.J. (1996): Comorbid substance use disorder: prevalence, patterns of use, and course. In: Dual diagnosis of major mental illness and substance use disorder II: Recent research and clinical implications (Drake, R.E., Mueser, K.T., eds.), Vol. 70, pp. 65–77. San Francisco: Jossey-Bass

Dickey, B. and Azeni, H. (1996): Persons with dual diagnoses of substance abuse and major mental illness: their excess costs of psychiatric care. American Journal of Public Health 86: 973–977

Dixon, L., Adams, C., and Lucksted, A. (2000): Update on family psycho-education for schizophrenia. Schizophrenia Bulletin 26(1): 5–20

Dixon, L., McNary, S., and Lehman, A. (1995): Substance abuse and family relationships of persons with severe mental illness. American Journal of Psychiatry 152: 456–458

Drake, R.E., Bartels, S.B., Teague, G.B., Noordsy, D.L., and Clark, R.E. (1993): Treatment of substance abuse in severely mentally ill patients. Journal of Nervous and Mental Disease 181: 606–611

Drake, R.E., Mueser, K.T., Clark, R.E., and Wallach, M.A. (1996): The course, treatment, and outcome of substance disorder in persons with severe mental illness. American Journal of Orthopsychiatry 66(1): 42–51

Edwards, D.V., Nikkel, B., and Coiner, B. (1991): Final report of the National Institute of Mental Health Young Adult Dual Diagnosis Oregon Demonstration Project. Salem, OR: Oregon Mental Health and Developmental Disability Division

Falloon, I.R.H., Boyd, J.L., and McGill, C.W. (1984): Family care of schizophrenia: A problem-solving approach to the treatment of mental illness. New York: Guilford

First, M.B., Spitzer, R.L., Gibbon, M., and Williams, J.B.W. (1996): Structured clinical interview for DMS-IV axis-I disorders - patient edition (SCID-I/P, Version 2.0). New York: Biometrics Research Department

Goldman, H.H. (1984): The chronically mentally ill: Who are they? Where are they? In: The chronically mentally ill: Research and services (Mirabi M., ed.), pp. 33–44. Spectrum Publications

Hatfield, A.B. and Lefley, H.P. (1987): Families of the mentally ill: Coping and adaptation. New York: Guilford Press

Haywood, T.W., Kravitz, H.M., Grossman, L.S., Cavanaugh, J.L., Jr., Davis, J.M., and Lewis, D.A. (1995): Predicting the 'revolving door': phenomenon among patients with schizophrenic, schizoaffective, and affective disorders. American Journal of Psychiatry 152: 856–861

Johnsen, J.A., Hall, H.E., Rhoades, M., and Harris, N. (1992): OASIS: Final report to the National Institute of Mental Health. Columbus, OH: Ohio Department of Mental Health

Lefley, H.P. and Johnson, D.L. (1990): Families as allies in treatment of the mentally ill: New directions for mental health professionals. Washington, DC: American Psychiatric Press

Mercer-McFadden, C., Drake, R.E., Brown, N.B., and Fox, R.S. (1997): The community support program demonstrations of services for young adults with severe mental illness and substance use disorders 1987–1991. Psychiatric Rehabilitation Journal 20(3): 13–24

Miller, W.R. and Rollnick, S. (1991): Motivational interviewing: preparing people to change addictive behavior. New York: Guilford Press

Miner, C.R., Rosenthal, R.N., Hellerstein, D.J., and Muenz, L.R. (1997): Prediction of compliance with outpatient referral in patients with schizophrenia and psychoactive substance use disorders. Archives of General Psychiatry 54: 706–712

Minkoff, K. (1991): Program components of a comprehensive integrated care system for serious mentally ill patients with substance disorders. In: Dual diagnosis of major mental illness and substance disorders (Minkoff, K., Drake, R.E., eds.). New Directions for Mental Health Services, Vol. 50, pp. 13–27. San Francisco: Jossey-Bass

Mueser, K.T., Bellack, A.S., Wade, J.H., Sayers, S.L., and Rosenthal, C.K. (1992): An assessment of the educational needs of chronic psychiatric patients and their relatives. British Journal of Psychiatry 160: 674–680

Mueser, K.T., Bennett, M., and Kushner, M.G. (1995a): Epidemiology of substance abuse among persons with chronic mental disorders. In: Double jeopardy: Chronic mental illness and substance abuse (Lehman, A.F., Dixon, L., eds.), pp. 9–25. New York: Harwood Academic Publishers

Mueser, K.T., Drake, R.E., Clark, R.E., McHugo, G.J., Mercer-McFadden, C., and Ackerson, T. (1995b): Toolkit for evaluating substance abuse in persons with severe mental illness. Cambridge, MA: Evaluation Center at HSRI

Mueser, K.T. Drake, R.E., and Noordsy, D.L. (1998): Integrated mental health and substance abuse treatment for severe psychiatric disorders. Journal of Practical Psychiatry and Behavioral Health 4(3): 129–139

Mueser, K.T. and Gingerich, S.L. (1994): Coping with schizophrenia: A guide for families. Oakland, CA: New Harbinger Publications

Mueser, K.T. and Glynn, S.M. (1999): Behavioral family therapy for psychiatric disorders. Oakland, CA: New Harbinger

Noordsy, D.L., Drake, R.E., Biesanz, J.C., and McHugo, G.J. (1994): Family history of alcoholism in schizophrenia. Journal of Nervous and Mental Disease 186: 651–655

Osher, F.C. and Kofoed, L.L. (1989): Treatment of patients with psychiatric and psychoactive substance use disorders. Hospital and Community Psychiatry 40: 1025–1030

Regier, D.A., Farmer, M.E., Rae, D.S., Locke, B.Z., Keith, S.J., Judd, L.L., and Goodwin, F.K. (1990): Comorbidity of mental disorders with alcohol and other drug abuse: Results from the Epidemiologic Catchment Area (ECA) study. Journal of the American Medical Association 264: 2511–2518

Ridgely, M.S., Goldman, H.H., and Willenbring, M. (1990): Barriers to the care of persons with dual diagnoses: Organizational and financing issues. Schizophrenia Bulletin 16(1): 123–132

Salyers, M.P., and Mueser, K.T. (in press): Social functioning, psychopathology, and medication side effects in relation to substance use and abuse in schizophrenia. Schizophrenia Research

Schooler, N.R., Keith, S.J., Severe, J.B., Matthews, S.M., Bellack, A.S., Glick, I. D., Hargreaves, W.A., Kane, J.M., Ninan, P.T., Frances, A., Jacobs, M., Lieberman, J.A., Mance, R., Simpson, G.M., and Woerner, M.G. (1997): Relapse and rehospitalization during maintenance treatment of schizophrenia: The effects of dose reduction and family treatment. Archives of General Psychiatry 54: 453–463

Sokolove, R.L. and Trimble, D. (1986): Assessing support and stress in the social networks of chronic patients. Hospital and Community Psychiatry 37: 370–372

Stanton, M.D. and Shadish, W.R. (1997): Outcome, attrition, and family-couples treatment for drug abuse: A meta-analysis and review of the controlled, comparative studies. Psychological Bulletin 122(2): 170–191

Steadman, H.J., Mulvey, E.P., Monahan, J., Robbins, P.C., Appelbaum, P.S., Grisso, T., Roth, L.H., and Silver, E. (1998): Violence by people discharged from acute psychiatric inpatient facilities and by others in the same neighborhoods. Archives of General Psychiatry 55: 393–401

Susser, E., Struening, E.L., and Conover, S. (1989): Psychiatric problems in homeless men: Lifetime psychosis, substance use, and current distress in new arrivals at New York City shelters. Archives of General Psychiatry 46: 845–850

Swartz, M.S., Swanson, J.W., Hiday, V.A., Borum, R., Wagner, H.R., and Burns, B. J. (1998): Violence and mental illness: The effects of substance abuse and nonadherence to medication. American Journal of Psychiatry 155: 226–231

Talbott, J.A. (1990): Current perspectives in the United States on the chronically mentally ill. In: Recent advances in schizophrenia (Kales, A., Stefanis, C.N., Talbott, J., eds.), pp. 279–295. New York: Springer

13
Illness Self-management Programs in Schizophrenia and Severe Affective Disorders

Annette Schaub

Introduction

Over the last 15 years there has been a remarkable change in how professionals treat patients with severe psychiatric illness and their relatives. It is now recognized that patients and families should be involved in the treatment process. They need information about the mental illness, its psychosocial and pharmacological treatment, as well as help in learning practical skills to cope with it. Up to now psychoeducational interventions have been developed for patients with schizophrenia and to a lesser extent for patients with depression. Whereas the efficacy of family interventions for schizophrenia (Goldstein, 1995; Pitschel-Walz et al., 2001) and severe affective disorders (e.g., Miklowitz et al., 2000) have been firmly established, illness self-management programs for patients have been less thoroughly investigated. This chapter provides an overview of these programs and of randomised controlled studies in this field. Two coping-oriented programs recently developed in Munich, one for schizophrenia, the other for depression are described as well as the results of randomised controlled trials for each. The chapter concludes with a discussion of which treatment elements in illness self-management programs may be critical for their effectiveness.

Defining Psychoeducation and Illness Self-management

The term "psychoeducation" was used by Anderson and colleagues (1980) to refer to workshops for relatives of persons with schizophrenia, later provided to relatives of persons with affective disorders (Anderson et al., 1986). These workshops were originally designed to reduce stress in all family members through enhanced education, and improved communication and problem-solving skills. Whereas the terms "psychoeducation" and "illness self-management" have much in common, the first term is more narrowly defined in this review and can be best described with regard to teaching methods. Psychoeducation refers to didactic, psychotherapeutic interventions intended to inform the patient and/or his or her relatives about the illness and its treatment. Illness self-management programs, on the other hand, include psychoeducation as well as cognitive-behavioral methods aimed at improving treatment adherence, coping with symptoms and stressors, developing relapse prevention skills, and modifying dysfunctional beliefs about the illness and self. The primary goals of these illness self-management programs are to enhance the patient's ability to manage his or her illness and to improve outcome. Programs that focus predominantly on cognitive therapy for persistent positive symptoms (see: Garety et al., 2000) were excluded as they attempt to modify psychosis without teaching skills per se.

Illness self-management programs are designed to be effective for primary, secondary, and tertiary prevention. The following components are common in these programs:

Education: Information is provided about the illness and its treatment based on the vulnerability-stress model. Topics cover diagnosis, etiology, symptoms, course of the illness, psychosocial and psychopharmacological interventions, effects and side-effects of medication, modes of action, and aftercare planning.

Enhancing the person's understanding and ability to manage the illness on his or her own: Patients are helped to improve their understanding of how they can influence the course of mental illness and to develop a concept of the self that is not exclusively defined in terms of the illness, but is based on a conception of their individuality and on the remaining possibilities of their life.

Teaching self-management skills: Procedures for taking medication and for evaluating individual responsivity to medication and level of dosage are taught. Patients are trained to monitor changes in symptoms and early warning signs of relapse as well as to develop strategies and problem solving skills to cope with stressors, deficits, and recurring symptoms.

Strategies for primary and secondary prevention: Developing a lifestyle which promotes health and well-being (e.g., scheduling leisure time activities), avoiding use of alcohol or drugs that provoke or worsen symptoms, and identifying and responding to early warning signs ("relapse prevention drill") are important strategies for preventing crises.

Learning assertiveness skills and strengthening the patient's social network: Patients learn how to talk about the illness and its effects, to ask for support from their social network as well as to express concerns and needs in treatment, and to negotiate with physicians about medication problems (e.g., side-effects).

Importance of Psychoeducational and Illness Management Programs

During the last decade, cognitive-behavioral treatment programs have gained prominence in the treatment of severe psychiatric illness. The limited effects of psychopharmacotherapy on specific symptoms (e.g., negative symptoms in schizophrenia) and psychosocial functioning, problems related to medication compliance, and the reduction of length of inpatient stay have intensified the search for more effective psychosocial treatment interventions. Vulnerability-stress models of schizophrenia (Zubin and Spring, 1977; Nuechterlein and Dawson, 1984) and bipolar disorder (Goodwin and Jamison, 1990) that highlight the interactions between biological vulnerability, stressors and protective factors, have played important roles in the development of these programs. The increasing focus on educating patients about mental illness and its management was fostered by several developments in psychiatry. Relatives and patients expressed their needs for more information and involvement in decision-making. Research on coping showed that the majority of patients are capable of understanding information about their illness, recognizing and coping with early warning signs of relapse, and learning effective strategies for coping with them (Schaub, 1994; Mueser et al., 1997). Whereas there used to be some reluctance to inform patients about their illness, especially in schizophrenia because of cognitive deficits and poor insight (Luderer and Böcker, 1993), psychoeducation is now widely accepted as a treatment standard (Schaub et al., 1999a).

Types of Illness Self-management Programs in Severe Psychiatric Illness

Formal approaches generally follow a fixed curriculum. The patient is seen as a partner in treatment process in which both the content of education and the process are important components. However, programs are quite diverse in their objectives, content, sophistication, structure, and time-frame. They focus on specific illnesses such as schizophrenia, or on specific aspects, such as medication management (e.g., Liberman, 1986), coping with symptoms (e.g, Liberman, 1988; Tarrier et al., 1993a), relapse prevention (e.g., Herz et al., 2000), or skills for dealing with various life problems (e.g., Liberman, 1988). Complex long-term programs cover psychoeducation, symptom management, social skills and problem solving modules in individual and/or group therapy (e.g., Hogarty et al., 1995).

Most programs are conducted in groups, but some are conducted on an individual basis (e.g., Süllwold and Herrlich, 1998). Whereas group treatment programs last for 8 to 25 sessions, individual treatment programs are more time-consuming on average (up to 94 sessions). Psychoeducational approaches often use supplemental teaching aids, such as working with flipcharts and handouts, in order to engage the patient more actively in learning information and to reinforce the concepts taught (Daley et al., 1992). Active learning techniques such as behavioral rehearsal and homework assignment are often used to help participants learn and practice new coping skills.

The highly-structured medication and symptom management modules of Liberman's group (1986, 1988) had a strong impact on the development of manualised psychoeducational programs in Germany (e.g., Kieserg et al., 1996; Wienberg et al., 1997) intended to help patients identify and manage warning signs of relapse, develop emergency plans and manage medication issues. The latter are short-term (14–16 sessions) compared to Liberman's programs (20–25 sessions), and put less emphasis on social skills and problem solving techniques. However, they provide more explicit information about schizophrenia (Schaub and Liberman, 1999). Hogarty's (1995) as well as Süllwold and Herrlichs' (1998) approach are the most comprehensive. They attempt to provide a growing awareness of personal vulnerability, including the 'internal cues' of affect dysregulation, by means of teaching graduated, internal coping strategies.

There is a broad range of programs for affective disorders ranging from basic psychoeducation to comprehensive cognitive-behavioral interventions (e.g., Perry et al., 1999). More complex programs, such as the manualised structured group psychotherapy for bipolar disorder (Bauer and McBride, 1996), strive to improve disease-specific self-management skills and assist individuals in achieving life goals. In contrast to schizophrenia and bipolar disorder, interventions for major depression focus more on self-help strategies (e.g., coping with depression; Lewinsohn et al., 1984) and only few provide information about medication for depression (e.g., Schaub, 2000).

Some techniques, such as short-term information about medication or developing strategies for incorporating medication into daily routine are considered to be part of illness self-management programs, however, they are not sufficient treatment programs for patients with cognitive deficits who are in need of more elaborate interventions.Very short-term programs that offered very few opportunities for discussion between patients and providers (e.g., in schizophrenia: Boczkowski et al., 1985; Brown et al., 1987; Kleinman et al., 1993; Angunawela and Mullee, 1998; in depression: Peet and Harvey, 1991; Mundt et al., 2001), and that showed no or only moderate effects (see overview: Merinder, 2000), were therefore excluded from this overview. Studies that focused only on compliance (e.g., Cochran, 1984; Razali and Yahya, 1995) and neglected psychosocial aspects of the illness in contrast to Anderson's definition of psychoeducation (1980) were also excluded.

Research on Illness Self-management Programs

In contrast to psychoeducational family interventions that have been found to be effective in numerous studies (Bustillo et al., 2001;

Pitschel-Walz et al., 2001), there are only few randomised controlled studies of illness management programs provided to the patients alone or in combination with their families that include long-term follow-up assessments. Table 1 and Table 2 give an overview of different illness self-management programs in severe psychiatric illness that have been found to be effective in randomised controlled studies. The patients involved were diagnosed as having schizophrenia, bipolar disorder or residual major depression.

Beneficial effects of a psychoeducational treatment program on relapse prevention were maintained at follow-ups ranging from one to seven years, especially when patients and relatives were involved in treatment, whereas the relapse rate in standard treatment increased (Kissling et al., 1995; Bäuml et al., 1996, 2001). Another study, which used the same program and design, could not replicate the favourable results at one year follow-up (Merinder et al., 1999). Controlled studies proved that patients who participated in illness self-management programs showed gains in knowledge, self-management skills, social functioning and quality of life as well as reduction in symptoms in schizophrenia compared to standard treatment (e.g., Eckman et al., 1992; Goldman and Quinn, 1988; Atkinson et al., 1996).

Complex treatment options including psychoeducation, cognitive therapy and key person counseling proved to be more effective at two and five year follow-up compared to placebo attention groups, whereas less comprehensive programs including only one or two of these elements, did not show significant differences (Buchkremer et al., 1997; Hornung et al., 1999). Comprehensive long-term programs (18 months) that focus on early personal signs of vulnerability (e.g., cues of affect dysregulation) as well as coping strategies (Herz et al., 2000; Hogarty et al., 1997a, b), proved to be effective in reducing relapses at postassessment compared to standard treatment. The first study also included multifamily groups and the latter showed differences in outcome depending on the patient's living situation: when the patient lived with his or her family he or she was more effective in preventing relapses in personal therapy than in standard treatment whereas patients living independently did better in standard treatment. Programs focusing on improving coping strategies as well as enhancing self-esteem (Lecomte et al., 1999) also showed beneficial results at six-month follow-up. With regard to affective disorders illness self-management programs are more effective in preventing

Table 1. Randomized controlled studies on group format psychoeducational and illness management programs in schizophrenia

Psychoeducation	Study design	Sample	Methods	Time frame	Results
Psychoeducational program (Kissling et al., 1995; Bäuml et al., 1996, 2001)	Psychoeducation (PE) vs. Standard Treatment (ST)	N = 163; 7th year: N = 48	Information session (presentation and discussion), handouts	8 sessions for patients and relatives in distinct groups for 3 months+	1-, 2-, 7-year follow-up: PE > ST: relapse rate 21%, 41%, 54% vs. 38%, 58%, 88% (p < .05)
Psychoeducational program (Merinder, 1999)	Psychoeducation (PE) vs. Standard Treatment (ST)	N = 46	Information session (presentation and discussion), handouts	8 sessions for patients and relatives in distinct groups for 3 months+	1-year follow-up: increase in knowledge in PE; no differences in outcome
Illness Management Patient Education Program (Goldman and Quinn, 1988)	Psychoeducation (PE) vs. Standard Treatment (ST)	N = 60	Information session, exercise sessions	25 hours per week for 3 weeks	10 days follow-up: PE > ST: gain in knowledge of illness; decrease in negative symptoms
Education program for schizophrenia (Atkinson et al., 1996)	Psychoeducation and Problem solving (PEPS) vs. Standard Treatment (ST)	N = 145	Information session (presentation and discussion), problem solving	20 weeks	3 months follow-up: no differences in compliance; PEPS > ST: social functioning and quality of life

Table 1. (Continued)

		N			
Illness Self-Management Modules (Eckman et al., 1992)	Symptom and Medication Management Modules (S+MMM) vs. Supportive Group Therapy (SGT)	N = 41	Clinician's manual, patient's workbook, videotape	2 weekly sessions for 6 months (50 sessions)	Posttreatment, 6 months, 1-year follow-up: S+MMM > SGT: attainment and retention of skills
Psychoeducational and cognitive program (Buchkremer et al., 1997; Hornung et al., 1999)	Psychoeducational Management Training (PMT), PMT + Cognitive Psychotherapy (CP), PMT + CP + Keyperson Counseling (KC), Leisure Time Activities (LTA)	N = 191	Psychoeducational sessions with patients and/or relatives, cognitive psychotherapy	PMT: 10 sessions CP: 10 sessions KC: 10 sessions+ LTA: 25 sessions	1-year follow-up: no sig. differences, 2- and 5-year follow-up: PMT+CP+KC > LTA: 24%, 41,7% vs. 50%, 68,6% (p < .05)
Self-esteem Module (Lecomte et al., 1999)	Self-esteem Module (SEM) vs. Standard Treatment (ST)	N = 95	Strategies to enhance empowerment (e.g., goal setting and coping)	2 × weekly sessions for 12 weeks	6-month-follow-up: SEM > ST in psychotic symptoms and coping skills; no diff. in negative symptoms
Early warning signs program (Herz et al., 2000)	Relapse Prevention (RP) vs. Standard Treatment (ST)	N = 82	Psychoeducation, focusing on early warning signs, multifamily group	Weekly groups for 18 months+	Posttreatment: relapse: RP (7%) > ST (34%)

*>= "better than"

+groups for relatives or family interventions provided

Table 2. Randomized controlled studies on individual illness management programs

Programs in schizophrenia	Study design	Sample	Methods	Time frame	Results
Cognitive therapy (Buchkremer and Fiedler, 1987; Lewandowski and Buchkremer, 1988)	Cognitive Therapy and relapse prevention (CT) vs. Social Skills Training (SST) vs. Extended Standard Treatment (EST)	N = 45	Psychoeducation on relapse prevention, training medication management skills.	10 weekly sessions	1-year follow-up: CT > SST > EST in relapse (p < .05), however, no significant differences at 2-year follow-up; 5 year follow-up: CT > SST (p<.05)
Coping Strategy Enhancement (Tarrier et al., 1993a,b)	Coping Strategy Enhancement (CSE vs. Problem Solving (PS) vs. Standard Treatment (ST)	N = 27	Behavioral analysis of psychotic symptoms and training coping strategies	2 × weekly sessions for 5 weeks	6-month follow-up: CS > PS > ST in symptom severity
Personal Therapy (Hogarty et al., 1997a,b)	Personal Therapy (PT) vs. Supportive Therapy (ST)	N = 151	Phasespecific psychoeducation and behavior therapy	Weekly sessions in one year, greater spacing in subsequent two years (94 sessions)+	Post-assessment: relapse rate: patients living with families: PT > ST; patients living independently: ST > ST; social adjustment: PT > ST

Table 2. (Continued)

Programs in affective disorders

Relapse Prevention program (Perry et al., 1999)	Relapse Prevention (RP) vs. Standard Treatment (ST) in bipolar disorder	N = 69	Identifying early warning signs and developing an action plan for crisis	7-12 sessions for 3 months	18-month follow-up: RP > ST in manic relapses and psychosocial functioning
Cognitive relapse prevention program (Paykel et al., 1999)	Cognitive therapy and relapse prevention (CRP) vs. Standard Treatment (ST) in residual depression	N = 127	Cognitive therapy and self-management techniques to prevent relapse	16 sessions plus 2 booster sessions for 6-7 months	18-months follow-up: CR > ST in relapse rate (29% vs. 47%)

>= "better than"

+groups for relatives or family interventions provided

manic episodes in bipolar disorder (Perry et al., 1999) as well as depressive episodes in residual depression (Paykel et al., 1999) at postassessment than standard treatment.

Coping-oriented Treatment Programs for Severe Psychiatric Illness in Munich

Since 1995 two coping-oriented group treatment programs that include psychoeducational and cognitive behavioral techniques were implemented at the Department of Psychiatry, University of Munich, for patients with schizophrenia (Schaub, 1998) or depression (Schaub, 2000). Both programs follow a similar format: psychoeducation (e.g., information about medical and psychosocial aspects), stress management (e.g., recognizing personal signs of stress and coping strategy enhancement) and teaching strategies for managing symptoms in schizophrenia and increasing rewarding activities and cognitive restructuring in depression. The patients of both groups are trained in relapse prevention and helped to develop a lifestyle which promotes health and well-being.

Both programs last for 12 sessions (twice a week) in the inpatient setting plus four booster sessions in the outpatient setting which last approximately 60–90 minutes. They are combined with eight psychoeducational sessions for relatives when the patient consents. There are guidelines for the therapists, handouts for the patients, and the groups are supervised on a regular basis to ensure treatment adherence. The programs are tailored to patients' level of cognitive functioning and their needs and interests. The groups include up to eight patients and are closed. Both programs were shown to be clinically feasible from 1995–1997 in 98 inpatients with schizophrenia and in 329 inpatients with depression (Schaub, 1998; Schaub et al., 1999b).

In 1997 and in 2000 randomized controlled trials were started to evaluate the programs. In the study on schizophrenia the coping-oriented group has been compared to a discussion group, in which the patients themselves chose the topics they wanted to discuss. In the study on depression three treatment options have been studied: (a) clinical management, (b) combined with coping-oriented group treatment, (c) the latter in combination with individual sessions.

Up to now 197 patients with schizophrenia have participated in the controlled trial (Schaub et al., 2000; Schaub and Mueser, 2000).

There were no significant differences in drop-out rate between the two treatment groups. Patients were asked to complete comprehensive feedback questionnaires about their satisfaction with treatment. Patients in the coping-oriented treatment program felt better informed about psychosis (N = 160, z = −3,487, p < .001) and showed greater gains in knowledge (F = 6,694, p = .011) from pre- to post-treatment than their counterparts. There was also a trend towards higher satisfaction with treatment. Topics most favoured were relapse prevention, coping with early warning signs, etiology and treatment options. The preliminary data showed no significant difference in relapses (18% in coping-oriented treatment vs. 28% in control treatment) at one-year follow-up, but there were differences in number of rehospitalisations favoring the treatment group (p < .05). The lower rate of rehospitalisations in the experimental group, compared to the control group, despite similar rates of relapse indicates that patients in the experimental group were more successful in coping with relapses while living in the community. The participants in the coping-oriented groups showed more improvement in symptoms (BPRS-E, Ventura et al. 1993), especially anxiety-depression (p < .021) and negative symptoms especially anhedonia (SANS, Andreason 1989; p = .05). At two year follow-up the difference in relapse rates (32% vs. 50%) was evident. The study including two year follow-up will be completed in November 2002.

Seventy-nine patients with depression have participated in the randomised controlled trial (Schaub et al., 2001). After randomisation the drop-out rate was highest in standard treatment. 100% of the patients who participated in the coping-orientated group treatment rated it as recommendable to others. More than 92% reported feeling well educated about depression and that their coping strategies had improved. About 90% rated it as helpful and as instilling hope and confidence. The patients in the illness self-management programs favoured similar topics to the patients with schizophrenia and showed greater gains in knowledge about depression. They also showed greater improvement in internal locus of control (cf. study in schizophrenia; Schaub et al., 1998a) and their dysfunctional attitudes and depressive thoughts decreased significantly compared to their counterparts. There were no significant differences in symptoms nor compliance between the two groups. At present it is expected that the study will be continued for another three years.

Discussion

While only few randomized controlled studies in illness self-management programs for patients with long-term follow-up have been conducted, results thus far have been encouraging. These programs are designed to meet patients' expressed needs for more information and involvement in decision-making. Psychoeducational interventions increase patients' satisfaction with treatment as they are rated as helpful and informative. Compared to standard treatment psychoeducational interventions result in greater gains in knowledge. However, these improvements are not associated with changes in self-management skills, social functioning, quality of life as well as reductions in symptoms that are mainly achieved by illness self-management programs, combining psychoeducation with cognitive-behavioral interventions (e.g., Eckman et al., 1992; Goldman and Quinn, 1988; Atkinson et al., 1996). Only one study showed beneficial effects of psychoeducational treatment on long-term outcome (Kissling et al., 1995, Bäuml et al., 2001) whereas, on the other hand, mainly comprehensive long-term illness self-management programs have beneficial effects in improving outcome at postreatment (e.g., Herz et al., 2000; Hogarty et al., 1997) or in preventing relapse at several years' outcome in schizophrenia (e.g., Hornung et al., 1999). The results seem to be most convincing when patients and relatives were involved in treatment at the same time. According to Goldstein (1992), psychoeducational programs tap deep-seated issues of personal identity and one's role in a family unit that cannot be ignored. Alternative therapeutic strategies have to be added in order to permit the psychoeducational approach to be effective at fostering coping skills.

What are the ingredients that make illness self-management programs effective? The results suggest that educating patients about their illness, training self-management skills, instilling hope and enhancing self-esteem as well as strengthening the patient's social network can be valuable components of a comprehensive approach to the treatment of schizophrenia. It appears that the capacity for taking an active part in managing one's illness enhances the experience of self-control and vice versa. The participants are treated as experts in their illness, taken seriously (Goldstein, 1996) and encouraged to develop better coping strategies (self-efficacy; Bandura, 1977) hoping for a better future. It is quite established that effective psychosocial interventions in schizophrenia do more than merely improve compliance (e.g., Hogarty et al., 1991). However, future studies could try to combine both aspects to be most effective.

Deficits in neuropsychological functioning in schizophrenia (Green, 1996; Schaub et al., 1998b) accentuate the importance of sound didactic and behavioral principles in illness management programs in severe psychiatric illness. Very short term interventions have not been found to be effective in psychiatric patients. Providing information about the illness and its treatment in an active long-term dialogue that compensates for the cognitive deficits of the patients lays the foundations for shared decision-making and treatment processes.

The group format provides opportunities for observational learning from other patients, sharing experiences and strategies that were evaluated as beneficial in coping with the illness. Participants also recognize that others share similar problems. Group interventions can help the patients attain knowledge as it is often much easier for the participant to listen to another patient and his experiences than to the expert's opinion. Groups are more effective in engaging the patient more actively in learning information. However, individual treatment programs are more easily tailored to the patients' level of functioning and needs (e.g., Hogarty et al., 1995).

In summary, there is still little replication work of established programs, and many programs differ substantially in what they teach and how they do it, however, results thus far have been encouraging. The need for quality standards in illness management programs and theory development are two main areas for future research.

Acknowledgements

The studies were supported by the Eli Lilly International Foundation, Homburg, the Federal Ministry of Education and Research for the competence-network "depression, suicidality" and SmithKline Beecham.

I want to thank Kim T. Mueser for being a critical, never hostile reader of this manuscript.

References

Anderson, C.M., Hogarty, G.E., and Reiss, D.J. (1980): Family treatment of adult schizophrenic patients: a psychoeducational approach. Schizophrenia Bulletin 6: 490–515

Anderson, C.M., Griffin, S., Rossi, A., Pagonis, I., Holder, D.P., and Treiber, R. (1986): A comparison study of the impact of education vs. process groups for families of patients with affective disorder. Family Process 25: 185–205

Andreason, N.C. (1989): Scale for the Assessment of Negative Symptoms (SANS). Br J Psychiatry 155(suppl. 7): 53–58

Angunawela, II., and Mullee, M.A. (1998) Drug information for the mentally ill: A randomised controlled trial. International Journal of Psychiatry in Clinical Practice 2: 121–127

Atkinson, J.M., Coia, D.A., Harper Gilmour, W., and Harper, J.P. (1996): The impact of education groups for people with schizophrenia on social functioning and qualify of life. British Journal of Psychiatry 168: 199–204

Bäuml, J., Kissling, W., and Pitschel-Walz, G. (1996): Psychoedukative Gruppen für schizophrene Patienten: Einfluss auf Wissensstand und Compliance. Psychoeducational groups for schizophrenic patients: Impact on knowledge and compliance. Nervenheilkunde 15: 145–150

Bäuml, J., Pitschel-Walz, G., Basahn, A., Kissling, W., and Förstl, H. (2001): Die Auswirkungen des protektiven Potentials von Angehörigen auf den Langzeitverlauf schizophrener Psychosen: Ergebnisse der sieben Jahres Katamnese der Münchner PIP-Studie (Effects of the protective strengths of relatives on long-term outcome in schizophrenia: Results of the seven year follow-up of the Munich PIP-Study). In: Angehörigenarbeit (Working with relatives) (Binder, W. und Bender, W., eds.). Köln: Claus Richter (forthcoming)

Bandura, A. (1977): Self-efficacy: towards a unifying theory of behavioral change. Psychological Review 84: 191–215

Bauer, M.S., and McBride, L. (1996): Structured group psychotherapy for bipolar disorder: The life goals program. New York: Springer

Boczkowski, J., Zeichner, A., and DeSanto, N. (1985): Neuroleptic compliance among chronic schizophrenic outpatients: An intervention outcome report. Journal of Consulting and Clinical Psychology 53: 666–671

Brown, C.S., Wright, R.G., and Christensen, D.B. (1987): Association between type of medication instruction and patients' knowledge, side effects, and compliance. Hospital and Community Psychiatry 38: 55–60

Buchkremer, G., and Fiedler, P. (1987): Kognitive versus handlungsorientierte Therapie (Cognitive versus action-oriented treatment). Nervenarzt 58: 481–488

Buchkremer, G., Klingberg, S., Holle, R., Schulze Mönking, H., and Hornung, W.P. (1997): Psychoeducational psychotherapy for schizophrenic patients and their key relatives or care-givers: results of a 2-year follow-up. Acta Psychiatrica Scandinavica 96: 483–491

Bustillo, J., Lauriello, J., Horan, W., and Keith, S. (2001): The psychosocial treatment of schizophrenia: An update. American Journal of Psychiatry 158: 163–175

Cochran, S.D. (1984): Preventing medical noncompliance in the outpatient treatment of bipolar affective disorders. Journal of Consulting and Clinical Psychology 52: 873–878

Daley, D.C., Bowler, K., and Cahalane, H. (1992): Approaches to patient and family education about affective disorders. Patient Education and Counseling 19: 162–174

Eckman, T.A., Wirshing, W.C., Marder, S.R., Liberman, R.P., Johnston-Cronk, K., Zimmerman, K., and Mintz, J. (1992): Technology for training schizophrenics in illness management: A controlled trial. American Journal of Psychiatry 149: 1549–1555

Garety, P.A., Fowler, D., and Kuipers, E. (2000): Cognitive-behavioral therapy for medication-resistant symptoms. Schizophrenia Bulletin 26: 73–86

Goldman, C.R., and Quinn, F.L. (1988): Effects of a patient education program in the treatment of schizophrenia. Hospital and Community Psychiatry 39: 282–286

Goldstein, M.J. (1992): Psychosocial strategies for maximizing the effects of psychotropic medication for schizophrenia and mood disorder. Psychopharmacological Bulletin 28: 237–240

Goldstein, M.J. (1995): Psychoeducation and relapse prevention. International Clinical Psychopharmacology (Suppl. 5) 59–69

Goldstein, M.J. (1996): Treating the person with schizophrenia as a person. Review in Contemporary Psychology 41: 256–258

Goodwin, F.K., and Jamison, K.R. (1990): Manic-depressive illness. New York: Oxford University Press

Green, M.F. (1996) What are the functional consequences of neurocognitive deficits in schizophrenia? American Journal of Psychiatry 153: 321–330

Herz, M.I., Lamberti, J.S., Mintz, J., Scott, R., O'Dell, S.P., McCartan, L., and Nix, G. (2000): A program for relapse prevention in schizophrenia: A controlled study. Archives of General Psychiatry 57: 277–283

Hogarty, G.E., Anderson, C.M., Reiss, D.J., Kornblith, S.J., Greenwald, D.P., Ulrich, R., and Carter, M. (1991): Family psychoeducation, social skills training and maintenance therapy in the aftercare treatment of schizophrenia: II. Two-year effects of a controlled study on relapse and adjustment. Archives of General Psychiatry 48: 340–347

Hogarty, G.E., Kornblith, S.J., Greenwald, D., Dibarry, A.L., Cooley, S., Flesher, S., Reiss, D., Carter, M., and Ulrich, R.F. (1995): Personal therapy: A disorder-relevant psychotherapy for schizophrenia. Schizophrenia Bulletin 21(3): 379–393

Hogarty, G.E., Kornblith, S.J., Greenwald, D., Dibarry, A.L., Cooley, S., Ulrich, R.F., Carter, M., and Flesher, S. (1997a): Three year trials of personal therapy among schizophrenic patients living with or independent of family, I: Description of study and effects on relapse rates. American Journal of Psychiatry 154: 1504–13

Hogarty, G.E., Kornblith, S.J., Greenwald, D., DiBarry, A.L., Cooley, S., Flesher, S., Reiss, D., Carter, M., and Ulrich, R.F. (1997b): Three year trials of personal therapy among schizophrenic patients living with or independent of family, II: Effects on adjustment of patients. American Journal of Psychiatry 154: 1514–1524

Hornung, W.P., Feldman, R., Klingberg, S., Buchkremer, G., and Reker, T. (1999): Long-term effects of a psychoeducational psychotherapeutic intervention for schizophrenic outpatients and their key-persons – results of a five-year follow-up. European Archives of Psychiatry and Clinical Neuroscience 249: 162–167

Kieserg, A., and Hornung, W.P. (1996): Psychoedukatives Training für schizophrene Patienten (PTS) (Psychoeducational training for schizophrenic patients). Materialie Nr. 27, überarbeitete und erweiterte Auflage. Tübingen: Deutsche Gesellschaft für Verhaltenstherapie

Kissling, W., Bäuml, J., and Pitschel-Walz, G. (1995): Psychoedukation und Compliance bei der Schizophreniebehandlung (Psychoeducation and compliance in the treatment of schizophrenia). Münchner Medizinische Wochenzeitschrift 137: 801–805

Kleinman, I., Schachter, D., Jeffries, J., and Goldhamer, P. (1993): Effectiveness of two methods for informing schizophrenic patients about neuroleptic medication. Hospital and Community Psychiatry 44: 1189–1191

Lecomte, T., Cyr, M.., Lesage, A.D., Wilde, J., Leclerc, C. and Ricard, N. (1999): Efficacy of a self-esteem module in the empowerment of individuals with schizophrenia. Journal of Nervous and Mental Disease 187: 406–413

Lewandowski, L. and Buchkremer, G. (1988): Bifokale therapeutische Gruppenarbeit mit schizophrenen Patienten und ihren Angehörigen – Ergebnisse einer 5jährigen Katamnese (Bifocal group therapy with schizophrenic patients and their relatives – results of 5-year follow-up). In: Die Schizophrenien: biologische und familiendynamische Konzepte zur Pathogenese (Schizophrenia: the aetiological role of biological factors and family dynamics). (Kaschka, W.P., ed), pp. 211–223. Berlin: Springer

Lewinsohn, P.M., Antonuccio, D.O., Steinmetz, J.L., and Teri, L. (1984): The coping with depression course. A psychoeducational intervention for unipolar depression. Eugene, OR: Castalia Publishing Company

Liberman, R.P. (1986): Social and independent living skills. The medication management module. Trainer's manual and patient handbook. Clinical Research Center for Schizophrenia and Psychiatric Rehabilitation, Los Angeles

Liberman, R.P. (1988): Social and independent living skills. The symptom management module. Trainer's manual and patient handbook. Clinical Research Center for Schizophrenia and Psychiatric Rehabilitation, Los Angeles.

Luderer, H.J., and Böcker, F.M. (1993): Clinicians' information habits, patients' knowledge of diagnoses and etiological concepts in four different samples. Acta Psychiatrica Scandinavica 88: 266–272

Merinder, L.B. (2000): Patient education in schizophrenia: A review. Acta Psychiatrica Scandinavica 102: 98–106

Merinder, L.-B., Viuff, A.G., Laugesen, H.D., Clemmensen, K., Misfelt, S., and Espensen, B. (1999): Patient and relative education in community psychiatry: a randomized controlled trial regarding its effectiveness. Social Psychiatry and Psychiatric Epidemiology 34: 287–294

Miklowitz, D.J., Simoneau, T.L., George, E.A., Richards, J.A., Kalbag, A., Sachs-Ericsson, N., and Suddath, R. (2000): Family-focused treatment of bipolar disorder: One-year effects of a psychoeducational program in conjunction with pharmacotherapy. Biological Psychiatry 48: 430–432

Mueser, K.T., Valentiner, D.P., and Agresta, J. (1997): Coping with negative symptoms of schizophrenia: patient and family perspectives. Schizophrenia Bulletin 23: 329–339

Mundt, J.C., Clarke, G.N., Burroughs, D., Brenneman, D.O., and Griest, J.H. (2001): Effectiveness of antidepressant pharmacotherapy: The impact of medication compliance and patient education. Depression and Anxiety 13: 1–10

Nuechterlein, K.H., and Dawson, M.E. (1984): A heuristic vulnerability/stress model of schizophrenic episodes. Schizophrenia Bulletin 10: 300–312

Paykel, E.S., Scott, J., Teasdale, J.D., Johnson, A.L., Garland, A., Moore, R., Jenaway, A., Cornwall, P.L., Hayhurst, J., Abbott, R., and Pope, M. (1999): Prevention or relapse in residual depression by cognitive therapy. Archives of General Psychiatry 56: 829–835

Peet, M. and Harvey, N.S. (1991) Lithium maintenance: 1. A standard education program for patients. British Journal of Psychiatry 158: 197–2000

Perry, A., Tarrier, N., Morriss, R., McCarthy, E., and Limb, K. (1999): Randomised controlled trial of efficacy of teaching patients with bipolar disorder to identify early symptoms of relapse and obtain treatment. British Medical Journal 318: 149–153

Pitschel-Walz, G., Leucht. S., Bäuml, J., Kissling, W., and Engel, R. (2001): The effect of family interventions on relapse and rehospitalisation in schizophrenia – A meta-analysis. Schizophrenia Bulletin 27: 73–92

Razali, M.S., and Yahya, H. (1995): Compliance with treatment in schizophrenia: A drug intervention program in a developing country. Acta Psychiatrica Scandinavica 91: 331–335

Schaub, A. (1994): Relapse and coping behaviour in schizophrenia. Schizophrenia Research 11: 188

Schaub, A. (1998): Cognitive-behavioral coping-orientated therapy for schizophrenia: A new treatment model for clinical service and research. In: Cognitive psychotherapy of psychotic and personality disorders: Handbook of theory and practice (Perris C, McGorry PD, ed.), p. 92–109. Chichester: Wiley

Schaub, A. (2000): Angehörigenarbeit und psychoedukative Gruppen in der Therapie affektiver Störungen (Working with relatives and psychoeducational groups in the treatment of affective disorders) (Möller, H.J., ed.), Therapie psychiatrischer Erkrankungen (Treatment of psychiatric disorders). Stuttgart New York: Thieme

Schaub, A., Behrendt, B., and Brenner, H.D. (1998a): A multi-hospital evaluation of the medication and symptom management module in Germany and Switzerland. International Review of Psychiatry 10: 42–46

Schaub, A., Behrendt, B., Brenner, H.D., Mueser, K.T., and Liberman, R.P. (1998b): Training schizophrenic patients to manage their symptoms: predictors of treatment response to the german version of the symptom management module. Schizophrenia Research 31: 121–130

Schaub, A., and Liberman, R.P. (1999): Training patients with schizophrenia to manage their illnesses: Experiences from Germany and Switzerland. Psychiatric Rehabilitation Skills 3(2): 246–268

Schaub, A., Luderer, H.J., Sibum, B., Hornung, P., Pitschel-Walz, G., and Bäuml, J. (1999a): Psychoeducation: An important intervention in schizophrenia. Current Opinion in Psychiatry 12 (Suppl. 1): 440

Schaub, A., and Mueser, K.T. (2000): Coping-oriented treatment in schizophrenia and schizoaffective disorder: Rationale and preliminary results. Proceedings of the 34th Annual Convention of the Association for Advancement of Behavior Therapy, New Orleans, p. 78

Schaub, A., Roth, L., Goldmann, U., Charypar, M., and Wiese, B. (2001): Impact of psychoeducation and coping on compliance and course of the illness in patients with depression. 2. Int. Workshop of the Competence-Network Depression at Tutzing

Schaub, A., Wolf, B., Gartenmaier, A., and Froschmayr, S. (1999b): Coping-orientated therapy in schizophrenia: Implementation and preliminary results. Proc. XI World Congress of Psychiatry at Hamburg, p. 169

Schaub, A., Wolf, B., Gartenmaier, A., and Möller, H.J. (2000) Bewältigungs-orientierte Therapie bei Patienten mit schizophrenen und schizoaffektiven Psychosen: Erste Ergebnisse der Ein- und Zwei-Jahres-Katamnese (Coping-oriented treatment in schizophrenia and schizoaffective psychosis). Proc. of Gfts – Jahrestagung Bonn, p. 5

Süllwold, L., and Herrlich, J. (1998): Psychologische Behandlung schizophren Erkrankter (Psychological treatment in schizophrenia). 2. überarb. Aufl. Stuttgart Berlin: Kohlhammer

Tarrier, N., Beckett, R., Harwood, S., Baker, A., Yusupoff, L., and Ugarteburu, I. (1993a): A trial of two cognitive behavioural methods of treating drug-resistant residual psychotic symptoms in schizophrenic patients: I. Outcome. British Journal of Psychiatry 162: 524–532

Tarrier, N., Sharpe, L., Beckett, R., Harwood, S., Baker, A., and Yusopoff, L. (1993b): A trial of two cognitive behavioural methods of treating drug-resistant residual psychotic symptoms in schizophrenic patients: II. Treatment-specific changes in coping and problem-solving skills. Social Psychiatry and Psychiatric Epidemiology 28: 5–10

Ventura, J., Green, M., Shaner, A., and Liberman, R.P. (1993): Training and quality assurance with the brief psychiatric rating scale. International Journal of Methods in Psychiatric Research 3: 221–244

Wienberg, D., Schünemann-Wurmthaler, S., and Sibum, B. (1997): Schizophrenie zum Thema machen. Manual und Materialien (Focusing on schizophrenia: manual and working sheets). 2. überarb. Aufl. Bonn: Psychiatrie-Verlag

Zubin, J., and Spring, B. (1977): Vulnerability - a new view of schizophrenia. Journal of Abnormal Psychology 86: 103–126

14
Drug Treatment of Schizophrenia: State of the Art and the Potential of the Atypical Neuroleptics

Hans-Jürgen Möller

Introduction

Based on the multifactorial etiopathogenesis of schizophrenia, a multi-dimensional therapy approach is suggested, in which psychophar-macological and psychosocial methods are combined (Deister and Möller, 1998; Möller and von Zerssen, 1995). The results of controlled group studies show that the efficacy of neuroleptics is very well proven for both treatment of the acute phase and relapse prevention (Möller et al., 2000). Supportive and educational approaches to increase compliance are widely used. Information about the complex causation of the disease and about its treatment requirements and possibilities are of great importance for the patient himself and also for his relatives, among others to increase the compliance.

Drug Treatment of the Acute Phase

The psychopharmacological treatment of psychotic symptoms can be performed principally with any neuroleptic (Kane and Marder, 1993). However, there is clinical experience with individual patients who appear to respond better to one medication than another (Gardos, 1974). The novel/atypical neuroleptics offer some important advan-tages compared to the classical neuroleptics. Therefore, they should increasingly be considered as the drugs of first choice in all conditions where they can guarantee sufficient management of the symptoms.

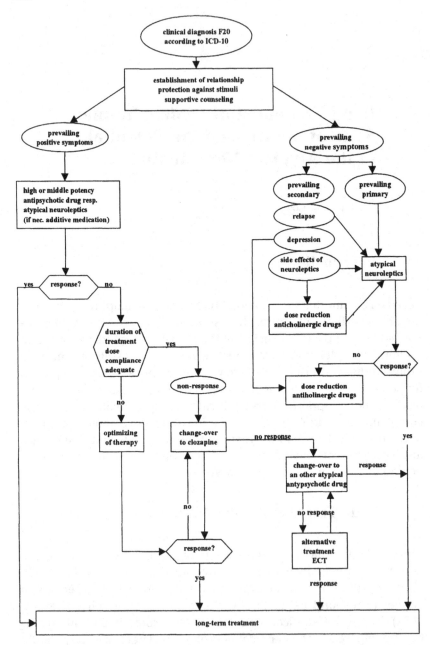

Fig. 1. Algorithm at pharmacotherapy (translated from the German guidelines of the German Association of Psychiatry, Psychotherapy and Neurology, Gaebel and Falkai, 1998)

As a general rule, a monotherapy should be applied (Fig. 1). A combination of different neuroleptics only seems rational under special conditions, for example if one wants to combine the highly potent antipsychotic effect of some butyrophenones with the sedative, or sleep-inducing effect of the potent neuroleptics from the phenothiazine group, or a benzodiazepine.

When choosing a neuroleptic, the psychopathological state of the patient, his reaction to previous drug treatment with respect to response and unwanted effects, as well as his individual risk for certain unwanted effects have to be taken into account.

When treating a patient suffering from a severe schizophrenic episode, one should begin with a sufficiently high dosage of the chosen neuroleptic. A much lower dosage may be used at first if the psychotic state is less severe. The adequate dosage can then be "titrated" by a stepwise increase. In extremely severe psychotic states, which can usually only be treated under inpatient conditions, particularly when there is a risk of endangerment for self or others, or when the patient's cooperation is insufficient, a parenteral initiation of treatment with a highly potent neuroleptic is indicated (Möller et al., 1982). In cases of agitation, excitement states or psychotic sleep problems, comedication with a low potency phenothiazine (e.g., levomepromazine or thioridazine) or a benzodiazepine (e.g., diazepam) may be administered as a single or multiple dosage in order to attain additional sedation. In the first four weeks of treatment, the neuroleptic dosage should not be further increased once dosages which are generally considered as being antipsychotic have been reached (Baldessarini et al., 1988) (500–1000 chlorpromazine equivalents) because it is well known from clinical experience that the full response to neuroleptic treatment is only seen after several weeks (Lieberman et al., 1993). If there is no sufficient partial response of the productive symptoms after 4–6 weeks, a dosage increase may be advisable, however, there is no sufficient evidence from controlled studies for such a procedure.

Stimulated by the increasing awareness for all types of extrapyramidal side effects and their troublesome consequences for the patient and his compliance, and based on PET and SPECT findings showing that striatal D_2-receptors are nearly completely blocked with relatively low dosages of highly potent neuroleptics (Nordstrom et al., 1993; Klemm et al., 1996) – e.g., 5 mg haloperidol –, there is a growing tendency, also by clinicians, to treat patients with relatively low dosages compared to those which were previously in widespread clinical use. Following this line, it was suggested that 350 to 700 mg chlorpromazine equivalents might be sufficient for the average schizophrenic patient (Reardon et al., 1989; Rifkin et al., 1991; Van et al., 1990). However, the PET findings should not be overinterpreted: it may be the case that the antipsychotic effect is not only a matter of D_2-blockade, but that other transmitter systems, e.g., the serotonergic system, are involved (Kane et al., 1983, 1996), and are influenced by higher dosages of a classical neuroleptic. Evidence for a comparatively low dosage, in this case titrated on an individual base according to the neuroleptic threshold concept (Bitter et al., 1991), comes from a study by McEvoy et al. (1991). They compared the treatment results of an individually titrated low dose which induced only very mild parkinsonian symptoms (3.7 ± 2.3 mg/d) with higher dosages (11.6 ± 4.7 mg/d). They did not find an improved efficacy in those patients who were switched to the higher dosage. However, a pitfall of this study might be too short a duration (14 days) of the control group design, and a possibly too small sample size to find differences.

Of special interest in this context is the 7-arm sertindole/haloperidol study, in which three different doses of haloperidol – 4, 8, 16 mg/day – were compared in the treatment of acute schizophrenia, under double-blind conditions (Zimbroff et al., 1997). There were no distinct differences in either efficacy or the extrapyramidal side effects between the various haloperidol dosage groups. Frequencies for administration of anticholinergics were between 40 and 50% for all three doses. This apparently means that in the dose range 4–16 mg we must not be too apprehensive about extrapyramidal side effects. On the other side, based on a group statistical approach, the higher dosage in this dosage range does not increase efficacy, at least not in such a sample of schizophrenic patients highly selected for a placebo-controlled phase III study.

The introduction of the novel/atypical neuroleptics overcomes most of these dosing problems related to extrapyramidal side effects since these drugs have no or only a low risk of extrapyramidal side effects.

For reasons of a flexible adaptation of the dosage to the individual clinical conditions, the treatment of the acute phase should not begin with a depot-neuroleptic, unless lack of patient compliance renders a therapy with a depot-neuroleptic advisable. In such a case, the depot-neuroleptics with a relatively short-term effect (e.g., 3 days) should be preferred to others, in order to keep at least some flexibility.

If after 6–8 weeks of therapy with the first neuroleptic, and inspite of increased dosages - a high dosage approach using up to tenfold higher dosages than the standard therapy is not further recommended (Fleischhacker, 1999) – *an unsatisfactory therapy result* has been achieved, another neuroleptic, if possible from another pharmacological class, should be administered. However, apart from Clozapine, this suggestion is only based on clinical evidence, but not on evidence from controlled clinical studies. There are only very few studies which focus on this issue. Kinon and coworkers (1993) found little benefit in switching from fluphenazine to haloperidol after four weeks, Shalev et al. (1993), however, reported that the great majority of patients improved after consecutive trials of different conventional antipsychotics, although they did not control for the time effect.

Well-founded empirical data support clozapine for the treatment of refractory patients. Among others, the excellent study by Kane and coworkers (1988) on severely refractory patients should be mentioned here. A clozapine treatment for such patients should last up to six months as it has been demonstrated that the treatment response can occur after a long delay (Meltzer et al., 1989), and the dosage should be increased up to 800 mg p.d.

Augmentation strategies such as the administration of carbamazepine, lithium or benzodiazepines have been reported as helpful in refractory patients (Schulz et al., 1990). However, the empirical evidence is weak (Meltzer, 1992) and apparently this is only meaningful in subgroups with special phenomenological features. Electroconvulsive therapy (ECT) should be considered as a final attempt, although only a small amount of data exists to support such an approach (Sagatovic and Meltzer, 1993).

In cases of therapy resistance, and when unexpected side effects are encountered, measures of serum levels should be made in order to better adapt the dosage of the medication. Among others, fast metabolizers (caused, for example, by genetic disposition or enzyme induction) and slow metabolizers can be detected in this way. Particularly the problem of enzyme induction during treatment with neuroleptics should be carefully considered. The problem whether there is a certain therapeutic range of serum concentration for certain neuroleptics still remains unsolved (Dahl, 1986).

In cases of *catatonic stupor*, if neuroleptic treatment does not lead to a clear therapeutic success already in the first days, ECT must be applied in order to avoid an endangerment of the patient's life by the development of febrile catatonia. Recently, high dosages of Lorazepam have been suggested as an alternative to the neuroleptic treatment of the catatonic stupor (Rosebush et al., 1990; Northoff et al., 1995; Ungvari et al., 1994).

The *schizoaffective psychoses* have a special position, under therapeutic aspects. Schizodepressive episodes are treated with a combination of a neuroleptic and an antidepressant (Möller and Morin, 1989; Goodnick and Meltzer, 1984). In schizomanic episodes, a monotherapy with a neuroleptic is usually regarded as sufficient. Because of the risk of neurotoxic complications, an additional dose of lithium may not be without risk, at least when relatively high dosages of the neuroleptic are administered. The efficacy of additional treatment with carbamazepine or valproate is not yet definitively proven. In milder cases, a monotherapy with carbamazepine or valproate is sufficient.

Although neuroleptic treatment traditionally focuses on positive symptoms as the outcome criteria, *negative symptoms* are an important part of schizophrenia and should be considered carefully during its treatment (Möller and Rao, 1996). Meanwhile, some evidence has been obtained showing that not only positive symptoms, but also negative symptoms respond to neuroleptics, especially to atypical neuroleptics (Möller, 1993; Möller, 1995; Möller, 1999a). However, in most studies only negative symptoms of patients suffering from an acute episode of schizophrenia have been addressed, while there is still some uncertainty whether negative symptoms of the chronic deficit syndrome can also be influenced by neuroleptics. Only very few studies supply evidence in this direction (Loo et al., 1997).

Particularly atypical neuroleptics, like amisulpride, clozapine, zotepine, and recently also risperidone and olanzapine, have demonstrated relatively good results in the treatment of negative symptoms (Möller, 1999a). An attempt can also be made with activating antidepressants, especially in cases of pure negative symptoms (Siris et al., 1978). However, an additional neuroleptic treatment is necessary to protect against a possible exacerbation of the schizophrenic psychosis. Possible causal factors for secondary negative symptoms have to be carefully considered and as far as possible eliminated, e.g., overdosage of neuroleptics, social understimulation, depression (Carpenter et al., 1985).

In cases of *postpsychotic depression*, a reduction of the neuroleptic dosage should be attempted, if clinically possible. Anticholinergics can be administered under the hypothesis of an akinetic depression, also if no clear parkinsonoid syndrome is detectable. Finally, an antidepressant treatment should be considered, although its efficacy in this indication is not as well established as for major depression without schizophrenia (Siris, 1995). To counter the risk of symptom provocation (Prusoff et al., 1979), which is attributed to antidepressants, a simultaneous neuroleptic medication should be administered. It is not well enough investigated which type of antidepressant is preferable under this condition. The classical tricyclics are problematic because of sedation and anticholinergic side effects, disturbances of vigilance and cognitive capacities (cognitive dysfunction is an important core symptom of schizophrenia). Selective serotonin re-uptake inhibitors (SSRI) and monoaminooxidase inhibitors (MAO-I) may be preferable under such aspects of effect, however, they are not well investigated in this indication.

After a clear improvement of the psychotic symptoms and a period of relative stability, the dosage can carefully be reduced in small steps over a relatively long period. Even if the symptoms completely disappeared under neuroleptic treatment, it is necessary to administer a maintenance therapy for at least 6 months, preferably one year, to prevent a reappearance of the psychotic symptoms.

Under treatment with neuroleptics, different undesirable side effects may appear, which can mostly be controlled by dosage adjustment, change of neuroleptic or additional medication, and which only very rarely (for example in cases of malign neuroleptic syndrome) necessitate a withdrawal of the medication. The different kinds of extrapyramidal motor symptoms are most frequently of clinical importance. Especially under this aspect, so-called atypical neuroleptics are advantageous (Möller, 1995; Möller, 1999b). However, even under these conditions there are still some problematic side effects, e.g., weight gain which seems to be a special problem under treatment with some atypical neuroleptics. Relative or absolute contraindications for a neuroleptic medication are rare.

Sufficient attention should be given to the side effects which are "only" subjectively disturbing, because they are of great relevance under compliance aspects (Fleischhacker et al., 1994). Among others, even a slight parkinsonoid or a slight akathisia should be avoided as far as possible. For this reason, it should be attempted to achieve a neuroleptic dosage which is adequate but as low as possible, if necessary (when using classical neuroleptics) through careful titration under exact clinical control. However, it may happen that a severe parkinsonism has to be tolerated, in order to obtain a sufficient therapeutic effect by a "classical", "typical" neuroleptic.

Regular laboratory monitoring is advisable in order to avoid particular medical complications of the neuroleptic therapy.

Long-term Medication

In particular after repeated remanifestations of the disease over the years prior to the current manifestation, a long-term relapse prevention is indicated (Möller, 1992; Möller, 1993). To this effect, neuroleptics have to be administered in a much lower dosage than during the acute treatment. It is particularly important that side effects be kept as low as possible by an adaptive treatment regimen. The optimal dosage has to be individually determined for each patient. According to recent reviews, the minimal effective dosage seems to be 6.5–12.5 mg every 2 weeks for fluphenazine decanoate, 20 mg every 2 weeks for flupenthixol decanoate, 50–60 mg every 4 weeks for haloperidol decanoate, 2.5 mg daily for oral haloperidol and 2.5 mg daily for oral fluphenazine hydrochloride (Kissling, 1994). Experience shows that the dosage which has been chosen at the end of treatment of the acute phase can be considerably reduced over the following months/years (Johnson, 1975).

Extrapyramidal symptoms, which may extremely impair the quality of life of the patient, and particularly the development of tardive dyskinesia – an incidence rate of 4% per year is reported in the prospective study by Kane et al. (1986) – have to be considered carefully. Particularly because of the risk of tardive dyskinesia, the dosage of neuroleptics should be kept as low as possible, or atypical neuroleptics should be applied, to avoid the risk of extrapyramidal side effects. One should avoid a long-term administration of anti-cholinergics in order not to conceal a chronic irritation of the extra-pyramidal system caused by too high a dosage of neuroleptics. When tardive dyskinesia appears, administration of the neuroleptic should be stopped and replaced by clozapine, since this is the only substance which as yet seems to carry no risk of tardive dyskinesia. Other atypical neuroleptics might have the same advantage, how-ever, the data are only preliminary.

Because of the well-known compliance problems, the use of depot neuroleptics (Barnes and Curson, 1994) for long-term prophylaxis has proven particularly useful. However, in controlled studies, the efficacy of depot neuroleptics compared to oral neuroleptics was not generally as superior as hypothesized (Möller, 1990). Advantages (reduction of the dosage due to absence of first-pass effect, relatively stable blood levels, guarantee that the patients take the drug) and disadvantages (lack of acute dose adjustment, "early peak"-phenomenon) of the depot-neuroleptics therapy have to be carefully balanced in the decision for the individual patient. Particularly when the patient's insight into the disease and the compliance are sufficient, and when the doctor-patient relation is good, oral long-term medication with its broad range of choice for different neuroleptics can have advantages. This is especially true for the oral long-term medication with novel/atypical neuroleptics, with their known advantage with respect to compliance.

As an alternative strategy to continuous neuroleptic long-term medication with a standard dose, the "*low dose strategy*" was studied. It appeared to be efficacious only when the dosage was not lowered too much (not more than about 1/5 of the standard dosage), and only when selected patients (among others those with a history of neuroleptic stabilization at relatively small dosages, no destabi-lization during change to these low dose treatments) were treated (Kane et al., 1983; Marder et al., 1987). Psychosocial therapies, including family-oriented intervention, can improve the relapse prevention efficacy of a low or standard dosage regimen (Goldstein et al., 1978; Hogarty et al., 1976). The "*early intervention strategy*", i.e., the discontinuation of the neuroleptic treatment after treatment of the acute manifestation, and renewed administration of neuro-leptics after the appearance of unspecific early warning symptoms (nervosity, insomnia etc.) could not prove sufficient efficacy com-pared to continuous neuroleptic long-term medication (Gaebel et al., 1995; Carpenter et al., 1992, Herz et al., 1991; Jolley et al., 1990). It should at the most be taken into consideration for patients who cannot be motivated to adhere to a standard or low-dose relapse prevention strategy.

For *schizoaffective psychoses*, at least for those with a strong affective component, relapse prevention with lithium, carbamazepin or valproate is indicated (Goodnick and Meltzer, 1984; Möller and Morin, 1989; Walden and Grunze, 1998). If the therapy is not successful enough, it is advisable to administer a neuroleptic long-term medication. If the patients do not respond to this, treatment should be tried with a combination of a neuroleptic and a mood stabilizer. In cases of patients suffering from a schizoaffective psychosis with a strong schizophrenic component, relapse prophylaxis with neuroleptics might be preferable.

In cases of *chronic productive psychoses*, a symptom suppressive maintenance therapy with neuroleptics has to be applied, with dosages that reduce the psychotic symptoms as far as possible on the one hand, whilst keeping the unwanted side effects as low as possible on the other. Especially with such patients, the benefit/risk ratio must be carefully considered and, under this condition, the reduction of the productive symptom-complex should not be overstressed. Chronic negative symptoms (chronic deficiency syndrome) should be treated according to the strategies mentioned above.

The Potential of Atypical Neuroleptics in the Drug Therapy of Schizophrenic Patients

The term "atypical neuroleptics" refers to antipsychotic drugs which, compared to typical neuroleptics, have a better relation of antipsychotic efficacy to extrapyramidal side effects. Furthermore, a greater efficacy in the treatment of negative symptoms in schizophrenia compared to traditional neuroleptics is also often implied in this definition (Möller, 1995). Altogether, the term atypical neuroleptics as referred to above is not clearly defined and may give rise to confusion.

Pharmacological screening shows some characteristics in atypical neuroleptics compared to traditional neuroleptics which may be found solely or in different combinations in the atypical neuroleptic under consideration. This field is too extensive to be described completely within this article, but is reviewed elsewhere (Möller et al., 1997). The most prominent features hypothetically implied with an atypical profile are:

– *Characteristics of binding to dopamine-receptors*

   • e.g., balanced relation between D_2- and D_1-blockade,
   • Preferential binding to D_4-receptors,
   • Preferential binding to D_3-receptors.

– *Preferential action at dopamine receptors of the limbic system*
– *Combined dopamine-D_2- and serotonin-5-HT_{2A}-antagonism with a predominance of the 5-HT_{2A} – blockade.*

There is one common characteristic in all atypical neuroleptics: The dose-response curves for antipsychotic efficacy and extrapyramidal side effects are widely separated from each other in animal tests. This means that low doses of the drug are able to exert antipsychotic efficacy, and only much higher doses will provoke extrapyramidal symptoms. This characteristic was first described for clozapine in animal screening tests.

The atypical neuroleptics have shown sufficient data suggesting efficacy in treating negative symptoms as well as a greatly reduced risk of extrapyramidal side effects. It goes without saying that these substances also showed a high efficacy in treating positive symptoms. These studies, mostly phase III studies, were performed according to the current methodological standards, and mostly in patients suffering from an acute episode of schizophrenia (Möller, 1997; Möller et al., 2000).

Despite the overall high standard of the different clinical phase III studies for new neuroleptics, there are differences in the design which have to be carefully considered in the interpretation of these results. For example, in both large phase III studies on risperidone (Peuskens, 1995; Marder and Meibach, 1994), only one dosage of the standard haloperidol was used, whereas risperidone was tested in different dosages. In the expert's opinion, this may lead to wrong conclusions as far as the advantages of the new substance are concerned. The advantages as seen with the new substance may occur only with a special dose compared to an undifferentiated dose of the standard neuroleptic. This is also true for most other new neuroleptics (Beasley et al., 1996, 1997; Tollefson et al., 1997; 1998). Some studies even test only one hypothetically equivalent dosage of the new substance against one dosage of haloperidol which is assumed to be a clinically used average dose (Tollefson et al., 1997; Tran et al., 1996; Petit et al., 1996). Many studies either use 10 or 20 mg/day of haloperidol. Some critics consider the 20 mg/day dosage of haloperidol as being too high and no longer a clinical standard. Furthermore, some critics point towards the fact that the high dosages of these standard substances were given under the assumption of optimal clinical efficacy, without keeping the higher rate of extrapyramidal side effects in mind. In principal, these arguments may be true. However, it has to be stated that 20 mg/day of haloperidol used to be common clinical practice at the time of planning of most of these studies, and that the assumption of a linear relationship between dose and extrapyramidal side effects has not been verified satisfactorily. In this context, the 7-arm sertindole/haloperidol study should be mentioned (Zimbroff et al., 1997), a study which overcomes most of the methodological pitfalls mentioned above. Under methodological aspects, it is also of importance in this context that the advantage of the atypical neuroleptics was not only demonstrated in comparison to high potency neuroleptics like haloperidol but also to the low potency chlorpromazine (Cooper et al., 1996).

To answer the question whether the atypical neuroleptics are also effective in negative symptoms of the chronic deficit syndromes, controlled studies should be performed in such patients. This is probably the most relevant clinical question, as chronic negative symptoms clearly predict the course of the disease. Ideally, the patients included in a study would be suffering from pure chronic negative symptoms, without any chronic positive symptoms, in order to avoid the difficulties in interpretation as mentioned above. Such patients could be best recruited from catamnestic studies but are rarely found within actual in- or outpatients. In order to fulfil the task of recruiting a set of patients with sufficient and predominating negative symptoms, it may be necessary to broaden inclusion criteria and to step down on exclusion criteria. Nevertheless, other possible factors which are capable of modulating negative symptoms should be excluded. Recommendations for such a design have been developed by a peer group of psychiatrists of university hospitals and specialised experts of the pharmaceutical industry (Möller et al., 1994). These consensus guidelines were mostly adopted for the CPMP guidelines for the evaluation of psychopharmacological effects on negative symptoms. However, studies which fully satisfy these standards have not yet been published. Apart from the clozapine studies on patients with refractory positive symptoms, which, in a narrow sense, do not follow these designs, only one amisulpride study comes close to these standards (Loo et al., 1997), when all published studies are considered. This study shows a clear-cut advantage of 100 mg amisulpride over placebo in treating negative symptoms.

In the search for differential benefits of the various new neuroleptics, further controlled group studies are currently being performed, comparing different atypical neuroleptics, e.g., an olanzapine versus risperidone and an amisulpride versus risperidone study.

Beside the evaluation of efficacy in acute episodes, it is also important to ensure efficacy and tolerability of a new neuroleptic in long-term treatment. Recently, the results of an open one-year trial of risperidone in about 400 patients have been published (Möller et al., 1997). It appears that risperidone shows high efficacy and good tolerability in long-term treatment. Most important is the observation that the drop-out rate due to side effects was very low (6% of the study population), especially the drop-out rate due to extrapyramidal side effects (2% of the study population).

Controlled long-term studies (up to one year) have also been conducted for olanzapine and sertindole, each in comparison to haloperidol. The results have mostly not yet been published, but it appears that patients receiving olanzapine or sertindole show clearly more favorable results than those receiving haloperidol (Satterlee et al., 1996; Street et al., 1996; Krystal et al., 1997; Tollefson and Sanger, 1997).

Atypical neuroleptics have a broad range of pharmacological profiles, ranging from the selective dopamine antagonist amisulpride, and the more or less selective D_2-$5HT_2$ receptor antagonists like risperidone, to pharmacologically non-selective "rich drugs" like clozapine or olanzapine with complex mechanisms of interaction. Clearly, this also results in different clinical profiles.

For example, olanzapine, zotepine and especially clozapine show a marked sedation, which is practically not observed with risperidone. Whereas sedation may not only be an unwanted side effect but an advantage in the acute treatment of excited psychotic patients, anticholinergic side effects frequently seen with zotepine, olanzapine and, to a lesser extent, with clozapine are clearly unwanted. Beside cognitive impairment and subjective side effects, they may also limit the use of these drugs in special patients at risk, e.g., patients with gastrointestinal problems, such as constipation, and patients with increased ocular pressure or cardiac problems. The last aspect is especially important for treatment with sertindole. Some cases of an increased QT-interval have been described, exceeding the critical limit of 500 ms. Therefore, patients with cardiac risk should be excluded and ECG controls should be carried out regularly during sertindole treatment.

Other drugs show a more pronounced α-adrenalytic profile, for example clozapine and sertindole. This may lead to a decrease of blood pressure and orthostatic problems, which can be avoided by a slow titration of the drug. However, this will limit its feasibility in the treatment of acutely psychotic patients. The occasional problem of a life-threatening agranulocytosis with clozapine, which led to restrictions of its use, does not seem to be apparent with olanzapine.

Compared to clozapine, zotepine and amisulpride, which have only medium antipsychotic potencies, making relatively high daily dosages necessary, risperidone, sertindole and olanzapine can be classified as high potency atypical neuroleptics.

When using non-sedating atypical neuroleptics in the treatment of acutely excited psychotic patients, a combination with sedatives such as benzodiazepines should be recommended in order to avoid an unneeded dosage increase of the neuroleptic to insure sufficient psychomotor calming. The combination of atypical neuroleptics with typical neuroleptics in order to increase efficacy in refractory patients or sedation is not evidence based and furthermore can be recommended only for a short period of time, as the advantage of a higher tolerability of atypical neuroleptics is otherwise at risk.

In conclusion, due to their better tolerability and partly better response of negative symptoms, atypical neuroleptics may increase the acceptance of neuroleptic treatment by patients and consequently also ensure compliance for short- and long-term treatment. This may in turn also improve the prognosis of schizophrenia.

References

Baldessarini, R.J., Cohen, B.M., and Teicher, M.H. (1988): Significance of neuroleptic dose and plasma level in the pharmacological treatment of psychoses. Archives of General Psychiatry 45: 79–91

Barnes, T.R., and Curson, D.A. (1994): Long-term depot antipsychotics. A risk-benefit assessment. Drug Safety 10: 464–479

Bitter, I., Volavka, J., and Scheurer, J. (1991): The concept of the neuroleptic threshold: An update. Journal of Clinical Psychopharmacology 11: 28–33

Carpenter, W.T.J, Stevens, J.H., and Rey, A.C. (1992): Early intervention vs. continuous pharmacotherapy in schizophrenia. Psychopharmacological Bulletin 18: 21–23

Carpenter, W.T.J., Heinrichs, D.W., and Alphs, L.D. (1985): Treatment of negative symptoms. Schizophrenia Bulletin 11: 440–452

Cooper, S.J., Raniwalla, J., and Wilch, C. (1996): Zotepine in acute exacerbation of schizophrenia: a comparison versus chlorpromazine and placebo. European Neuropsychopharmacology 6 (Suppl. 3): p. 148

Dahl, S.G. (1986): Plasma level monitoring of antipsychotic drugs. Clinical utility. Clinical. Pharmacokinetics 11: 36–61

Deister, A., and Möller, H.J. (1998): Schizophrenie und verwandte Psychosen Stuttgart: Wissenschaftliche Verlagsgesellschaft

Fleischhacker, W.W. (1999): The pharmacotherapy of schizophrenic disorders. Depressive disorders (in press)

Fleischhacker, W.W., Meise, U., Gunther, V., and Kurtz, M. (1994): Compliance with antipsychotic treatment, influence of side-effects. Acta Psychiatrica Scandinavica 89(Suppl. 382): 11–15

Gaebel, W., and Falkai, P. (1998): Praxisleitlinien in Psychiatrie und Psychotherapie, Band 1: Behandlungsleitlinie Schizophrenie. Dentsche Gesellschaft für Psychiatrie, Psychotherapie und Nerrenheilkunde. Darmstadt: Steinkopff

Gaebel, W., Frick, U., Köpcke, W., Linden, M., Müller, P., Müller-Spahn, F., Pietzcker, A., and Tegeler, J. (1995): Early neuroleptic intervention in schizophrenia: are prodromal symptoms valid predictors of relapse? British Journal of Psychiatry 163 (Suppl. 21): 8–12

Gardos, G. (1974): Are antipsychotic drugs interchangeable? Journal of Nervous and Mental Disease 159: 343–348

Goldstein, M.J., Rodnick, E.H., Evans, J.R., May, P.R., and Steinberg, M.R. (1978): Drug and family therapy in the aftercare of acute schizophrenics. Archives of General Psychiatry 35: 1169–1177

Goodnick, P.J. and Meltzer, H.Y. (1984): Treatment of schizoaffective disorders. Schizophrenia Bulletin 10: 30–48

Herz, M.I., Glazer, W.M., Mostert, M.A., Sheard, M.A., Szymanski, H.V., Hafez, H., Mirza, M., and Vana, J. (1991): Intermittent vs maintenance medication in schizophrenia: Two-year results. Archives of General Psychiatry 48: 333–339

Hogarty, G.E., Ulrich, R., Goldberg, S., and Schooler, N. (1976): Sociotherapy and the prevention of relapse among schizophrenic patients: An artifact of drug? Proceedings of the Annual Meeting of the American Psychopathological Association 285–293

Johnson, D.A.W. (1975): Observations on the dose regimens of fluphenazine decanoate in maintenance therapy of schizophrenia. British Journal of Psychiatry 126: 457–461

Jolley, A.G., Hirsch, S.R., Morrison, E., McRink, A., and Wilson, L. (1990): Trial of brief intermittent neuroleptic prophylaxis for selected schizophrenic outpatients: Clinical and social outcome at two years. British Journal of Medicine 301: 837–842

Kane, J.M., Honigfeld, G., Singer, J., and Meltzer, H.Y. (1988): Clozapine for the treatment-resistant schizophrenic: A double-blind comparison versus chlorpromazine/benztropine. Archives of General Psychiatry 48: 789–796

Kane, J.M. and Marder, S.R. (1993): Psychopharmacologic treatment of schizophrenia. Schizophrenia Bulletin 19: 287–302

Kane, J.M., Möller, H.J., and Awouters, F. (1996): Serotonin in antipsychotic treatment – Mechanisms and clinical practice. New York Basel Hong Kong: Marcel Dekker

Kane, J.M., Rifkin, A., Woerner, M., Reardon, G., Sarantakos, S., Schiebel, D., and Ramos Lorenzi, J. (1983): Low-dose neuroleptic treatment of outpatient schizophrenics. I. Preliminary results for relapse rates. Archives of General Psychiatry 40: 893–896

Kane, J.M., Woerner, M., Borenstein, M., Wegner, J., and Lieberman, J. (1986): Integrating incidence and prevalence of tardive dyskinesia. Psychopharmacological Bulletin 22: 254–258

Kinon, B.J., Kane, J.M., Johns, C., Perovich, R., Ismi, M., Koreen, A., and Weiden, P. (1993): Treatment of neuroleptic-resistant schizophrenic relapse. Psychopharmacological Bulletin 29: 309–314

Kissling, W. (1994): Compliance, quality assurance and standards for relapse prevention in schizophrenia. Acta Psychiatrica Scandinavica 89 (Suppl. 382): 16–24

Klemm, E., Grünwald, F., Kasper, S., Menzel, C., Broich, K., Danos, P., Reichmann, K., Krappel, C., Rieker, O., Briele, B., Hotze, A.L., Möller, H.J., and Biersack, H.J. (1996): IBZM SPECT for imaging of striatal D_2 Dopamine receptors in 56 schizophrenic patients taking various neuroleptics. American Journal of Psychiatry 153: 183–190

Krystal, J., D'Souza, D.C., Holgate, K.L., Staser, J.A., Silber, C.J., and Mack, R.J. (1997): Sertindole: A multi-center, one year, haloperidol controlled trial assessing the long term safety, efficacy and quality of life in stable schizophrenic patients. Paper presented at the 10th ECNP, Vienna

Lieberman, J., Jody, D., Geisler, S., Alvir, J., Loebel, A., Szymanski, S., Woerner, M., and Borenstein, M. (1993): Time course and biologic correlates of treatment response in first-episode schizophrenia. Archives of General Psychiatry 50: 369–376

Loo, H., Poirier, L.M., Theron, M., Rein, W., and Fleurot, O. (1997): Amisulpride versus placebo in the medium-term treatment of the negative symptoms of schizophrenia. British Journal of Psychiatry 170: 18–22

Marder, S.R. and Meibach, R.C. (1994): Risperidone in the treatment of schizophrenia. American Journal Psychiatry 151: 825–835

Marder, S.R., Van, P.T., Mintz, J., Lebell, M., McKenzie, J., and May, P.R. (1987): Low- and conventional-dose maintenance therapy with fluphenazine decanoate. Two-year outcome. Archives of General Psychiatry 44: 518–521

McEvoy, J.P., Hogarty, G.E., and Steingard, S. (1991): Optimal dose of neuroleptic in acute schizophrenia. A controlled study of the neuroleptic threshold and higher haloperidol dose. Archives of General Psychiatry 48: 739–745

Meltzer, H.Y. (1992): Treatment of the neuroleptic-nonresponsive schizophrenic patient. Schizophrenia Bulletin 18: 515–542

Meltzer, H.Y., Bastani, B., Kwon, K.Y., Ramirez, L.F., Burnett, S., and Sharpe, J. (1989): A prospective study of clozapine in treatment-resistant schizophrenic patients. I. Preliminary report. Psychopharmacology (Suppl. 99), S68–S72

Möller, H.-J. (1999a): Atypical antipsychotics: a new approach in the treatment of negative symptoms? European Archives of Psychiatry and Clinical Neuroscience 249 (Suppl. 4): IV99–IV107

Möller, H.-J. (1999b): State of evaluation and clinical benefits of atypical neuroleptics. The treatment of schizophrenia: Status and emerging trends. (Brenner, H.D. Böker, W. and Genner, R., eds.), Göttingen Seattle Toronto: Hogrefe and Huber

Möller, H.-J., Müller, N., and Bandelow, B. (2000): Neuroleptika. Stuttgart: Wissenschaftliche Verlagsgesellschaft

Möller, H.-J., and Rao, M.L. (1996): Negative symptoms of schizophrenia: Methodological issues, biochemical findings and efficacy of neuroleptic treatment. In: Implications of psychopharmacology to psychiatry. Biological, nosological, and therapeutical concepts (Ackenheil, M., Bondy, B., Engel, R., Ermann, M., and Nedopil, N., eds.), pp. 158–178. Berlin Heidelberg New York: Springer

Möller, H.J. (1990): Neuroleptische Langzeittherapie schizophrener Erkrankungen. In: Leitlinien neuroleptischer Therapie (Heinrich, K., ed.), pp. 97–115: Berlin Heidelberg New York: Springer

Möller, H.J. (1992): Neuroleptische Rezidivprophylaxe und Langzeitbehandlung schizophrener Psychosen. In: Neuroleptika, pp. 153–168. Wien: Springer

Möller, H.J. (1993): Neuroleptic treatment of negative symptoms in schizophrenic patients. Efficacy problems and methodological difficulties. European Neuropsychopharmacology 3: 1–11

Möller, H.J. (1995): Extrapyramidal side effects of neuroleptic medication: focus on risperidone. In: Critical issues in the treatment of schizophrenia (Brunello, N., Racagni, G., Langer, S.Z., and Mendlewicz, J., eds.), pp. 142–151. Basel: Karger

Möller, H.J. (1997): Atypische Neuroleptika: Ist der Begriff gerechtfertigt? Psychopharmakotherapie 4: 130–132.

Möller, H.J., Bäuml, J., Ferrero, F., Fuger, J., Geretsegger, C., Kasper, S., Kissling, W., and Schubert, H. (1997): Risperidone in the treatment of schizophrenia: Results of a study of patients from Germany, Austria, and Switzerland. European Archives of Psychiatry and Clinical Neuroscience 247: 291–296

Möller, H.J., Kissling, W., Lang, C., Doerr, P., Pirke, K.M., and von Zerssen, D. (1982): Efficacy and side effects of haloperidol in psychotic patients: oral versus intravenous administration. American Journal of Psychiatry 139: 1571–1575

Möller, H.J., and Morin,C. (1989): Behandlung schizodepressiver Syndrome mit Antidepressiva. In: Schizoaffektive Psychosen. Diagnose, Therapie und Prophylaxe (Marneros, A., ed.), pp. 159–178. Berlin Heidelberg New York: Springer

Möller, H.J., van Praag, H.M., Aufdembrinke, B., Bailey, P., Barnes, T.R., Beck, J., Bentsen, H., Eich, F.X., Farrow, L., Fleischhacker, W.W., Gerlach, J., Grafford, K., Hentschel, B., Hertkorn, A., Heylen, S., Lecrubier, Y., Leonhard, J.P., McKenna, P., Maier, W., Pedersen, V., Rappard, A., Rein, W., Ryan, J., Sloth Nielsen, M., Stieglitz, R.D., Wegener, G., and Wilson, J. (1994): Negative symptoms in schizophrenia: Considerations for clinical trials. Working group on negative symptoms in schizophrenia. Psychopharmacology 115: 221–228

Möller, H.J., and von Zerssen, D. (1995): Course and outcome of schizophrenia. In: Schizophrenia (Hirsch, S.R. and Weinberger, D.R., eds.), pp. 107–127. Oxford: Blackwell Science

Nordstrom, A.-L., Farde, L., and Wiesel, F.A. (1993): Central D – dopamine receptor occupancy in relation to antipsychotic drug effects: A double-blind PET study of schizophrenic patients. Biological Psychiatry 33: 227–235

Northoff, G., Wenke, J., Demisch, L., Eckert, J., Gille, B., and Pflug, B. (1995): Catatonia: short-term response to lorazepam and dopaminergic metabolism. Psychopharmacology 122: 182–186

Petit, M., Raniwalla, J., Tweed, J., Leutenegger, E., Dollfus, S., and Kelly, F. (1996): A comparison of an atypical and typical antipsychotic, zotepine versus haloperidol in patients with acute exacerbation of schizophrenia: A parallel-group double-blind trial. Psychopharmacological Bulletin 32: 81–87

Peuskens, J. (1995): Risperidone in the treatment of patients with chronic schizophrenia: a multi-national, multi-centre, double-blind, parallel-group study versus haloperidol. Risperidone Study Group. British Journal of Psychiatry 166: 712–726

Prusoff, B.A., Williams, D.H., Weissman, M.M., and Astrachan, B.A. (1979): Treatment of secondary depression in schizophrenia. Archives of General Psychiatry 36: 569–575

Reardon, G.T., Rifkin, A., Schwartz, A., Myerson, A., and Siris, S.G. (1989): Changing patterns of neuroleptic dosage over a decade. American Journal of Psychiatry 146: 726–729

Rifkin, A., Doddi, S., Karajgi, B., Borenstein, M., and Wachpress, M. (1991): Dosage of haloperidol for schizophrenia. Archives of General Psychiatry 48: 166–170

Rosebush, P.I., Hildebrand, A.M., Furlong, B.G., and Mazurek, M.F. (1990): Catatonic syndrome in a general psychiatric inpatient population: frequency, clinical presentation, and response to lorazepam. Journal of Clinical Psychiatry 51: 357–362

Sagatovic, M., and Meltzer, H.Y. (1993): The effect of short-term electroconvulsive treatment plus neuroleptic in treatment-resistant schizophrenia and schizoaffective disorder. Convulsive Therapy 9: 167–175

Satterlee, W., Dellva, M.A., Beasley, C., Tran, P., and Tollefson, G. (1996): Effectiveness of olanzapine in long-term continuation treatment. Psychopharmacological Bulletin 32: 509

Schulz, S.C., Kahn, E.M., Baker, R.W., and Conley, R.R. (1990): Lithium and Carbamazepine. Augmentation in treatment-refractory schizophrenia. In: The neuroleptic-nonresponsive patient: Characterization and treatment (Angrist, B. and Schulz, S.C., eds.), pp. 111–136. Washington London: American Psychiatric Press

Shalev, A., Hermesh, H., Rothberg, J., and Munitz, H. (1993): Poor neuroleptic response in acutely exacerbated schizophrenic patients. Acta Psychiatrica Scandinavica 87: 86–91

Siris, S.G. (1995): Depression and schizophrenia. In: Schizophrenia (Hirsch, S.R. and Weinberger, D.R., eds.), pp. 128–145. Oxford: Blackwell Science

Siris, S.G., Kammen, v.P., and Docherty, J.P. (1978): Use of antidepressant drugs in schizophrenia. Archives of General Psychiatry 35: 1368–1377

Street, J.S., Tamura, R., Sanger, T., and Tollefson, G. (1996): Long-term treatment-emergent dyskinetic symptoms in patients treated with olanzapine and haloperidol. Psychopharmacological Bulletin 32: 522

Tollefson, G.D., Beasley C., Tran, P.V., Street, J.S., Krueger, J.A., Tamura, R.N., Graffeo, K.A., and Thieme, M.E. (1997): Olanzapine versus haloperidol in the treatment of schizophrenia and schizoaffective and schizophreniform disorders: results of an international collaborative trial. American Journal of Psychiatry 154: 457–465

Tollefson, G.D. and Sanger, T.M. (1997): Negative symptoms: a path analytic approach to a double-blind, placebo- and haloperidol-controlled clinical trial with olanzapine. American Journal of Psychiatry 154: 466–474

Tollefson, G.D., Sanger, T.M., Lu, Y., and Thieme, M.E. (1998): Depresive signs and symptoms in schizophrenia: A prospective blinded trial of olanzapine and haloperidol. Archives of General Psychiatry 55: 250–258

Tran, P., Beasley, C. and Tollefson, G. (1996): Acute and long-term results of the dose ranging double-blind olanzapine trial. Melbourne

Ungvari, G.S., Leung, C.M. and Chiu, H.M. (1994): Lorazepam in stupor. British Journal Clinical Practise 48: 165–166

Van, P.T., Marder, S.R., and Mintz, J. (1990): A controlled dose comparison of haloperidol in newly admitted schizophrenic patients. Archives of General Psychiatry 47: 754–758

Walden, J. and Grunze, H. (1998): Bipolare affektive Störungen: Ursachen und Behandlung. Stuttgart New York: Thieme

Zimbroff, D.L., Kane, J.M., Tamminga, C.A., Daniel, D.G., Mack, R.J., Wozniak, P.J., Sebree, T.B., Wallin, B.A., and Kashkin, K.B. (1997): Controlled, dose-response study of sertindole and haloperidol in the treatment of schizophrenia. Sertindole Study Group. American Journal of Psychiatry 154: 782–791

List of Contributors

Altorfer Andreas, Ph.D.,
*Psychiatric Institutions, University of Berne, Bolligenstr. 111,
3000 Berne 60, Switzerland*

Dingemans Peter, Ph.D.,
*Academic Medical Center, University of Amsterdam,
Psychiatric Center, Tafelbergweg 25, 1105 BC Amsterdam,
The Netherlands*

Dominiak George, M.D.,
*Department of Psychiatry, Mount Auburn Hospital, MA 02138,
U.S.A.*

Fox Lindy, M.A.,
*New Hampshire-Dartmouth, Psychiatric Research Center, State
Office Park South, 105 Pleasant Street, Concord, New
Hampshire 03301, U.S.A.*

Hahlweg Kurt, Ph.D.,
*Technical University Braunschweig, Institut of Psychology,
Spielmannstr. 12A, 38106 Braunschweig, Germany*

Hooley Jill, D.Phil.,
*Department of Psychology, Harvard University, 33 Kirkand
Street Cambridge, MA 02138, U.S.A.*

Käsermann Marie-Luise, Ph.D.,
*Psychiatric Institutions, University of Berne, Bolligenstr. 111,
3000 Berne 60, Switzerland*

Leff Julian, Ph.D.,
*Institute of Psychiatry, Social Psychiatry Section, De Crespigny
Park, London SE5 8AF, Great Britain*

Lenior Maria E., Ph.D.,
*Academic Medical Center, University of Amsterdam,
Psychiatric Center, Tafelbergweg 25, 1105 BC Amsterdam,
The Netherlands*

Linszen Don H., M.D., Ph.D.,
Academic Medical Center, University of Amsterdam,
Psychiatric Center, Tafelbergweg 25, 1105 BC Amsterdam,
The Netherlands

Mercer Carolyn, Ph.D.,
New Hampshire-Dartmouth, Psychiatric Research Center, State
Office Park South, 105 Pleasant Street, Concord, NH 03301,
U.S.A.

Miklowitz David J., Ph.D.,
Department of Psychology, University of Colorado, Muenzinger
Building, Campus Box 345, Boulder, CO 80309-0345, U.S.A.

Möller Hans-Jürgen, M.D.,
Department of Psychiatry, Ludwig Maximilian University of
Munich, Nußbaumstrasse 7, 80336 Munich, Germany

Mueser Kim T., Ph.D.,
New Hampshire-Dartmouth, Psychiatric Research Center, State
Office Park South, 105 Pleasant Street, Concord, NH 03301,
U.S.A.

Nuechterlein Keith H., Ph.D.,
UCLA Department of Psychiatry and Biobehavioral Sciences,
300 UCLA Medical Plaza, Rm. 2240, Los Angeles,
CA 90095-6968, U.S.A.

Richards Jeffrey A., M.A.,
Department of Psychology, University of Colorado, Muenzinger
Building, Campus Box 345, Boulder, CO 80309-0345, U.S.A.

Schaub Annette, Ph.D.,
Department of Psychiatry, Ludwig Maximilian University of
Munich, Nußbaumstrasse 7, 80336 Munich, Germany

Subotnik Kenneth L., Ph.D.,
UCLA Department of Psychiatry and Biobehavioral Sciences,
300 UCLA Medical Plaza, Rm. 2240, Los Angeles,
CA 90095-6968, U.S.A.

Tompson Martha C., Ph.D.,
Department of Psychology, Boston University, 64 Cummington
Street, Boston, MA 02215, U.S.A.

Ventura Joseph, Ph.D.,
UCLA Department of Psychiatry and Biobehavioral Sciences,
300 UCLA Medical Plaza, Rm. 2240, Los Angeles,
CA 90095-6968, U.S.A.

Weisman Amy G.,
Department of Psychology, Boston University, 64 Cummington Street, Boston, MA 02215, U.S.A.

Wiedemann Georg, M.D.,
Department of Psychiatry, University of Tuebingen, Osianderstr. 22, 72076 Tuebingen, Germany

Editor and Contributors

Editor

Annette Schaub is Assistant Professor and head of Applied Clinical Psychology in the Department of Psychiatry, University of Munich, Germany, which she joined in 1995. She has been principal investigator of controlled treatment studies in schizophrenia and depression and her research has been supported by the Swiss National Funds, the German Ministry of Education and Research and Eli Lilly Foundation. She is a behavioral and family therapist and licensed supervisor. She has published articles and book chapters on coping and treatment, including research on coping-oriented therapy in schizophrenia. At the University of Munich she is responsible for the training of medical doctors and psychologists in behavior therapy. Before joining the faculty at the University of Munich Dr. Schaub worked as a research fellow in Bonn (Germany) and Berne (Switzerland). In 1992, at the invitation of Michael J. Goldstein, she traveled to the U.S.A. to learn more about his work on the treatment of families of persons with bipolar disorder. Under Mike's mentorship in Los Angeles she honed her clinical and research skills, and participated in numerous stimulating discussions with him and his research team. This fruitful experience in Los Angeles established the basis for a rich collegial friendship that continued at international conferences after Dr. Schaub returned to Europe, until Mike's untimely death in 1997.

The following bio sketches and comments were added by the contributors themselves.

Contributors

Andreas Altorfer is research psychologist at the Psychiatric Institutions (Department of Theoretical and Evaluative Psychiatry) of the University of Berne (Switzerland). His main interests concern verbal interaction, nonverbal communication, and analyses in psychophysiology (cardiovascular activity). Several methodological approaches were developed which allow for measuring nonverbal behavior and psychophysiological variables during conversation. After attending schools in Basle and studies in Berne (Psychology, Musicology and Psychopathology) he received his Ph.D. at the University of Berne in 1986. Supported by a grant of the Swiss National Science Foundation in 1987 he was visiting scientist at the University of California Los Angeles (UCLA) working with the Family-Project Group of Prof. Michael J. Goldstein.

Peter M. Dingemans is Associate Professor at the University of Amsterdam and a Clinical and Research Psychologist at the Academic Medical Center, division of Psychiatry in Amsterdam. He has (co-)authored articles and books about the various aspects of schizophrenia. In 1988 he was a Fulbright fellow in the UCLA Family project and started to work with Mike Goldstein on his various projects. This was continued when Mike was appointed a Spinoza professorship at the University of Amsterdam in 1992; a period when the first wave results of the Amsterdam schizophrenia project were analyzed. Through all this work he got to know Mike as an astute scholar, a much loved teacher, and a gregarious, warm person.

George Dominiak is Chief of Psychiatry at the Mount Auburn Hospital in Cambridge, MA and Assistant Professor of Psychiatry at the Harvard Medical School. He is actively involved in the teaching and supervision of psychiatrists and specializes in the clinical management of difficult to treat patients. His research interests include eating disorders, and personality disorders, including borderline personality disorder.

Lindy Fox, M.A., L.A.D.C., is a Research Associate at the New Hampshire-Dartmouth Psychiatric Research Center. She has worked extensively on research projects examining the effectiveness of treatment for people with serious mental illnesses and substance use disorders. She also has a great deal of clinical experience providing group and individual treatment to consumers with dual diagnoses. Ms. Fox's expertise has been gained through a combination of formal education, personal experience, and professional focus. She has been a recipient of the services she now participates in designing and evaluating. As a result of this unusual combination of personal and professional experience, Ms. Fox brings sensitivity, humor, and extensive knowledge to this challenging field of working with people with both serious mental illnesses and substance use disorders. Ms. Fox has consulted throughout the United States and in other countries including Australia, Canada, England, and Sweden. She has co-authored several articles, and is on faculty at Dartmouth Medical School in the Department of Family and Community Medicine.

Kurt Hahlweg is full professor for Clinical Psychology, Psychotherapy, and Assessment at the Technical University of Braunschweig. His main interests are: behavioral marital and family therapy, in particular in psychoeducational family management in schizophrenia; expressed emotion; family interaction research; prevention of marital and child behavior problems. He received his doctorate from the University of Hamburg in 1977 and was a senior research fellow at the Max-Planck-Institut for Psychiatry in Munich from 1974 till 1988, when he became professor at the Technical University of Braunschweig. His professional and social relationship with Mike Goldstein began in 1981. In 1983 till 1984 he was a visiting scholar at the University of California, Los Angeles, working with the Family Project Group headed by Dr. Goldstein. The two organized several international conferences, shared platforms at various meetings, edited books, and published several papers in peer reviewed journals.

Jill Hooley is Professor of Psychology in the Psychology Department at Harvard University. She is also head of the Experimental Psychopathology Program and Director of Clinical Training. In 1980 she began to study Expressed Emotion and has explored the concurrent and predictive validity of EE in depression, schizophrenia, and borderline personality disorder. More recently she has become involved in basic research involving self-harming behavior and has also been investigating the link between pain insensitivity and psychosis. Her association with Michael Goldstein dates back to the mid 1980s. They frequently met at research meetings, exchanged ideas, and enjoyed lively discussions.

Marie-Louise Käsermann is research psychologist at the Psychiatric Institutions (Department of Theoretical and Evaluative Psychiatry) and Professor at the Department of Psychology of the University of Berne (Switzerland). Her main interests concern verbal communication, emotions during conversation, and evaluations of psychophysiological variables. After attending schools in Solothurn and studies in Fribourg and Berne (Psychology, Zoology and Psychopathology) she received her Ph.D. at the University of Berne in 1978. 1978–1980 Marie-Louise Käsermann was research scientist at the Max-Planck-Institute of Psycholinguistics in Nijmegen (Holland). Since 1980 she had been the head of the Human Communication Lab of the Psychiatric Institutions, conducting basic research in verbal and nonverbal interaction, emotion, and psychophysiological measures.

Julian Leff is Professor of Social and Cultural Psychiatry at the Institute of Psychiatry, London, and is a full time researcher for the Medical Research Council. He has also been Honorary Director of the Team for the Assessment of Psychiatric Services for the past 14 years, involved in evaluating the national policy of replacing psychiatric hospitals with community services. He began research on Expressed Emotion with Dr. Christine Vaughn in the early 1970s and progressed from naturalistic studies to family interventions. His recent research includes an extension of the schizophrenia family work to depressed patients with a partner, and a social and biological exploration of the possible causes for the high incidence of schizophrenia in African-Caribbeans in the UK. His professional and social relationship with Mike Goldstein began in the early 1980s. They shared the platform at numerous meetings and enjoyed many relaxed hours together.

Don H. Linszen is a psychiatrist and Head of the Adolescent Clinic, Academic Medical Center, University of Amsterdam, Amsterdam. After acquiring his M.D. (1976) Don Linszen studied philosophy and medicine at the University of Amsterdam. He completed his internship and psychiatric residency at the Academic Hospital of University of Amsterdam and residencies in neurology at the St. Elisabeth Hospital in Amersfoort and in social psychiatry at the Mental Health Centre in Amsterdam. He acquired his specialty certification in 1981 and became staff psychiatrist at the Academic Medical Centre (AMC) of the University of Amsterdam. From 1986 he leads as chef de clinique the adolescent clinic of the Psychiatric Centre of the AMC, a model agency for adolescent and young adults patients with first psychotic episodes of schizophrenia and related disorders. Don Linszen has published many articles, abstracts, chapters of books on biopsychosocial aspects of psychosis and schizophrenia and lectured on leading congresses in that domain.

Carolyn Mercer, Ph.D. was a senior researcher, public policy specialist at the New Hampshire-Dartmouth Psychiatric Research Center. Dr. Mercer received her A.B. degree from Harvard College in 1963 and her Ph.D. in Social Research from Brandeis University in 1978. In a long career in social welfare, Ms. Mercer most recently served as Long-Range Planning Director of the New Hampshire-Dartmouth Psychiatric Research Center. She had previously been associated with the State of New Hampshire Division of Mental Health, the United States Department of Health and Human Services, and her own company, Social Planning Services, Inc., of Watertown, Massachusetts. In the last decade, Ms. Mercer had developed a separate career in environmental protection, receiving awards from the New Hampshire Sierra Club, Renew America, and the United States Department of Agriculture. Dr. Mercer died in 1999.

David J. Miklowitz, Ph.D. is Professor of Psychology, Department of Psychology (Clinical Area), University of Colorado at Boulder. Dr. Miklowitz did his undergraduate work at Brandeis University and his doctoral (1979–1985) and postdoctoral work (1985–88) at UCLA. He has been at the University of Colorado, Boulder since 1989. His specialty is in the family environmental factors associated with bipolar and schizophrenic disorders, and in the family and individual treatment of bipolar disorder. He has received Young Investigator Awards from the International Congress on Schizophrenia Research and the National Alliance for Research on Schizophrenia and Depression. He has received funding for his research from the National Institute for Mental Health and the MacArthur Foundation. He has published 75 research papers on bipolar disorder and schizophrenia. His articles have appeared in high ranking peer-reviewed journals (e.g., Archives of General Psychiatry). His book with Michael J. Goldstein, published by Guilford Press, "Bipolar Disorder: A Family-Focused Treatment Approach," won the 1998 Outstanding Research Publication Award from the American Association of Marital and Family Therapy.

Hans-Jürgen Möller is Chairman of the Psychiatric Clinic of the University of Munich and President of the World Federation of Societies of the Biological Psychiatry (WFSBP), President of the "Arbeitsgemeinschaft für Neuropsychopharmakologie" (Association of Neuropsychopharmacology), President of the "Arbeitsgemeinschaft für Methodik und Dokumentation in der Psychiatrie" (Association of Methodology and Documentation in Psychiatry), member of several national and international psychiatric societies, main editor of "European Archives of Psychiatry and Clinical Neuroscience", of "Nervenarzt", of "Psychopharmakotherapie" and Chief editor of "The World Journal of Biological Psychiatry". His main research fields are: methodology of clinical research, follow-up research, clinical psychopharmacology, psychogeriatry. He is author of more than 400 German and international publications, author and editor of several books, editor of several textbooks on psychiatry and on psychopharmacology. His professional and social relationship with Prof. Michael J. Goldstein goes back to a schizophrenia meeting in the early 1980s. From this time a close communication on problems of drug treatment of schizophrenic patients started.

Kim T. Mueser, Ph.D., is a clinical psychologist and a Professor in the Departments of Psychiatry and Community and Family Medicine at the Dartmouth Medical School in Hanover, New Hampshire. Dr. Mueser received his Ph.D. in clinical psychology from the University of Illinois at Chicago in 1984 and was on the faculty of the Psychiatry Department at the Medical College of Pennsylvania in Philadelphia, Pennsylvania until 1994. In 1994 he moved to Dartmouth Medical School. Dr. Mueser's clinical and research interests include the psychosocial treatment of schizophrenia and other severe mental illnesses, dual diagnosis, and posttraumatic stress disorder. He has published extensively and given numerous lectures and workshops on psychiatric rehabilitation. Dr. Mueser's association with Dr. Michael Goldstein dates back to the mid 1980s, when he was a psychology intern and postdoctoral fellow at the UCLA Research Center for Severe Mental Illness.

Keith H. Nuechterlein, Ph.D., is Professor in the Departments of Psychiatry and Biobehavioral Sciences and of Psychology, University of California, Los Angeles, and is Principal Investigator of the Developmental Processes in Schizophrenic Disorders project. He also serves as the Director of the UCLA Aftercare Research Program and of the Cognition, Psychophysiology, and Neuropsychology Laboratory for Schizophrenia. Dr. Nuechterlein has directed longitudinal research that examines a vulnerability-stress model of influences on the early course of schizophrenia, including particularly enduring neurocognitive and psychophysiological vulnerability factors, psychosocial stressors, and their potential interactions. He also continues family genetic research to identify the nature and transmission of neurocognitive vulnerability factors for schizophrenia in biological relatives of individuals with schizophrenia.

Jeffrey A. Richards, M.A., is a graduate student in clinical psychology working with Dr. David J. Miklowitz in the Department of Psychology at the University of Colorado at Boulder. His research interests include statistical design issues relevant to psychological treatment studies of bipolar disorder.

Kenneth L. Subotnik, Ph.D., is Adjunct Associate Professor and Associate Research Psychologist in the Department of Psychiatry and Biobehavioral Sciences, University of California, Los Angeles, and project coordinator for the Developmental Processes in Schizophrenic Disorders project. Dr. Subotnik's research interests have included the identification of vulnerability factors in schizophrenic patients and family members that predispose to schizophrenia, with a focus on psychometric measures such as the MMPI, the examination of formal thought disorder and its neurocognitive and neuroanatomical correlates, and the study of the course of negative symptoms and their clinical correlates.

Joseph Ventura, Ph.D., is Associate Research Psychologist in the Department of Psychiatry and Biobehavioral Sciences, University of California, Los Angeles (UCLA), and the Director of the Diagnosis and Psychopathology Unit of the UCLA Center for Research on Treatment and Rehabilitation of Psychosis. Dr. Ventura's longstanding interests in the effects of stress on the early course of schizophrenia are reflected in the publication of several papers from prospective studies showing that life events are "triggers" of psychotic relapse. His recent work has included a survival analysis showing that stressful life events were associated with a significantly increased risk for depressive exacerbation in schizophrenia. Currently, he is conducting research on the influence of psychological and neurocognitive factors on coping behavior in the early course of schizophrenia and in individuals at high risk for psychosis.

Amy Weisman earned her doctorate from the University of Southern California in 1994, completing her pre-doctoral internship at the UCLA neuropsychiatric institute. From 1994–1996 she served as a post-doctoral fellow at the UCLA Family Project under the mentorship of Michael J. Goldstein, who made a tremendous impact on her career. Dr. Weisman is currently an assistant professor at the University of Massachusetts Boston. Her research focuses primarily on family and cultural factors that influence the course of severe mental illness. She has published several articles specifically examining and comparing differences in Anglo and Latino family members' reactions to a relative with schizophrenia.

Georg Wiedemann is associate professor for Psychiatry, Psychotherapy, and Psychosomatic Medicine at the University Hospital of Psychiatry and Psychotherapy Tuebingen. After studies at the

Universities in Bochum, Regensburg and Munich he received his MD at the University of Munich in 1984. He worked in the first behavior therapy oriented hospital of Psychosomatic Medicine in Germany, and afterwards in a psychoanalytically oriented Department of Psychosomatic Medicine of a general hospital and the Technical University of Munich. Then he was a senior research fellow at the Max-Planck-Institute of Psychiatry in Munich. Since 1993 he has been consultant psychiatrist at the University Hospital of Psychiatry and Psychotherapy in Tuebingen. He began research on Expressed Emotion with Prof. Kurt Hahlweg at the Max-Planck-Institute in Munich in the late 1980s and progressed to family interventions in schizophrenia. His main interests concern family therapy, in particular family management in schizophrenia. His recent research includes an extension of schizophrenia family work to other psychiatric disorders and to relatives' groups in various areas of psychiatry and psychosomatic medicine, as well as a psychological and psychophysiological exploration of anxiety disorders and pain.

SpringerPhilosophie

Leonhard Bauer, Klaus Hamberger (Hrsg.)

Gesellschaft denken

Eine erkenntnistheoretische Standortbestimmung
der Sozialwissenschaften

2002. XIV, 375 Seiten. 20 Abbildungen.
Format: 16,5 x 24,2 cm
Broschiert **EUR 34,90**, sFr 54,–
ISBN 3-211-83733-7
Politische Philosophie und Ökonomie

„Gesellschaft denken" nimmt aus erkenntnistheoretischer
Perspektive eine Standortbestimmung der Sozialwissenschaften am Beginn des neuen Jahrhunderts vor. Die Bei-
träge internationaler Wissenschaftler aus den verschieden-
sten Disziplinen und Denkrichtungen ergeben ein kompaktes
Bild des derzeitigen Stands sozialwissenschaftlicher Selbst-
reflexion und vermitteln einen Eindruck der wesentlichen
Schnittlinien, an denen sich der Dialog zwischen den Tra-
ditionen und Disziplinen zur Zeit konzentriert. Der Leser kann
sich sowohl einen Überblick über den gegenwärtigen Stand
der Debatte verschaffen, als auch durch die heterogene Viel-
zahl der in diesem Band versammelten Gedanken zu weite-
rer Reflexion anregen lassen.

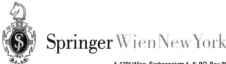
Springer WienNewYork

A-1201 Wien, Sachsenplatz 4–6, P.O. Box 89, Fax +43.1.330 24 26, e-mail: books@springer.at, **www.springer.at**
D-69126 Heidelberg, Haberstraße 7, Fax +49.6221.345-229, e-mail: orders@springer.de
USA, Secaucus, NJ 07096-2485, P.O. Box 2485, Fax +1.201.348-4505, e-mail: orders@springer-ny.com
EBS, Japan, Tokyo 113, 3–13, Hongo 3-chome, Bunkyo-ku, Fax +81.3.38 18 08 64, e-mail: orders@svt-ebs.co.jp

SpringerMedicine

Christian Behl

Estrogen – Mystery Drug for the Brain?

The Neuroprotective Activities of the Female Sex Hormone

2001. XV, 228 pages. 50 figures.
Hardcover **EUR 65,–**
(Recommended retail price)
Net-price subject to local VAT.
ISBN 3-211-83539-3

It is well known that estrogen is "somehow" a protective hormone for various age-related disorders. This book provides a solid knowledge of estrogen's neuroprotective activities in the brain with a special emphasis on neurodegenerative disorders such as Alzheimer's Disease. The focus is (1) to describe the biochemical, molecular, and cellular basis of the protective activity of estrogen and (2) to transfer this knowledge into the hospitals by discussing preventive and therapeutic approaches such as estrogen replacement therapy for post-menopausal women.

Besides up-to-date information on estrogen and the brain, this book explains in a highly understandable manner molecular and cellular techniques by which basic data have been collected. The reader, which may include the professional specialist as well as the interested non-specialist, will also gain insight into the scientific transfer process of knowledge from basic science to the clinical situation and therefore "from bench to bed".

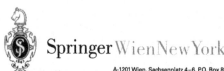

Springer Wien New York

A-1201 Wien, Sachsenplatz 4–6, P.O. Box 89, Fax +43.1.330 24 26, e-mail: books@springer.at, **www.springer.at**
D-69126 Heidelberg, Haberstraße 7, Fax +49.6221.345-229, e-mail: orders@springer.de
USA, Secaucus, NJ 07096-2485, P.O. Box 2485, Fax +1.201.348-4505, e-mail: orders@springer-ny.com
EBS, Japan, Tokyo 113, 3–13, Hongo 3-chome, Bunkyo-ku, Fax +81.3.38 18 08 64, e-mail: orders@svt-ebs.co.jp